DICTIONARY OF AMERICAN NURSING BIOGRAPHY

DICTIONARY OF AMERICAN NURSING BIOGRAPHY

Martin Kaufman, Editor-in-Chief

Joellen Watson Hawkins, Loretta P. Higgins, and Alice Howell Friedman, Contributing Editors

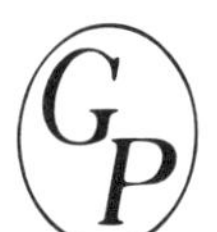

GREENWOOD PRESS
New York • Westport, Connecticut • London

Library of Congress Cataloging-in-Publication Data

Dictionary of American nursing biography.

Companion v. to: Dictionary of American medical biography.
1. Nurses—United States—Biography—Dictionaries.
2. United States—Biography—Dictionaries. I. Kaufman, Martin, 1940- . II. Dictionary of American medical biography. [DNLM: 1. History of Nursing—United States. 2. Nursing—United States—biography.
WZ 112.5.N8 D554]
RT34.D53 1988 610.73'092'2 [B] 87-25454
ISBN 0-313-24520-7 (alk. paper)

British Library Cataloguing in Publication Data is available.

Library of Congress Catalog Card Number: 87-25454
ISBN: 0-313-24520-7

First published in 1988

Greenwood Press, Inc.
88 Post Road West, Westport, Connecticut 06881

Printed in the United States of America

The paper used in this book complies with the Permanent Paper Standard issued by the National Information Standards Organization (Z39.48-1984).

10 9 8 7 6 5 4 3 2 1

Contents

Preface

In 1984, while the *Dictionary of American Medical Biography* was in production, Martin Kaufman and Joellen Hawkins began to discuss the possibility of producing a companion volume on nursing. Although the *Dictionary of American Medical Biography* did include sixteen persons of importance in the history of nursing, it was clear that a separate book on nursing would be required to provide information on the large number of women whose contributions resulted in the development of nursing as a profession and who are largely unknown even to members of their own profession. Since there was no reference work similar to the *Dictionary of American Medical Biography* with a focus on American nurses, we decided to devote the next four years to the project. After recruiting Loretta Higgins and Alice Friedman to complete the research and writing team, we began work on the book.

We believe that a new biographical dictionary is a welcome addition to reference collections in the history of American medicine and public health, as well as to collections with a focus on the history of women and their changing role in American society.

This book contains a total of 196 biographical sketches of persons who were important in the history of American nursing, from the early pioneers of the mid-nineteenth century to those who entered the scene after the process of professionalization had clearly begun and who carried on the work of their foremothers in transforming nursing from a trade to a profession based on scientific research and formal education in a college or university setting. A large number of biographies focus on women who contributed to the development of military nursing, as well as nurse-educators and nurse-administrators.

The selection process was difficult; it clearly was impossible to include everyone mentioned in the leading histories of American nursing.

We developed a lengthy listing of persons who should be researched to determine both their importance and whether sufficient biographical information could be found to provide a relatively complete biographical sketch. In order to maintain historical perspective, we established a cutoff date of January 31, 1987. Any important figures who died after that date were not included in this book, although we assume that eventually they may be included in new editions. Also subsequent editions will certainly include new information which may be located after publication of this book. We are well aware that, despite our best efforts, subjects who might merit inclusion in the *Dictionary of American Nursing Biography* have been omitted. In some cases they have been omitted because of our inability to find enough information to provide anything resembling a complete biographical sketch, at least without extensive travel to obscure collections in various parts of the country, collections which may not have provided more than an additional clue to the detective work of historical research on persons who have not been the focus of biographical study by others, either during their lives or after their deaths.

As any author or editor is well aware, the research process can be a never-ending task, and this book would never have been published if we waited until we had found every last bit of information on every person under study. We have made every effort to locate books, articles, dissertations, and personal papers which may cast light on the background and contributions of the individuals under study, and for those who have not been the subject of prior historical study, we have sent countless queries to college and university archives, personnel directors of hospitals, and the organizations in which a subject was active in the hope of locating a resume or finding a colleague who might be able to provide information which would enable us to prepare as complete sketches as possible.

Our work began with the traditional biographical reference works and with books and articles on the history of American nursing. With few exceptions, books and articles provided little biographical information, although they contained specific information on a person's contributions, information which then could be followed up by correspondence with individuals and repositories which might have further material on the subject.

Traditional reference works were of little use; only a small number of nurses were included in *Notable American Women* or in the *Dictionary of American Biography* or *Who Was Who in America.* In many cases we began with a name, which led us to an obituary in a nursing journal, which in turn led us to other sources of information, all eventually resulting in the sketches published here.

After the selection process was completed, we established a format for the biographical sketches, and it was decided that the format of the *Dictionary of American Medical Biography* was ideal, providing necessary biographical information, adequate description of contributions and significance, important or representative writings by the subjects, and references which would enable readers to locate more detailed information. When the sketches were completed, we checked as much information as possible for accuracy. The following format is used in this book:

NAME OF SUBJECT (last name, first name, middle name). (date of birth, place of birth -- date of death, place of death). *Area of specialization.* Parents' names and occupations. Marital information (names of spouses, dates of marriages, number of children by each marriage). EDUCATION: Beginning with high school, nursing school, college or university, post-graduate studies. CAREER: Information, including dates and positions.
CONTRIBUTIONS. WRITINGS: A maximum of five important or representative works and, where available, the location of a bibliography. REFERENCES.

If a sketch mentions another individual who is included in this book, the reference has been marked by (q.v.), indicating that the reader who wants more information on that individual should consult the biographical sketch elsewhere in the book. In some cases, information could not be located by the editors. The most common omissions are parents' names and occupations, spouse's names, and number of children. Since marriage normally resulted in a nurse's retirement, and until the modern era relatively few nurses married, lack of information on spouse or number of children clearly is not a major problem. The editor-in-chief would ask persons with such information to write to him so the biographies in question can be changed in subsequent editions of this book.

In order to make the information in the sketches more readily available, the editor-in-chief has included several appendices which list the biographical subjects by birth, state where prominent, and specialty or significant area of work within nursing. In addition, there is an index which can provide a handy reference to all information on specific individuals, organizations, and so forth. It should be noted that the index does not duplicate the appendices; states and specialties are not included in the index, but may be found in the appendices.

As those who have worked in teams are aware, the success of a team depends on all the members. This work represents the combined efforts of not only the editors, but also the assistance provided by a large number of librarians, archivists, friends, colleagues, persons in alumni offices, agencies, or institutions where the individuals in this dictionary were trained, received their degrees, and/or spent their professional lives. We are most appreciative of their assistance, which substantially improved this book by filling in thousands of gaps and by enabling us to provide as complete biographical sketches as possible.

The editor-in-chief, Martin Kaufman, would like to express his thanks and appreciation to Dr. John Nevins, Vice President for Academic Affairs at Westfield State College, who provided encouragement and assistance, and who helped to locate funds needed for the purchase of the laser printer on which this volume was typeset. In addition, it should be noted that much of the initial planning of this volume was completed during a sabbatical leave, which was crucial for the success of the project. Finally, it must be acknowledged that Lee Mangiaratti, secretary to the Westfield State College department of history, provided service far beyond the call of duty, including having to learn a new word-processing system necessary for the use of the laserprinter.

We must express our thanks and appreciation to Mary Pekarski of the Boston College O'Neill Library and to the staff at O'Neill Library responsible for interlibrary loan and the microfilm collection. We received extensive assistance also from the reference librarians and the staff of the interlibrary loan department of University Library, University of Massachusetts, Amherst. We are also indebted to Helen Sherwin and Margaret Goostray at the Nursing Archives, Mugar Memorial Library, Boston University, who gave us access to the papers of various organizations and individuals, papers which were indispensable for the completion of this project. We are indebted to Elizabeth Schneider of the Treadway Library of the Massachusetts General Hospital, Boston; to the staff of the Francis Countway Library of Medicine, Boston; and to Nancy McCall and Gerard Shorb of the Alan Mason Chesney Medical Archives of the Johns Hopkins Medical Institutions, Baltimore, Maryland. We thank the staff of the Computer Center of Westfield State College, for providing their expertise, and especially to Kenneth Haar and Morgan Wheelock, who provided help with the use of the laser printer on which this book was printed.

Martin Kaufman
Joellen Watson Hawkins
Loretta P. Higgins
Alice Howell Friedman

A

AIKENS, CHARLOTTE A. (?--October 20, 1949, Detroit, Michigan). *Author; hospital administrator.* Never married but adopted two children, including a daughter who became a physician. EDUCATION: Attended Alma College, Ontario, Canada; 1897, graduated from Stratford City Hospital training school for nurses; post-graduate study in ward administration, Polyclinic Hospital, New York City. CAREER: 1898, served as a Spanish-American War nurse; c. 1899-1901, superintendent, Sibley Memorial Hospital, Washington, D.C., and then superintendent, Methodist Hospital, Des Moines, Iowa; c. 1901-1911, superintendent, Columbia Hospital, Pittsburgh, Pennsylvania; 1911-1916, associate editor, *Trained Nurse and Hospital Review*; 1916-1922, editor, *Trained Nurse and Hospital Review.*

CONTRIBUTIONS: Charlotte Aikens was well known as an author of nursing textbooks, for her pioneering work on nursing ethics, and for her service as editor of two important nursing journals. Her textbooks ranged from studies of hospital management to clinical studies and ethics, and practical nursing. In 1916 the first edition of her book on nursing ethics was published (*Ethics for Nurses*; it was reprinted numerous times until 1943 and was translated into fourteen languages. The book undoubtedly played a major role in strengthening the professionalism of countless nurses, who often read the book as part of their training school requirements. From 1902 to 1907, Aikens served as associate editor of the *International Hospital Record*, and in 1908 she joined the staff of the *Trained Nurse and Hospital Review.* In 1911 she gave up her administrative career to devote full time to her work as associate editor of that journal, and in 1916 she succeeded Annette Sumner Rose as its editor, serving until 1922, when she retired to raise her adopted children.

She was an active member of the American Hospital Association (AHA), and it was reported that when she spoke at committee or director's meetings, she was listened to with great respect. She served as chairperson of the AHA committee to study nurse-training schools, and the committee published several reports which were highly praised by the *American Journal of Nursing*. Although not diagnosing the problems facing America's nursing profession, the report did point out many of the symptoms which had to be addressed. As a hospital administrator, Aikens supported the use of subsidiary workers (now known as nursing assistants or nurses' aides), but when the idea was advocated by the AHA's study committee, it met with a great deal of opposition from hospital administrators, who tended to view the nursing school as a source of cheap labor and did not want to spend money on aides when student nurses were readily available (and who even paid for the right to learn nursing while working in the hospital's wards).

She encouraged registration for all nurses who accepted payment for their services, and she believed that a system of national registration and reciprocity among states was of vital importance in ensuring nationwide standards of nursing education and care.

She was involved in the development of the Detroit Home Nursing Association in 1913. In 1920, at the request of the Methodist Church mission board, she made a survey of South America in order to make recommendations about establishing and maintaining medical missions on that continent. Before she began her career in hospital administration, Aikens had planned to become a missionary, and working with the Methodist mission board undoubtedly helped satisfy her need to serve humanity on the world scene. She was intensely religious; in the first pages of her books, she customarily included religious poems which she apparently hoped would serve to inspire her readers.

WRITINGS: *Hospital Housekeeping* (1906 and three subsequent editions); *Hospital Training School Methods and the Head Nurse* (1907); *Primary Studies for Nurses* (1909 and four subsequent editions); *Hospital Management* (1911); *The Home Nurse's Handbook for Practical Nursing* (1912, many editions until 1932); *Ethics for Nurses* (1916, reprinted many times until 1943); *Training School Methods for Institutional Nurses* (1919); and many articles in the *Trained Nurse and Hospital Review* and the *International Hospital Record*.

REFERENCES: *American Journal of Nursing* (December 1949), p. 818; Mary M. Roberts, *American Nursing: History and Interpretation* (1954); *Trained Nurse and Hospital Review* (December 1949), p. 279.

LORETTA P. HIGGINS

ALCOTT, LOUISA MAY (November 29, 1832, Germantown, Pennsylvania--March 6, 1888, Roxbury, Massachusetts). *Volunteer nurse in Civil War; author.* Daughter of A{mos} Bronson Alcott, teacher and philosopher, and Abigail (May) Alcott, seamstress, teacher, and charity worker. Never married. EDUCATION: Studied at home under the tutelage of her parents and also with Henry David Thoreau when the family moved in April 1840 to Concord, Massachusetts; attended Concord Academy, run by Henry and John Thoreau; 1844, attended Maria Chase's district school in Still River; 1845, after return to Concord, was taught by Sophia Foord, a teacher who joined the family and taught Louisa and her sisters; late summer of 1845, Charles Lane, a member of the Fruitlands communal experiment, took over the task of teaching the sisters; fall of 1845, attended the local Concord school, taught by John Hosmer.
CAREER: 1848, taught adult Negroes in Boston to read and write; 1849, assisted her older sister Anna in her school at Canton Street, Boston; 1851, served briefly as a companion to a woman in Dedham, Massachusetts, then returned to teaching; September 1851, her first literary work was published, a poem "Sunlight," in *Peterson's Magazine*; May 8, 1852, her first story, "The Rival Painters," was published in *Olive Branch*, a paper devoted to Christianity, literature, the arts, agriculture, and general intelligence; 1852-1855, taught in a school she operated with her sister Anna, at 20 Pinckney Street, Boston; December 19, 1854, her first book, *Flower Fables*, was published; July 10, 1855, moved to Walpole, New Hampshire, and with her sister Anna founded Walpole's first Amateur Dramatic Company; November 1855, moved alone to Boston, where she worked as a seamstress and housekeeper and continued to write; 1857, returned with her family to Concord and was active in the Concord Dramatic Union; fall 1858, took a position as a governess, continuing to write and publish and to act in amateur theatrical productions; 1860, appointed to a vigilance committee in Concord to protect Frank Sanborn, abolitionist friend of John Brown; May 4, 1860, her first play, *Nat Bachelor's Pleasure Trip*, was produced at the Howard Athenaeum, Boston; 1860-1862, wrote stories and worked on a novel in Concord; June 1862, sewed for Union soldiers; December 14, 1862-January 7, 1863, served as a volunteer nurse in the Civil War; July 20, 1865, sailed to Europe as a paid companion to an invalid woman, returning July 5, 1866; from 1863 to her death in 1888 (two days after her father's death), supported herself and her family with the royalties from her writing; 1867, began to edit *Merry's Museum*, a magazine for children; spent her last days at Dunreath Place, Roxbury, Massachusetts, a nursing home run by Dr. Rhoda Lawrence.
CONTRIBUTIONS: Louisa May Alcott's most important contribution to nursing history was *Hospital Sketches*, a firsthand view of volunteer

nursing during the Civil War. She had volunteered as a nurse, and on December 14, 1862, she was assigned to the Union Hotel Hospital in the Georgetown section of Washington, D.C., working under the supervision of Hannah Ropes (q.v.), the matron. In preparation for her role as a nurse, she studied Florence Nightingale's *Notes on Nursing*. Alcott felt that she fulfilled the regulations Dorothea Dix (q.v.) had established for volunteer nurses, and she believed that the hours she had devoted to caring for her sister Lizzie during the last days of her life would be put to good use during the Civil War.

In January 1863 Alcott became ill and at the urging of Dorothea Dix returned to Concord on January 23, accompanied by her father. During her convalescence, she wrote *Hospital Sketches*, which was first serialized in the *Commonwealth* in 1863 and published as a book (for which she received $200) in the same year. In the book, she drew on her recollections of the hospital and on the letters she had written to her relatives during her stay at the hospital. The book described her experiences through the eyes of "Nurse Periwinkle." The large doses of calomel she was administered during her illness in Georgetown were to shape the rest of her life. The mercury poisoning that resulted racked her body with pain and caused deterioration to the end of her life, often preventing her from writing and from other work necessary to provide for her family. One of her biographers, Martha Saxton, states that had it not been for the mercury poisoning and the physical toll that it took, Alcott might well have continued in nursing or in some other expression of her humanitarianism as an alternative to marriage and motherhood.

WRITINGS: *Flower Fables* (1854); *Hospital Sketches* (1863); *Moods* (1864); *Little Women* (1869); *An Old Fashioned Girl* (1870); *Little Men* (1871); *Work* (1873); *Eight Cousins* (1875); *Rose in Bloom* (1876); *Silver Pitchers* (1876); *A Modern Mephistopheles* (1877); *Under the Lilacs* (1878); *Jack and Jill* (1880); *Aunt Jo's Scrap Bag* (6 vols., 1872-1882); *Proverb Stories* (1882); *Spinning Wheel Stories* (1884); *Jo's Boys* (1886); *Lulu's Library* (3 vols., 1886-1889); *A Garland for Girls* (1888).

REFERENCES: Louisa May Alcott, *Hospital Sketches* (1863); Katharine Anthony, *Louisa May Alcott* (1938); Gamaliel Bradford, *Portraits of American Women* (1919); Ednah D. Cheney, ed., *Louisa May Alcott: Her Life, Letters, and Journals* (1925); *Dictionary of American Biography*, I: 141-142; Cornelia Meigs, *Invincible Louisa* (1933); Belle Moses, *Louisa May Alcott: Dreamer and Worker* (1942); *National Cyclopedia of American Biography*, I: 204; Martha Saxton, *Louisa May* (1977); Madeleine B. Stern, *Louisa May Alcott* (1950); Marjorie Worthington, *Miss Alcott of Concord* (1958).

JOELLEN WATSON HAWKINS

ALLINE, ANNA LOWELL (1864, East Machias, Maine--December 16, 1935, Iowa). *Nurse-educator.* Married E. Wilton Brown, 1923.
EDUCATION: Attended public schools and state normal school in Iowa; 1893, received diploma from Brooklyn Homeopathic Hospital Training School for Nursing, Brooklyn, New York; 1896, six months of post-graduate study, General Memorial Hospital, New York City; 1900, enrolled in hospital economics course, Teachers College, Columbia University, New York City.
CAREER: c. 1884-1890, taught public school, Plymouth County, Iowa; 1893-1900, various nursing positions, including assistant to the superintendent, Brooklyn Homeopathic Hospital; 1900-1906, directed the Home Economics Program, Teachers College; 1906-1909, inspector, Board of Registration in Nursing, New York State; 1910-1912, superintendent, Buffalo Homeopathic Hospital, Buffalo, New York; 1917-1918, Red Cross work; 1918-1923, in charge of laboratory work and the out-patient department, Albany Homeopathic Hospital, Albany, New York.
CONTRIBUTIONS: Anna Alline was a pioneer in nursing education. After having studied under Linda Richards (q.v.) at the Brooklyn Homeopathic Hospital School of Nursing and serving as Richards' assistant, she went on to teach at Teachers College, Columbia University. She was one of the first two students enrolled in the newly established (1900) course in hospital economics at Teachers College. Upon completion of the course, she was urged to stay as director of the Teachers College program in home economics. She supplemented the work of visiting lecturers and conducted fieldwork excursions. At that time (1903), the course was extended to two years. Her work did much to ensure the continuity of the program, which was the forerunner of the nursing education department at Teachers College. She was the first inspector of nursing schools for a state board of nurse examiners. In that capacity, she oversaw the operation of nursing schools in New York State and monitored their compliance with the mandated rules of the new Board of Registration. She worked tirelessly to secure an understanding of training school problems and to inspire standardization of methods and practices, in spite of the opposition of many school superintendents who resented and resisted state inspection of their schools. From 1900 to 1909, she served as treasurer of the American Society of Superintendents of Training Schools for Nurses, and from 1916 to 1923 she served as chairman of the Albany Red Cross. She was a life member of the National League of Nursing Education.
WRITINGS: "Inspection of Nurse Training Schools: Its Aims and Results," *Transactions* of the American Hospital Association, tenth annual conference (1911); also many articles in the *American Journal of Nursing*

regarding state supervision of nursing schools, including new aspects of nursing curriculum, i.e., "Training School Libraries" (1905), p. 853, "Supply and Demand of Students" (1907), p. 758, and "State Supervision of Nursing Schools in New York" (1909), p. 1911.
REFERENCES: The American Journal of Nursing and Sophia F. Palmer Historical Collections, Nursing Archives, Mugar Library, Boston University; Helen E. Marshall, *Mary Adelaide Nutting* (1972), pp. 102, 106, 109-110, and 135; National League of Nursing Education, *Leaders of American Nursing* (February 1923); Mary M. Roberts, *American Nursing: History and Interpretation* (1954), pp. 28 and 75.

ALICE HOWELL FRIEDMAN

AMY MARGARET, SISTER (?, England--March 6, 1941, Boston, Massachusetts). *Educator and administrator.* Never married. EDUCATION: c. 1900, graduated from Children's Hospital School of Nursing, Boston, Massachusetts. CAREER: Emigrated to the United States at the age of seventeen, when she entered the Order of the Sisters of Saint Margaret of the Episcopal church; 1886, began work as a nurse in the private hospital of the Order of Saint Margaret; during summer months, in charge of sick infants at Seashore Home, now Floating Hospital, Boston; 1889, general nursing and maternity work, St. Barnabas Hospital, Newark, New Jersey; 1890, assisted another sister of her order in organizing Christ Hospital, Jersey City, New Jersey; c. 1890-1891, private duty nursing, Halifax, Nova Scotia; c. 1891-1895, superintendent of nursing, St. Barnabas Hospital, Newark, New Jersey; 1896 (while a nursing student), taught at Children's Hospital School of Nursing, Boston; 1903-1906, assistant superintendent, Children's Hospital, Boston; 1906-1912, superintendent of nurses and director of the Children's Hospital School of Nursing, Boston (retiring due to illness); mistress of novices in the mother house of the Order of St. Margaret, Boston.
CONTRIBUTIONS: Sister Amy Margaret was recognized in her day as one of the foremost nurse-educators whose career in that field began before she received her diploma from Boston's Children's Hospital. In 1903, she became assistant superintendent of the hospital, and in 1906 was appointed superintendent of nurses and director of the hospital. As superintendent, she arranged new affiliations for her students, including a novel program begun in 1904 to send nursing students to Simmons College, Boston, for preliminary science courses. In addition, she arranged for students to gain experience (beginning in 1909) in the social service department of the Massachusetts General Hospital (MGH), probably the first time such an affiliation was arranged by any diploma

nursing school in the United States. Sister Amy Margaret also established an affiliation at the MGH for a course in adult nursing, as well as an elective course at the Corey Hill Private Hospital, Boston. In 1906, with a colleague, Sister Caroline, she met with physicians from the Boston Lying-in Hospital to arrange an obstetrical rotation for nurses, an affiliation which began the following year. In addition, she established an eight-hour day for nursing students, required a high-school diploma for admission, and charged tuition fees. By 1908, the nursing program at Children's Hospital was recognized as one of the best in the country, and Stella Goostray (q.v.), the early nursing historian, described Sister Amy Margaret as one of the most outstanding teachers who ever taught at the Children's Hospital.

Sister Amy Margaret was also active in nursing organizations. She was an early member of the Society of Superintendents of Training Schools for Nurses (now the National League for Nursing). From 1909 to 1911, she served as a counsellor of that group, the first religious to do so. She attended conventions and often was a featured speaker. She served on the society's program committee and as chairperson of the committee on infants and children. She retired because of illness, and after recuperating she became mistress of novices for her order and then infirmarian.

WRITINGS: "Artificial Feeding," *American Journal of Nursing* (April 1907), p. 521.

REFERENCES: *American Journal of Nursing* (April 1941), p. 509; Children's Hospital School of Nursing Collection, Nursing Archives, Mugar Memorial Library, Boston University; Stella Goostray, *Fifty Years: A History of the School of Nursing, The Children's Hospital, Boston* (1940); M. Adelaide Nutting Collection, Teachers College, Columbia University (microfiche number 0934).

LORETTA P. HIGGINS

ANDERSON, LYDIA ELIZABETH (January 16, 1863, New York City--April 11, 1939, Brooklyn, New York). *Leader in nursing administration.* Daughter of Rev. Thomas D. Anderson, D.D., Baptist clergyman, and Lucy (Spence) Anderson. Never married. EDUCATION: Attended private schools, then graduated from Rutgers Female College, New Brunswick, New Jersey; 1895-1897, attended New York Hospital Training School for Nurses, graduating in 1897; 1909-1910, post-graduate courses at Teachers College, Columbia University, New York City.

CAREER: 1897, superintendent, Homeopathic Hospital, Providence, Rhode Island; 1897-1902, associate superintendent, Sloane Maternity

Hospital, New York City; 1903-c. 1904, private duty nursing; c. 1905, assistant superintendent, Long Island Hospital; c. 1905-1909, Mt. Sinai Hospital, New York City; 1910-1936, taught at Mt. Sinai Training School and New York Hospital Training School; taught at thirty-two schools in New York State and New Jersey.

CONTRIBUTIONS: Lydia Anderson's principal contribution was to the development of hospitals and their schools of nursing. All but a brief period of her career was devoted to serving as a faculty member, superintendent, or assistant superintendent for many hospital training schools in Rhode Island, New York, and New Jersey. She was acclaimed by her students as an outstanding teacher and an understanding and wise faculty member. She was a friend to her students, with wit and a spontaneous sense of humor which put them at ease.

In addition to her professional posts, Anderson was very much involved in professional organizations and activities. She was an active member of the New York Hospital School of Nursing Alumnae, and in 1927 she was selected to write the history of the school, serving also on a committee for reorganization of the school and hospital in 1930. At the school's fiftieth anniversary in 1927, she delivered a speech which eloquently and graphically described the early days. She was enrolled as a Red Cross nurse, was an early member of the American Nurses' Association (then the Associated Alumnae), and was a member of the National League of Nursing Education. She was interested in the history of nursing and was a charter member of the History of Nursing Society of New York. From 1910 to 1927, she was a member of the New York State Board of Nurse Examiners, serving as secretary for one year and president for seven. Legend has it that during her tenure she signed 27,000 state certificates.

Over the course of her career, she received numerous honors in recognition of her exceptional work on behalf of the nursing profession. In 1927, her friends and former students gave a dinner in her honor in recognition of her thirty years of nursing service. The money presented to her at the dinner she turned over to the New York League of Nursing Education to be administered as the Lydia E. Anderson Instructors' Loan Fund, for nurses preparing to be instructors in nursing schools. On March 4, 1941, the forty-fourth anniversary of her graduation, the New York Hospital School of Nursing library was named the Lydia E. Anderson Library, and at that time a case was unveiled which contained her nursing insignia, her class pin, the Canadian and U.S. flags, the New York Hospital gold medal, and her Red Cross badge number 3580. A bronze tablet affixed to the wall indicated that it was "The Lydia E. Anderson Library."

WRITINGS: *History of the New York Hospital School of Nursing* (1927).

REFERENCES: *American Journal of Nursing* (June 1927), p. 499, (May 1939), pp. 585-586, and (June 1941), p. 736; Helene Jamieson Jordan, *Cornell University-New York Hospital School of Nursing, 1877-1952* (1952); Bertha H. Lehmkuhl, "Lydia E. Anderson, R.N., B.S.," *American Journal of Nursing* (February 1929), pp. 201-202; Anna D. Wolf and Margaret E. Wyatt, *National League of Nursing Education Biographical Sketches* (1940).

JOELLEN WATSON HAWKINS

ANGELA, MOTHER (born Eliza Maria Gillespie, February 21, 1824, West Brownsville, Pennsylvania--March 4, 1887, Notre Dame, Indiana). *Civil War nurse; hospital administrator.* Daughter of John Purcell Gillespie and Mary Madeleine (Miers) Gillespie. Never married. EDUCATION: Attended a private school in Brownsville until 1836; 1836-1838, School of the Dominican Sisters, Somerset, Ohio; 1838-1842, Academy of the Visitation, Washington, D.C., graduating in 1842; studied in France during her novitiate. CAREER: 1842, went to Lancaster, Pennsylvania, where her mother and stepfather lived, doing parish work, raising money for Irish famine victims, and caring for cholera patients; before entering the Convent, taught at Mount St. Mary's Seminary, St. Mary's City, Maryland; helped to organize a Catholic school for girls, where she taught from 1847 to 1851; 1853, became a Sister of the Holy Cross, becoming director of studies at St. Mary's Academy, and was appointed mother superior of the Bertrand Convent, a position she held for about thirty years. 1855, St. Mary's Academy moved to South Bend, Indiana, near Notre Dame University, and it became St. Mary's College.

CONTRIBUTIONS: Although she was a pioneer in the education of women, Mother Angela is best remembered for her work during the Civil War. At the outbreak of the war, she led sixty nuns in the care of over 1,400 wounded at the Mound City Hospital, in Illinois. During the war, Mother Angela and other nuns of the Order of the Holy Cross cared for the wounded in hospitals and ships that transported the wounded. Under her direction, the hospital at Mound City was considered the best military hospital in the United States. She raised supplies and clothing for the wounded, cared for Northern and Southern soldiers alike, and supervised work of sisters in military hospitals at Paducah, Louisville, Memphis, Cairo, and Mound City. Mary Livermore (q.v.) described the hospital at Cairo as the epitome of cleanliness, order, and good nursing care. While she was mother superior of the Sisters of the Holy Cross, the order developed from humble origins and became a strong organization of Catholic women. As director of studies at St. Mary's Academy, she

supervised the school's move to Indiana and the transition to one of the earliest Catholic women's colleges. Her brother was the Reverend N. H. Gillespie, the first graduate of Notre Dame University, who later became vice-president of that college.
WRITINGS: Edited a series of Catholic school books; with Father Sorin, founded the *Ave Maria*, a Catholic publication.
REFERENCES: George Barton, *Angels of the Battlefield* (1898); *Dictionary of American Biography*, I: 302-303; Mary H. Gardner Holland, *Our Army Nurses* (1897); Ellen Ryan Jolly, *Nuns of the Battlefield* (1927); Mary A. Livermore, *My Story of the War: A Woman's Narrative of Four Years Personal Experiences* (1889); *Notable American Women*, II: 34-35; *A Story of Fifty Years: Sisters of the Holy Cross, 1855-1905* (n.d.); Agatha Young, *The Women and the Crisis: Women of the North in the Civil War* (1959).

LORETTA P. HIGGINS

ANTHONY, SISTER (born Mary O'Connell, August 15, c. 1814, Limerick, Ireland--December 8, 1897, Norwood, Ohio). *Civil War Nurse.* Daughter of William and Catherine (Murphy) O'Connell. Never married.
EDUCATION: Attended Ursaline Academy, Charlestown, Massachusetts.
CAREER: 1835, entered order of Sisters of Charity, Emmitsburg, Maryland; 1837, took vows of profession; 1837-1880, transferred to Cincinnati, Ohio; 1852, placed in charge of St. John's Hospital for Invalids, Cincinnati; 1862-1865, Civil War nurse, assigned to the Army of the Cumberland; 1866, founded, and 1866-1880, managed the Good Samaritan Hospital, Cincinnati; 1873-1880, managed St. Joseph's Foundling and Maternity Hospital; 1880, retired at the request of Bishop William Henry Elder and spent her remaining years at St. Joseph's Hospital.
CONTRIBUTIONS: Sister Anthony became famous as a result of her work during the Civil War. During the war, St. John's Hospital for Invalids, Cincinnati, was turned over to the care of the wounded who often arrived after being transported from the battlefields on boats on the Ohio River. Sister Anthony and other Sisters of Charity often accompanied those wounded soldiers on board what in effect were floating hospitals. The decks of those boats became surgical amphitheaters where limbs were amputated. She cared for the wounded with unceasing devotion and selflessness. Although many nurses performed meritoriously during those difficult times, the name of Sister Anthony continues to stand out as giving exceptional service to the

wounded of both the North and the South. She is especially remembered for her ministrations to the wounded on the battlefield of Shiloh.

On September 1, 1862, Sister Anthony was officially appointed to service with the nurse corps, following the Army of the Cumberland to Stone's River, where she was assigned to a base hospital. She ministered primarily to the soldiers in Tennessee and Kentucky, often jeopardizing her own life in the care of the wounded, as the sobriquets describing her indicate. She was called "Angel of the Battlefield," the "Florence Nightingale of America," the "Ministering Angel of the Army of the Tennessee," and "Angel of Goodness." She was reportedly highly respected by the Confederates as well as by Union soldiers, and by Protestants as well as Catholics.

After the war, in 1866, as a result of donations from two Protestant men who were impressed by the charitable work done by the Sisters of Charity, she founded and managed the Good Samaritan Hospital. Also donated to her were funds to establish a home for unmarried mothers and orphans, called St. Joseph's Foundling and Maternity Hospital, which opened in 1873. She was an indefatigable fund-raiser to benefit the sick, orphans, and the poor, and one result of her fund-raising was an orphanage at Cumminsville, Ohio.

REFERENCES: George Barton, *Angels of the Battlefield* (1898); *Dictionary of American Biography*, I: 319; Ellen Ryan Jolly, *Nuns of the Battlefield* (1927); Otto Juettner, *Daniel Drake and His Followers* (1909); Sister Mary Agnes McGann, *The History of Mother Seton's Daughters* (1923); John Francis Maguire, *The Irish in America* (1876); *Notable American Women*, pp. 647-648.

LORETTA P. HIGGINS

ARNSTEIN, MARGARET GENE (October 27, 1904, New York City--October 8, 1972, New Haven, Connecticut). *Public health nurse; nurse-educator*. Daughter of Leo Arnstein and Elsie (Nathan) Arnstein. Never married. EDUCATION: 1921, graduated from the preparatory school of the Ethical Culture Society, New York City; 1925, A.B., Smith College, Northampton, Massachusetts; 1928, graduated from Presbyterian Hospital School of Nursing, New York City; 1929, A.M., Teachers College, Columbia University, New York City; 1934, M.S., Johns Hopkins University, Baltimore, Maryland. CAREER: 1929-1934, staff nurse, then supervisor, Westchester County Hospital, White Plains, New York; 1934-1937, consultant nurse, communicable disease division of the New York State Department of Health; 1938-1940, associate professor, University of Minnesota, Minneapolis; 1940-1946, consultant, New York

State Department of Health (on leave 1943-1946); 1943-1945, nurse-advisor to the Balkan countries, United Nations Relief and Rehabilitation Administration; 1946, senior nurse, U.S. Public Health Service; 1949-1957, chief, bureau of nurse resources, U.S. Public Health Service; 1958, visiting professor, Yale University School of Nursing, New Haven, Connecticut; 1960, chief, division of nursing, U.S. Public Health Service; 1965-1967, professor of nursing, University of Michigan; 1967-1972, dean, Yale University School of Nursing.

CONTRIBUTIONS: Margaret Arnstein was a distinguished leader and educator in public health nursing, in both the United States and abroad. Following in the footsteps of parents who were active in social and public health activities in New York City, Arnstein continued their example by way of her public health nursing involvement. She was encouraged to do so by Lillian Wald (q.v.), a close friend of the family whose work at Henry Street Settlement was supported by the Arnsteins.

Arnstein was a nurse-researcher before that became a popular designation. She devised field studies to analyze and systematize the observations and insights of nurses as early as 1940, when she was a consultant for the New York State Department of Health. Under her direction (1946-1966), the nursing division of the U.S. Public Health Service was able to increase its provision of statistical information as well as assistance when requested by those doing research in nursing. She added considerable knowledge of nursing resources within the country as a result of her consultation and her participation in many state surveys. This knowledge was useful for the planning of nursing education and for utilization of nursing services. On the global level, she directed the first International Conference on Nursing Studies, Sevres, France. In 1952, she worked with the World Health Organization staff in Geneva, Switzerland, to prepare a guide for surveying nursing services in individual countries, an important first step toward relieving the postwar shortages of trained nurses.

Arnstein was influential in improving health care in the Balkan region of Europe following World War II. She was responsible for developing nursing services for the war-ravaged countries of Albania, Greece, and Yugoslavia. For this assignment, she was employed by the United Nations Relief and Rehabilitation Administration. She wrote many articles in American and international journals in which she described the health needs of refugees. In 1945, she was appointed a senior nursing advisor for international health (U.S. Public Health Service), and in that capacity she participated in a joint Rockefeller Foundation/Administration for International Development study of health manpower training requirements of developing countries. This study was to determine whether in countries with differing characteristics, there was a need for alternative systems for the preparation of health personnel. For the study, she travelled to Guatemala, Jamaica, Senegal, and Thailand.

During her twenty-year career with the U.S. Public Health Service, Arnstein helped to launch the emergency program of support to nursing education which was the precursor of the Cadet Nurse Corps of World War II. This plan to increase the number of nursing students, as a solution to the nursing shortage, was adopted by Congress, and she was brought from her position with the New York State Department of Health to be one of the consultants administering the cadet nurse program.

One of her projects while serving with the U.S. Public Health Service was to establish a new nursing unit to serve the health programs of the Agency for International Development, emphasizing the training of nurses and midwives for new programs of nutrition and population control. She urged workers in the field to observe the practices of the countries they were serving and, as Western health workers, to come to understand the Eastern approach to family life and to learn from the native health-care workers.

Over the years, Arnstein received a number of awards in recognition of her contributions to public health nursing. She was the first woman to receive the Rockefeller Public Service Award, recognizing the distinguished service of career employees in the upper levels of the federal government. She was the first visiting professor on the Annie W. Goodrich (q.v.) Endowment, a faculty post established in memory of the founder and first dean of the Yale School of Nursing. In 1925, during her senior year at Smith College, she was inducted into Phi Beta Kappa. In 1950, Smith College awarded her an honorary doctor of science degree. Five years later, in 1955, she received the Lasker Award for Nurses (with Pearl McIver {q.v.} and Lucille P. Leone). In 1962, Wayne State University, Detroit, Michigan, awarded her an honorary doctorate. In 1964, she received the U.S. Public Health Service's Public Health Distinguished Service Medal. In 1965, she received the Rockefeller Public Service Award. In 1971, the American Public Health Association bestowed upon her its highest honor, the Sedgwick Memorial Medal. In 1972, the year of her retirement as dean of the Yale School of Nursing, and the year of her death, she received an honorary doctorate from the University of Michigan.

WRITINGS: *Communicable Disease Control* (1962, with Gaylor Anderson and Mary Lasker); many articles in professional journals.

REFERENCES: *New York Times* (October 9, 1972), p. 34; *Notable American Women* (1971), pp. 37-38 and (1980), p. 39; unpublished material, in Nursing Archives, Mugar Memorial Library, Boston University; Mary M. Roberts, *American Nursing: History and*

Interpretation (1954), pp. 309, 494, 502 and 627; unpublished material, Smith College Archives; Myron Wegman, "Tribute to Margaret Arnstein," *American Journal of Public Health* (1973), p. 97; *Who Was Who in America* (vol. 5, 1969-1973), p. 22.

ALICE HOWELL FRIEDMAN

AUSTIN, ANNE L. (August 7, 1891, Ischus, Cattaguagus County, New York--September 1986, Philadelphia, Pennsylvania). *Nurse-historian.* EDUCATION: 1910, graduated from Lockport, New York, High School where one of her teachers was Belva Lockwood, the first woman admitted to practice before the U.S. Supreme Court and the first woman to run for the presidency on a national ticket; c. 1915, graduated from Homeopathic Hospital Training School for Nursing, Buffalo, New York; 1927, B.S. in nursing and teaching certificate, Teachers College, Columbia University, New York City; 1932, A.M. in sociology, University of Chicago; 1934, post-graduate studies in summer school, Teachers College, Columbia University. CAREER: 1915-1917, private duty nursing in Buffalo, New York; 1917-1919, member of the Army Nurse Corps; 1919-1920, taught home hygiene and care, American Red Cross, Lockport, New York; 1920, night supervisor and instructor, Lockport Hospital, Lockport, New York; 1921-1927, assistant principal, Buffalo Homeopathic Hospital School of Nursing; 1927-1934, instructor, Harper Hospital School of Nursing, Detroit, Michigan; 1930, taught in the summer session, Loyola University, Chicago; 1934-1948, assistant professor, associate professor, then professor of nursing, Frances Payne Bolton School of Nursing, Western Reserve University, Cleveland, Ohio; 1948-retirement, taught nursing at the University of California at Los Angeles, and at the University of Pennsylvania School of Nursing, Philadelphia.

CONTRIBUTIONS: Anne Austin is best remembered for her work on the history of nursing. In the first issue of the *Journal of Nursing History*, Josephine Dolan, a leading nurse-historian of the 1980s, wrote a glowing tribute, calling Austin "a scholar, master teacher, and noted nurse historian." Austin is best known for her *History of Nursing Source Book* (1957), and for collaborating with Isabel M. Stewart (q.v.) on *A History of Nursing from Ancient to Modern Times: A World View* (fifth edition, 1962). She also wrote numerous articles for the *American Journal of Nursing*, *Nursing Research*, and even for *Notable American Women: 1607-1950* (1971). After World War II, when the teaching of nursing history began to lose its place in the curriculum to the new specialties and subspecialties, Austin contributed valuable textbooks and important articles which maintained among many nurses an interest in understanding the place of nursing in history. In addition to original works on nursing history, Austin lectured widely on the historical method as applicable to nursing research. Her leadership was inspiring to those who continued to study and do research on the history of the profession.

In addition to writing about the history of nursing, Austin's second greatest contribution was her enthusiasm for the preservation of historical documents related to the profession. She spearheaded several state committees which devoted time and energy to locating source materials in nursing and to ensure that they were deposited in a repository in which they would be properly preserved. She was one of the first members appointed to the National League of Nursing's committee on historical source materials in nursing and served on the committee from 1947 to 1967. She also was a member of the California League for Nursing's committee on historical sources and a member of the University of Pennsylvania's committee on historical resources in schools of nursing. In the early 1970s, she became a member of the advisory committee of the section on nursing history of the Medical Heritage Society (1970s).

Austin's career provided her a unique set of experiences which undoubtedly served to give her a broad view of the profession. She worked as a public health nurse in Lockport, New York, served with the Army Nurse Corps in France during World War I (with Base Hospital Number 23, of Buffalo), and taught at diploma and baccalaureate schools of nursing from coast to coast.

Over the course of her career, Austin received a number of honors in recognition of her contributions to nursing history. In 1938, she was made an honorary member of the Frances Payne Bolton School of Nursing, Western Reserve University; in 1975, she was made an honorary member of the Millard Fillmore Hospital School of Nursing, Buffalo, New York; and in 1974, she received from the alumni association of Columbia University Teachers College an award for distinguished achievements in research and scholarship.

WRITINGS: *The History of the Farrand Training School for Nurses* (co-author with Agnes G. Deens, 1936); *History of Nursing Source Book* (1957); *A History of Nursing from Ancient to Modern Times: A World View*; *The Woolsey Sisters of New York: A Family's Involvement in the Civil War and a New Profession*, vol. 85 of the *Memoirs of the American Philosophical Society* (1971); numerous articles in journals.

REFERENCES: Manuscript materials in the personal papers of Anne Austin, Nursing Archives, Mugar Memorial Library, Boston University; Josephine Dolan, "A Tribute to Anne L. Austin," *Journal of Nursing History* (1985), pp. 7-10.

ALICE HOWELL FRIEDMAN

B

BANFIELD, EMMA MAUD (c. 1870, South Wales--September 22, 1931, Wadestown, New Zealand). *Administrator; educator.* Married A. R. Atkinson, c. 1923. EDUCATION: Attended convent school in Bruges, Belgium, where she converted to Catholicism and learned French; late 1880s, attended St. Bartholomew's Hospital School of Nursing, London. CAREER: Reorganized nursing service at St. Agnes Hospital, London; 1895-1897, superintendent of nurses and assistant superintendent, Polyclinic Hospital, Philadelphia; 1897-1910, superintendent, Polyclinic Hospital; 1898, supervised the reception and care of wounded soldiers evacuated from Puerto Rico and Cuba at the conclusion of the Spanish-American War; 1910-1914, retirement in England; 1914-1915, served with British Red Cross unit in France during World War I; 1915-1918, continued working for the British War Office, London, while working as staff nurse and then as matron of the Lord Derby War Hospital, Warrington; 1918, served at the front; c. 1919, incapacitated by a bicycle accident; c. 1923, married A. R. Atkinson, an attorney who was her childhood friend, and moved with him to New Zealand, where she died of cancer in 1931.

CONTRIBUTIONS: During her tenure as superintendent of the Philadelphia Polyclinic Hospital, Emma Banfield lengthened the course of study from two to three years, she was instrumental in the development of the alumni association, and she instituted a post-graduate course for nurses. She removed the tuberculosis and obstetrical patients from the general wards, in spite of strong opposition. In 1902, land was acquired, and under her supervision a nurses' home was constructed. In 1903, she moved into a newly acquired residence next to the hospital which had been purchased by the hospital as the superintendent's quarters. Her annual reports included recommendations that stressed the concept of prevention. She also consistently urged visiting-nurse services for patients with tuberculosis. Under her leadership, the Polyclinic grew in number of patients as well as nursing students. In 1909, it was combined with the University of Pennsylvania and became the post-graduate department of that university. The fact that she was a hospital superintendent at the turn of the century, a time when few women held such positions, was testament to her knowledge and leadership skills.

She was active in the Association of Hospital Superintendents and did much to promote nursing in the United States and Canada. As a member of the Society of Superintendents of Training Schools for Nurses, she participated in the historic beginning of the department of nurses at Teachers College, Columbia University. The first course that was offered was in hospital economics, under the department of domestic science. The education committee of the society took the responsibility for screening candidates applying to the college and for the expenses incurred in the teaching of the course. Banfield was involved in screening applicants, as well as in the appropriation of funding for the course. In 1899, she was a member of the first board of examiners at Teachers College and participated in teaching the course in hospital economics. In 1901, she became chairperson of the Hospital Economics Committee of the Society of American Superintendents.

In addition to her position as a hospital administrator and her participation in the Teachers College course, she conducted a department of home nursing for the *Ladies Home Journal.* In addition to writing numerous articles, she answered letters from readers seeking advice. For her fearless service during World War I, she was decorated by the Royal Red Cross and was mentioned in dispatches for her "gallant and distinguished conduct in the field." During her last days when she was losing her fight to cancer, she was described by visitors as possessing quiet heroism and gracious patience.

WRITINGS: Numerous articles in various professional journals and in the *Ladies Home Journal.*

REFERENCES: Teresa E. Christy, *Cornerstone for Nursing Education* (1969); M. Adelaide Nutting Collection, Teachers College, Columbia University, New York City (microfiche 2425, 2426).

LORETTA P. HIGGINS

BARTON, CLARISSA HARLOWE (December 25, 1821, North Oxford, Massachusetts--April 12, 1912, Glen Echo, Maryland). *Civil War nurse; founder of the American Red Cross.* Daughter of Stephen Barton, farmer, soldier, and sawmill owner, and Sarah (Stone) Barton, farmer. Never married. EDUCATION: Taught at home by her schoolteacher siblings; at three, was sent to district school, Oxford, Massachusetts, at eight, sent to board for high school, but homesickness prevailed, and she returned home to be taught by her family; at thirteen, attended Lucian Burleigh's school in her home town and was tutored by Jonathan Dana, a local teacher; 1850-1851, studied at the Liberal Institute, Clinton, New York.

CAREER: Beginning in May 1839, served as a schoolteacher in District 9, North Oxford, Massachusetts, then taught at Millbury, Massachusetts, and in 1852 started her own school for the children of mill workers in Hightstown, New Jersey; 1852-1854, started a school in Bordentown, New Jersey; 1854-1857 and 1860-1861, served as copyist in the Patent Office, Washington, D.C.; 1861-1865, volunteer nurse, Civil War; 1865-1868, served as general correspondent for the Friends of Paroled Prisoners, locating missing soldiers and marking graves at Andersonville Prison, Georgia; 1866-1868, lecturer on the Civil War; 1869-1873, travelled in Europe to study care of soldiers in the Franco-Prussian War, the International Red Cross movement, and served as a volunteer relief worker; after four years of illness (1873-1877), began work to establish the American Red Cross, which was realized on May 21, 1881; 1881-1904, president, American Red Cross; 1883 (for six months), served as superintendent, Woman's Reformatory Prison, Sherborn, Massachusetts; 1906, organized the National First Aid Association.

CONTRIBUTIONS: Clara Barton's most important contribution to nursing was as the first woman to take to the battlefield as a volunteer nurse and relief worker during the Civil War. Her two years (from age eleven to thirteen) of nursing her brother David after a bad accident apparently laid the foundation for her nursing career. Beginning in 1861, while still in Washington, D.C., she began to collect supplies and bring comfort and relief to the men tented around Washington and to those in the Washington Infirmary. In August 1862, she succeeded in receiving permission to go to the field as a nurse, and thereafter often followed the line of battle. She was present at a number of battles, including Second Bull Run, Antietam, Fredericksburg, and the siege of Charleston. Again and again she appeared at the sites of major battles, with supplies to care for the wounded. Soldiers called her the "Angel of the Battlefield."

With the support of President Abraham Lincoln, in 1865 she set up an office at Annapolis, Maryland, to attempt to locate the 80,000 men who were missing at the end of the war. Her official title was general correspondent for the friends of paroled prisoners. She was able to send word to 22,000 families of missing soldiers and served at Andersonville Prison, to help mark as many as possible of the 13,000 graves of Union soldiers.

Between 1866 and 1868, she lectured on the Civil War to over 300 audiences in the North and West to replenish her depleted resources in order to continue her work of locating missing soldiers. Her work took a toll on her health, however, and in 1869 she went abroad at the urging of friends and family. While in Europe, Barton studied the work of the International Red Cross, served as a volunteer nurse during the Franco-Prussian War, and recuperated in England and at home until 1877. In 1877, with the same fervor that had characterized her work during the Civil War, she undertook to convince the federal authorities and the nation of the need for an American Red Cross organization. In 1881, she was successful, and through her efforts she earned recognition as the founder of the American Red Cross. She persevered through several administrations to persuade the United States to ratify the Geneva Treaty, which was approved at last with the signature of President Chester Allan Arthur (March 1, 1882). In keeping with her approach to most challenges, she was an active participant in the work of the Red Cross during her tenure as president. She took to the field during numerous disasters to which the Red Cross responded, including the 1881 Michigan forest fire, the 1884 Ohio and Mississippi River floods, the 1888 Florida yellow fever epidemic, the Mt. Vernon, Illinois, tornado of the same year, the 1889 Johnstown, Pennsylvania, flood, the 1891-1892 Russian famine, the 1893 and 1894 South Carolina Sea Islands hurricane and tidal wave, the 1900 Galveston hurricane, and the 1904 Butler, Pennsylvania, typhoid fever epidemic. She served in the Armenian crisis of 1896 to bring relief to the persecuted Armenians and in the 1898 Cuban crisis. She represented the United States at the 1887 convention of the International Red Cross (at Karlsruhe), at the 1897 Vienna convention, and at the 1902 convention at St. Petersburg, Russia. She served as president of the American Red Cross until May 14, 1904, when she resigned amid controversy which included a communication from President Theodore Roosevelt withdrawing his support and that of his cabinet from their positions on her Board of Consultation.

During her lifetime, Barton received more than twenty-five honors, including the Iron Cross of Germany (1871), recognition from the Serbian Red Cross (1876), the Medal of the International Red Cross (1882), and the sultan's decoration of Shefaket, Turkey (1883). For many years, she served as national chaplain of the Woman's Relief Corps and as guest of honor at encampments of the Grand Army of the Republic. She was a friend of Susan B. Anthony, was present at the first suffrage meeting in Washington, D.C., in 1869, and she had a lifelong association with the woman's suffrage movement. She died at Glen Echo, Maryland, in the house that served as her home during the later years of her life

and as the headquarters of the American Red Cross from 1897 to 1904. She was buried in North Oxford, Massachusetts, near her birthplace.
WRITINGS: *The Red Cross: A History of This Remarkable International Movement in the Interest of Humanity* (1898); *The Red Cross in Peace and War* (1899); *The Story of My Childhood* (1907); *A Story of the Red Cross* (1918); and numerous articles. She also prepared official reports for her various positions and kept more than forty diaries and a copious correspondence.
REFERENCES: *American Journal of Nursing* (November 1905), p. 95 and (May 1912), p. 621; Clara Barton, *The Red Cross in Peace and War* (1898) and *The Story of My Childhood* (1907); William E. Barton, *The Life of Clara Barton* (2 vols., 1922); *Dictionary of American Biography*, II: 18-21; Bertha S. Dodge, *The Story of Nursing* (1954); Patrick F. Gilbo, "Candid Cranky Clara Barton Gave Us the Red Cross," *Smithsonian* (May 1981); Mary E. Gardner Holland, *Our Army Nurses* (1897); Portia B. Kernodle, *The Red Cross Nurse in Action, 1882-1948* (1949); Robin McKown, *Heroic Nurses* (1966); *National Cyclopedia of American Biography*, XV: 314-315; National Park Service, *Clara Barton* (1981); Jeannette Covert Nolan, *The Story of Clara Barton of the Red Cross* (1941); *Notable American Women*, I: 103-108; Ishbel Ross, *Angel of the Battlefield* (1956); Blanche Colton Williams, *Clara Barton: Daughter of Destiny* (1941).

JOELLEN WATSON HAWKINS

BATTERHAM, MARY ROSE (c. 1870, England--April 4, 1927, Asheville, North Carolina). *First American registered nurse.* Never married. EDUCATION: 1893, graduate of Brooklyn City Hospital, Brooklyn, New York. CAREER: 1893-1927, private and public health nursing, Asheville, North Carolina, and head nurse, Oakland Heights Sanitarium, North Carolina, and Metropolitan nurse, Asheville, North Carolina.
CONTRIBUTIONS: Mary Rose Batterham is credited with being the first nurse to be registered in the United States. In 1902 North Carolina became the first state to enact legislation requiring the registration of nurses, and on June 5, 1903, Batterham registered in Buncombe County. Her position as the first, however, is denied by Mary L. Wyche (q.v.), who stated in a footnote in her book on the history of nursing in North Carolina that one day before Mary Rose Batterham registered, Josephine Burton did so in Craven County. In spite of that discovery, however, Mary Rose Batterham continues to be credited with being the first registered nurse in the United States.

Regardless of whether Josephine Burton registered before Mary Rose Batterham, the fact is that Batterham can be viewed as a pioneer in more than the act of submitting to the county evidence of her nursing education and practice. She attended the 1901 meeting in Raleigh, North Carolina, at which nurses discussed the need to establish a statewide organization, and on October 28, 1902, she served as chairperson of the meeting at which the North Carolina Nurses' Association was founded. She was a charter member of the association, and served as its first vice-president.

In April 1916, she was one of twelve nurses to organize a public health section in the state nurses' association and in 1917 was elected chairperson of that section. She was also a charter member of her alumnae association (1895) and a member of the North Carolina Red Cross Nursing Committee.

She wrote a number of articles for nursing journals, expressing her ideals and her sense of professional ethics. She believed that a private duty nurse occasionally should nurse those who could not afford professional care and that the nurse should not be selective of her patients, instead serving all. As a nurse, she was a health educator, and in that role she encouraged nurses to be aware of social problems such as the underfed school child and the unnecessary death of women and their infants. She believed nurses should be concerned about civic needs and engage in welfare work. For students, she advocated shorter hours and improved living quarters and working conditions. She believed that nurses should have superior educational and cultural backgrounds and should be offered a broad curriculum.

WRITINGS: Numerous articles for professional journals.

REFERENCES: *American Journal of Nursing* (September 1926), p. 700 and (May 1927), p. 410; Minnie Goodnow, *Nursing History* (7th ed., 1943); Mary L. Wyche, *History of Nursing in North Carolina* (1938); copy of original certificate of registration, North Carolina Board of Nursing, Raleigh, North Carolina (June 5, 1903).

JOELLEN WATSON HAWKINS

BEARD, MARY (November 14, 1876, Dover, New Hampshire-December 4, 1946, New York City, New York). *Administrator, educator, public health nurse.* Daughter of Ithamar Warren Beard, Episcopal rector, and Marcy (Foster) Beard. Never married. EDUCATION: Attended public schools of Dover, New Hampshire; 1899-1903, attended New York Hospital School of Nursing, New York City. CAREER: 1904-1909, staff nurse, then director, Visiting Nurse Association of Waterbury,

Connecticut; 1910-1912, worked at Laboratory of Surgical Pathology, College of Physicians and Surgeons of Columbia University, New York City; 1912-1922, director of the Boston Instructive District Nursing Association, Boston; 1922-1924, director of the Community Health Association, which resulted from a merger of the Boston Instructive District Nursing Association and the Baby Hygiene Association; 1924-1938, various posts with the Rockefeller Foundation, including 1925-1927, special assistant to the director of the division of studies, 1927-1930, assistant to the director of the division of medical education, and 1930-1938, associate director of the international health division; 1938-1944, director of the newly consolidated nursing service of the American Red Cross; 1944, due to ill health, resigned from the Red Cross.

CONTRIBUTIONS: Mary Beard was one of the best-known nurses of her time. An advocate of preventive health services, she was responsible for many projects whose goals were to advance the causes of education and public health in the United States and abroad. Under her leadership, the Boston Instructive District Nursing Association merged in 1922 with the Baby Hygiene Association, forming the Community Health Association. Her success in that endeavor obviously impressed interested observers, and she became a member of the Rockefeller Foundation Committee for the Study of Nursing and Nursing Education, which prepared a significant report published in 1923, *Nursing and Nursing Education in the United States*, popularly known as the Goldmark Report. That report advocated high standards in nursing education, and it was ultimately responsible for the closing of many schools unable to meet those standards.

In 1924, Beard began a fourteen-year relationship with the Rockefeller Foundation, and under her influence, it donated four million dollars to nursing and in the process helping encourage nursing schools to implement the Goldmark Report. During her years with the foundation, she travelled internationally, learning about nursing in other countries and helping many countries to develop schools of nursing.

In 1938, at the age of sixty-two, Beard accepted what would prove to be a challenging position as director of the newly consolidated nursing service of the American Red Cross. During the twenty years since World War I, the nursing service of the Red Cross had lost prestige and standing as the "backbone of the Red Cross." During World War II, much confusion existed about the route nurses were to take to join the army. The Red Cross had traditionally provided the means by which nurses were recruited and processed into the military. In 1942, after consultation with the army and navy, the Red Cross, under Mary Beard, again took full responsibility for the recruitment, processing, and certification of nurses for those branches of the armed forces.

Other programs that flourished under the directorship of Mary Beard were the Red Cross nurse's aide educational program and the home nursing program. Another program begun during the war years, was Camp Community Emergency Nursing Services, whose primary contribution was maternal and child care for the families of servicemen, who without these Red Cross services were left without health care.

In addition to contributing to nursing and public health through her positions in Boston, with the Rockefeller Foundation, and with the Red Cross, she was active in various nursing organizations. She was one of the founders of the National Organization for Public Health Nursing, serving as its president during World War I. She was also a member of that organization's board of directors for a total of eighteen years between 1912 and 1946 and as its vice-president in 1915-1916. At various times during her career, she served as a member of the Nursing Committee of the Henry Street Nursing Service and of the Advisory Committee on Nursing of the New York City Department of Health. She served as chairwoman of the Subcommittee on Public Health Nursing of the General Medical Board of the Council of National Defense. She had a reputation as a humanitarian, a person who worked well with groups, but who took an individual interest in each person she met.

Beard received numerous honors, including honorary degrees from the University of New Hampshire (doctor of humanities, 1934), and Smith College (doctor of laws, 1945), and honorary membership in the council of the International Council of Nurses and the Association of Collegiate Schools of Nursing.

WRITINGS: *The Nurse in Public Health* (1929) and numerous articles in professional nursing journals.

REFERENCES: *American Journal of Nursing* (December 1931), pp. 1411-1413 and (October 1938), pp. 1161-1163; *Dictionary of American Biography*, supplement 4: 64-66; Alan Gregg, "Mary Beard: Humanist," *American Journal of Nursing* (February 1947), pp. 103-104; *National Cyclopedia of American Biography*, XXXV: 183; *Public Health Nursing* (January 1947), p. 3.

LORETTA P. HIGGINS

BECK, SISTER M. BERENICE (Born Annetta Beck, October 19, 1890, St. Louis, Missouri--March 1, 1960, Racine, Wisconsin). *Educator.* Never married. EDUCATION: 1910, joined the Franciscan Sisters; 1915, received diploma, St. Anthony's Hospital School of Nursing, St. Louis,

Missouri; 1927, B.A., and 1931, M.A., Marquette University, Milwaukee, Wisconsin; 1935, Ph.D., Catholic University of America, Washington, D.C. CAREER: 1916-1929, instructor then assistant director, Saint Joseph's Hospital School of Nursing, Milwaukee, Wisconsin; 1929-1932, director, St. Joseph's Hospital School of Nursing; 1932-1936, instructor, Catholic University of America; 1936-c. 1952, taught at Marquette University College of Nursing, and 1936-1942, dean; 1946-1948, assistant administrator, St. Anthony's Hospital, St. Louis; 1952, because of failing health, went into semi-retirement at St. Mary's Hospital, Racine, Wisconsin, where she died at the age of seventy.
CONTRIBUTIONS: Undoubtedly, Sister Beck will always be remembered in the nursing world for her role as chairperson of the ethics committee of the American Nurses' Association (ANA) that was successful in the development of the Code for Professional Nurses, the association's first code of ethics (adopted by the ANA House of Delegates in 1950). Before she became its chairperson, the committee had worked diligently to develop a code that would be acceptable to the ANA board, but to no avail. She was also one of the first nurses to receive a doctorate (1935), as well as the first in Wisconsin to do so. The year after she received her doctorate from the Catholic University of America, she became the first dean of the newly established Marquette University School of Nursing (1936), one of the first baccalaureate programs for nurses in the country. At Catholic University, she helped to develop the nursing education department while she was an instructor and completing requirements for her doctorate.

She was a visionary as demonstrated by some of her controversial positions. In the 1930s she foresaw that by about the mid-1950s the hospital school of nursing would no longer exist and she supported the development of university-education of nurses. Although she was overly optimistic as to the time involved for such a momentous change, she was correct in her prediction. She also was supportive of staff nurses and encouraged their participation in professional organizations and staff development, the latter a relatively new concept in nursing.

She believed in the stratification of nursing into two tiers, the professional nurse and the subsidiary worker, and she also foresaw the need for nurse-specialists and for further education for head nurses, administrators, and educators.

During her career, she was active in the major nursing organizations. She was a member of the board of directors of the ANA, the American Journal of Nursing Company, the Wisconsin State Nurses' Association, and the District of Columbia League of Nursing Education. She was a member of the National League of Nursing Education's sisters committee and curriculum committee, and in 1946 she was selected by the ANA to be its representative to the Committee on the Structure of National Nursing Organizations, which was made up of representatives of the six national nursing organizations. From 1943 to 1948, she was an educational consultant to the U.S. Cadet Nurse Corps. She was a member of the council on nursing education of the Catholic Hospital Association. She served as vice-president and president of the Wisconsin League of Nursing Education. She also was vice-president of the ANA counseling and placement service. While she was semi-retired and serving at St. Mary's Hospital in Racine, Wisconsin, she established a hospital library.

On January 23, 1960, she celebrated her golden jubilee in the Order of St. Francis. In June of 1986, she was inducted into the nursing hall of fame of the American Nurses' Association. She was remembered by her colleagues as being a strong presence at nursing meetings during which she kept her fingers busy tatting (making lace). When she spoke, people listened, and her words often swayed a decision. She was outspoken in her opinions, however, and occasionally alienated those with different ideas.

WRITINGS: *The Nurse, Handmaid of the Divine Physician* (1945); many articles in professional journals including "Coordinating the Teaching of Sciences and Nursing Practice," *American Journal of Nursing* (June 1934), pp. 579-586; "Analysis of Nursing Service," *Hospital Progress* (August 1935), pp. 304-306; and "Hospital or Collegiate Schools of Nursing," *American Journal of Nursing* (July 1936), pp. 716-725.

REFERENCES: *American Journal of Nursing* (May 1960), p. 638; *The American Nurse* (June 1986), p. 10; Signe S. Cooper, *Wisconsin Nursing Pioneers* (1968); Cordelia W. Kelly, *Dimensions of Professional Nursing* (1962); archives of the Marquette University School of Nursing (including a speech by Mary Paquette, October 6, 1983); *Nursing Outlook* (April 1960), p. 82; information provided by the staff of the State Historical Society of Wisconsin, Madison, Wisconsin; *Wisconsin State Nurses Association Bulletin* (March-April 1960), p. 9.

LORETTA P. HIGGINS

BEEBY, NELL V. (August 1, 1896, Secundrabad, India--May 17, 1957, Jackson Heights, New York). *Editor.* Daughter of William Henry Beeby and Clara (Bridge) Beeby, missionaries. Never married. EDUCATION: 1916, graduated from Urbana High School, Illinois; 1919, graduated from St. Luke's Hospital School of Nursing, Chicago; 1932-1934, attended University of Chicago; 1936, B.S., Teachers College, Columbia University, New York City. CAREER: 1919-1924, private duty nursing; 1924-1927, faculty member and supervisor of obstetrical and surgical departments, Hunan-Yale Hospital, Yale-in-China, Changsha, China; 1928-1934, private duty obstetrical nursing and then supervisor of obstetrics, St. Luke's Hospital, Chicago; 1936-1949, member of the editorial staff, *American Journal of Nursing*, 1936-1949; April 1, 1949-1956, editor, *American Journal of Nursing*; 1949-1957, executive editor, American Journal of Nursing Company.

CONTRIBUTIONS: Throughout her life, including the last five months when she was in the terminal stage of cancer, Nell Beeby exhibited the characteristics that made her a special person in the nursing profession: she was described as being charming and witty, generous with her advice and wisdom, always busy yet serene, and interested in everything from politics to the latest fashions. Her greatest contribution came as a result of her strong leadership of the *American Journal of Nursing*. Her association with the *Journal* began when she wrote four articles on obstetrical nursing. When her studies at Teachers College brought her to New York in 1934, she joined the editorial staff as a part-time news editor. After graduation in 1936, she assumed a full-time position as assistant editor. She was credited with revitalizing the news section of the journal, developing a network of reliable sources for news of professional organizations, as well as international, national and local nursing activities. During World War II, she served as war correspondent for the journal, visiting nurses in military installations in France, England, and Germany.

When Mary M. Roberts (q.v.) retired in 1949, Nell Beeby not only became editor of the *Journal* but also the first executive editor of the American Journal of Nursing Company. Under her leadership, the company expanded its work from one publication with a circulation of 99,000 to three publications with over 175,000 monthly circulation. Under her guidance, *Nursing Outlook* and *Nursing Research* joined the *American Journal of Nursing* as the publications of the company.

Perhaps her missionary roots or her extensive travel through war-torn Europe during World War II convinced her of the need for closer ties among nurses around the world. She maintained an extensive correspondence with nursing editors and nursing leaders throughout the world, using those ties to provide readers with up-to-date information on worldwide nursing activities. Editors around the world valued her expertise and advice and sought them often. She won the respect of not only the nursing profession but the wider health-care community.

Shortly after Nell's birth, her missionary parents returned to the United States, and she grew up in Illinois. It is not surprising, then, that she attended a school of nursing in Chicago. Even as a student, her primary clinical interest was in maternity nursing, and so she chose to specialize in it as a private duty nurse. She hoped to return to India in missionary service, but there were no openings there so she accepted appointment at the Hunan-Yale School of Nursing in China, again specializing in maternity. After her experience in China, she returned to Chicago, where she became supervisor of St. Luke's Hospital obstetric department, developing methods for correlating classroom teaching and ward experience, as well as instituting an additional clinical experience for nursing students in the out-patient department. Her first four published articles grew out of her experience in obstetrical nursing in China and Chicago. Interestingly, those articles represented her past experience in maternal nursing and her future endeavor as a writer.

Beeby's contributions were not confined to the *Journal* company and to the institutions she served in China and Chicago. Throughout her life, she was active in nursing organizations, including her alumnae association, the National League for Nursing, the American Nurses' Association, the American Hospital Association, the American Public Health Association, and the Christian Medical Council for Overseas Work. She was on the board of the American Bureau for Medical Aid to China, helping to arrange for scholarships for Chinese nurses to study in the United States and for procurement of books and equipment for Chinese nursing schools.

In 1957, the last year of her life, Beeby was relieved of responsibility for editing the *Journal* in order to concentrate her energies on the work needed for managing the American Journal of Nursing Company. Characteristically, she had just completed a survey of the world's nursing publications and was compiling and writing up the information for a presentation at the International Council of Nurses' assembly in Rome, Italy, when she suddenly died. In February 1957, three months before she died, the National League for Nursing awarded her the M. Adelaide Nutting Award for Leadership in Nursing.

WRITINGS: Countless articles and editorials in professional journals.

REFERENCES: *American Journal of Nursing* (September 1936), p. 954, (June 1949), pp. 330-331, (April 1957), p. 469, (June 1957), pp. 728-736; *Canadian Nurse* (September 1949), pp. 680-681, (July 1957), p. 628; *Nursing Outlook* (June 1957), pp. 340-343; *Public Health Nurse* (June 1949), p. 366; *South African Nursing Journal* (May 1957), p. 29; *Who's Who of American Women* (1959), p. 101.

JOELLEN WATSON HAWKINS

BERTHOLD, JEANNE (SAYLOR) (June 4, 1924, Kansas City, Missouri--July 6, 1983, Downey, California). *Leader in nursing research.*

Daughter of Carl Richard Saylor and Anna Elizabeth (Wolfe) Saylor. EDUCATION: 1945, graduated from Highland School of Nursing, Oakland, California; 1953, B.S., 1955, M.S. in psychiatric nursing, and 1961, Ph.D. in counseling psychology, University of California, Berkeley. CAREER: 1945-1946, public health staff nurse, Visiting Nurse Association, Los Angeles; 1946-1947, school nurse, Los Angeles; 1947-1951, staff assistant, Sonoma County Hospital, Santa Rosa, California; 1955-1961, psychiatric nurse, Langley Porter Neuro-Psychiatric Institute, San Francisco; 1955-1961, instructor and lecturer, School of Nursing, University of California Medical Center, San Francisco; 1961-1963, assistant professor, 1963-1964, associate professor, and 1964-1971, professor, Francis Payne Bolton School of Nursing, Case Western Reserve University, Cleveland, Ohio; 1971-1973, professor adjoint, University of Colorado School of Nursing, Denver; 1973-1983, professor of community and family medicine, University of Southern California School of Medicine, Los Angeles; 1973-1975, director of nursing research, and 1975-1983, director of nursing research and education, Rancho Los Amigos Hospital, Downey, California; 1977-1983, adjunct professor, California State University, Long Beach.
CONTRIBUTIONS: Jeanne Saylor Berthold was a leader in nursing research. In the 1950s, when few nurses were engaged in research, she was already leading the way, preparing herself with education and practical experience for a career of clinical research. Her first funded investigation focused on sensory deprivation and effective nursing interventions. She served as principal investigator for a study of concept attainment and nurses' preferences, and she was on the program staff for a faculty research development grant, a nurse-scientist training grant, and a grant for development of nursing education technology at Case Western Reserve University. From 1971 to 1973, she was principal investigator and program director for a regional program for nursing research and development under the auspices of the Western Interstate Commission for Higher Education. Later, she served as director of research and education at Rancho Los Amigos Hospital.

Concerned with theory development in nursing, Berthold was also interested in the ethics of clinical research, the protection of human rights and values. One of her research projects focused on patient care and nursing service responsibilities in a rehabilitation facility. Her research efforts reached an apex in the position she held at the time of her death. At the world-famous rehabilitation hospital, she was responsible for a dynamic and active nursing service department. Committed to continuing education, Berthold was a lifelong student as well as a teacher. As technology changed the practice of nursing, she updated her skills and knowledge, learning about computer technology and incorporating it into her practice, research, and teaching. A number of her publications reflect her ability to integrate computer technology into the nursing profession.

Berthold's professional contributions were not limited to her roles as practitioner, teacher, administrator, and researcher, however. She was a member of many professional organizations, including the National League for Nursing (NLN), the American Nurses' Association (ANA), the American Psychological Association, the American Educational Research Association, the National Council of Measurement in Education, the New York Academy of Sciences, the American Association for the Advancement of Science, the Center on Evaluation, Development, and Research of Phi Delta Kappa, the Hastings Center, the American Congress of Rehabilitation Medicine, and the Association of Rehabilitation Nurses.

She was the secretary (1955) and a member of various professional organizations and committees, including the steering committee (1956-1958), of the California League for Nursing interdivisional council of psychiatric and mental health nursing, the volunteer advisory committee of the California Mental Health Association (1957-1959), the workshop planning committee for the California State Board of Nurse Examiners (1957-1958), a board member and membership chairperson of Pi Lambda Theta (1959-1961), chairperson of the interdivisional council on research of the NLN (1965-1967), member of the board of trustees of the American Nurses' Foundation (1965-1971) and president (1969-1971), the ANA standing committee on research and studies (1965-1970), serving as chairperson the last two years. From 1969 to 1971, she was vice-chairperson of the NLN department of baccalaureate and higher degree programs. For the ANA, she chaired the commission on nursing research (1970-1975), was a member of the executive commmittee of the council of nurse researchers (1970-1975), served as a resource person for the committee on interrelationships (1972-1975), and chaired the advisory committee for research conferences (1969-1973). From 1976 to 1979, she chaired or was a member of a number of committees for the American Congress of Rehabilitation Medicine, including president of rehabilitation resources from 1979 to 1980 and chairperson of the rehabilitation nursing institute research committee in 1979. From 1969 to 1973, she was a member of the editorial board of *Nursing Research*, serving as chairperson from 1972 to 1973.

Berthold presented papers at local, regional, and national conferences from 1956 to 1980. She was widely sought as a speaker and consultant. For both the schools and service institutions where she held positions and also for the state of California, Berthold gave time to numerous committees and participated in educational and policy analysis conferences.

Over the course of her career, she received a large number of honors in recognition of her accomplishments and contributions to her profession. She graduated with honors from the University of California at Berkeley in 1953, and was elected to Pi Lambda Theta in 1958 and to Sigma Theta Tau in 1966. She was listed in *Who's Who of American Women* (from 1966 on), *American Men of Science* (1968), *American Men and Women of Science* (1972), *Who's Who in American Education: Leaders in American Science Education* (1971), *International Scholars Directory* (1971-1973), *2000 Women of Achievement* (1972), *Who's Who in America* (from 1974 on), and many similar publications.

WRITINGS: Numerous articles in professional journals, and monographs, including *Human Rights Guidelines for Nurses in Clinical and Other Research* (1975); produced numerous computer programs for use in practice settings, as well as several films of nursing activities.

REFERENCES: *American Journal of Nursing* (October 1983), p. 1490; unpublished curriculum vitae and memorial tribute, Rancho Los Amigos Medical Center archives, Downey, California; *Who's Who of American Women* (1972-1973), p. 63.

JOELLEN WATSON HAWKINS

BICKERDYKE, MARY ANN (BALL) (July 19, 1817, Knox County, Ohio--November 8, 1901, Bunker Hill, Kansas). *Civil War nurse.* Daughter of Hiram Ball, farmer, and Anna (Rodgers) Ball, a distant relative of Mary Ball Washington, mother of the first president. Married Robert Bickerdyke, a widower with children, a musician and housepainter, April 27, 1847 (he died in March 1859); three children, two sons and a daughter, the last dying at the age of two. EDUCATION: Early education in a one-room log schoolhouse in Ohio; 1833-1837, she claimed to have gone to Oberlin College, although the college has no record of her attendance (she did move to Oberlin in 1833, and it has been theorized that she worked in the household of a professor and was allowed to audit courses); 1837, sources indicate that she attended a course for nurses under Dr. Reuben D. Mussey, Cincinnati, Ohio (this is questionable, for at that time, twenty-year-old unmarried women generally could not be nurses; more probably she studied under a Dr. Hussey, who ran the Physio-Botanic Medical College in Cincinnati). CAREER: 1837-1847 and 1859-1861, possibly served as a botanic physician; 1847-c. 1851, lived in Cincinnati, where she took fugitive slaves into her home and passed them on to a Quaker group in Hamilton,

Ontario, Canada; 1851-1861, lived in Galesburg, Illinois, presumably as a wife and mother; June 9, 1861-March 20, 1865, worked in regimental hospitals during the Civil War; 1866-1867, worked at the newly constructed Cairo (Illinois) Soldiers' Home; 1867, was housekeeper in the Chicago Home for the Friendless and in that same year sponsored a homestead project in Kansas for "her boys"; she led a group of homesteaders (veterans and their families) to Kansas and filed a claim for herself and her sons; under the auspices of the Kansas-Pacific Railroad, ran a hotel in Salina, which came to be known as Bickerdyke House; 1870-1874, missionary in New York under the Board of City Missions, participating in a slum clearance program and teaching Sunday school in a Salvation Army mission; 1874, returned to Kansas and travelled extensively to raise funds to help the sufferers during the locust plague of that year; 1876, went to the West Coast, where she worked as a pension attorney to help veterans and nurses secure their pensions; when the pension problem was resolved to her satisfaction, she took a position in the U.S. Mint in San Francisco; continued to provide volunteer social work, helping to organize the first Woman's Relief Corps in California, including an attempt to rescue prostitutes in San Francisco; 1887, at the urging of her son, returned to Kansas to nurse her dying stepdaughter, Mary; maintained contact with the home and hospital at Ellsworth, Kansas, which was known as Mother Bickerdyke Home (in 1941, the home housed fifty women, mostly elderly and disabled World War I nurses); she died in Kansas, and was buried in Galesburg, Illinois.

CONTRIBUTIONS: Known as "Mother Bickerdyke," and to others as "General Bickerdyke," she nursed Union soldiers during the Civil War. She was also known as the "cyclone in calico" because of the gray calico dress she wore. In 1859, her husband died just a few years after their move to Illinois, and in order to support her family, she hung out her shingle as a botanic physician (treating ailments through the use of drugs made from herbs, roots, and barks). In 1861, when the Civil War broke out, her church congregation voted that she go to Cairo, Illinois, to see how the Union troops were doing. She went on June 9, 1861, and set to work in the hospital tents at Cairo and five other army tent hospitals in the area, bathing the men, cleaning out the tents, and reorganizing the preparation of food. In the process, she enraged the first of many presiding physicians. In February 1862, she went to Fort Donelson on the *City of Memphis* hospital ship and then followed General Ulysses Grant's troops to Savannah. After one battle, she worried that some wounded might have been left on the field, so it became her custom to go out with a lantern and make a survey before she could sleep. She was at the Battle of Shiloh, and took over at the Savannah Hospital, then at Farmington, arriving there on July 9, 1862. From there she went to Corinth to set up a hospital in what had been a young lady's seminary.

In November 1862, she returned to Galesburg for a brief rest, then proceeded to Chicago where she met with Mary Livermore (q.v.) of the U.S. Sanitary Commission. At Livermore's urging, Mother Bickerdyke launched a speaking campaign in Illinois and Wisconsin to raise funds for the U.S. Sanitary Commission and was successful in persuading people to give money and supplies. One story has it that she asked for live cattle and chickens in Chicago and was given 200 head of cattle and a great many chickens. In January 1863, she accepted an assignment at Fort Pickering and at General Grant's suggestion served in other hospitals in and around Memphis. By May, she went on to Vicksburg. Thereafter, at General William Tecumseh Sherman's request, she was permanently assigned to his corps, the fifteenth. She had a confrontation with General Sherman over his orders concerning non-military use of the railroad, and she won the right to have Sanitary Commission supplies carried for her patients. Perhaps the most famous incident of her career occurred when she procured the discharge of a surgeon who had been on a drinking spree. When the surgeon complained to General Sherman, Sherman was reported to have replied that he could do nothing as she outranked him.

Much of her time as a volunteer nurse was spent campaigning for women nurses in the army. She appealed directly to General Ulysses S. Grant, who overruled the physicians' disapproval of women nurses. Gravely concerned that supplies from the U.S. Sanitary Commission were not reaching the wounded, she undertook to remedy the situation, again with General Grant's support. She moved to the hospital in Huntsville and rode in the ambulance wagon with Sherman's march to Atlanta in May 1864. While the battle for Atlanta raged, Mother Bickerdyke oversaw the tent hospital outside Marietta. After another fund-raising trip, this time to New York and Pennsylvania, she was summoned south by Sherman, who wanted her to care for the men released from the Andersonville prisoner-of-war camp in Georgia. She celebrated the surrender of Robert E. Lee with Sherman at Beaufort, South Carolina, on April 9, 1865. On May 24, she rode in the victory parade in Washington, D.C., and sat on the reviewing stand with General Sherman.

Mary Livermore included Bickerdyke in her book and referred to her as an uneducated and illiterate woman. Perhaps it was Mother Bickerdyke's persistent use of the word aint that prompted that conclusion. On July 19, 1897, her eightieth birthday, Kansas honored her with a statewide celebration of Mother Bickerdyke Day. In 1906, a statue was erected on the courthouse lawn in Galesburg, Illinois, honoring "Mother Bickerdyke, Army Nurse." In 1920, the renewal certificate for registered nurses in the state of Illinois included a reproduction of that statue. In 1943, the "victory freighter" *S.S. Mary A. Bickerdyke* was launched, making twenty-eight trips to the Pacific carrying supplies to island outposts during World War II.

WRITINGS: Voluminous correspondence.

REFERENCES: Nina Brown Baker, *Cyclone in Calico: The Story of Mary Ann Bickerdyke* (1952); L. P. Brackett, *Woman's Work in the Civil War* (1867); *Dictionary of American Biography*, II: 237-238; Margaret B. Davis, *Mother Bickerdyke and the Soldiers* (1886); E. V. Erlandson, "The Story of Mother Bickerdyke," *American Journal of Nursing* (May 1920), pp. 628-631; Marjorie Barstow Greenbie, *Lincoln's Daughters of Mercy* (1944); Mary A. G. Holland, *Our Army Nurses* (1897); correspondence with Irene Matthews, R.N., Holmes, Pennsylvania, April 20, 23, August 19, 1987; Mary A. Livermore, *My Story of the War* (1889); Robin McKown, *Heroic Nurses* (1966); Frank Moore, *Women of the War: Heroism and Self Sacrifice* (1867); *National Cyclopedia of American Biography*, XXI: 131-132; Julia C. Stimson and Ethel C. S. Thompson, "Women Nurses with the Union Forces during the Civil War," *Military Surgeon* (January-February 1928); Agatha Young, *The Women and the Crisis: Women of the North in the Civil War* (1959).

JOELLEN WATSON HAWKINS

BLAKE, FLORENCE GUINNESS (November 30, 1907, Stevens Point, Wisconsin--September 10, 1983, Madison, Wisconsin). *Pediatric nursing leader; author.* Daughter of Reverend Blake, Baptist minister and missionary to the Belgian Congo, and Thelma (Dunlap) Blake, music teacher and church organist. Never married. EDUCATION: 1925, graduated from Emerson High School, Stevens Point, Wisconsin; 1925-1928, attended Michael Reese Hospital School of Nursing, Chicago; 1928, attended summer term at the University of Chicago; 1929-1930 and 1933-1934, attended Teachers College, Columbia University, New York City, graduating with a B.S. in 1934 and with a diploma in supervision in schools of nursing; 1934, recognizing her need for more clinical preparation before returning to a position as supervisor of pediatric nursing at Michael Reese Hospital, she spent one month in nursery school and convalescent wards at Bellevue Hospital, two months of bedside nursing at Boston Children's Hospital, and two weeks at the Charles V. Chapin Hospital for Communicable Diseases, Providence, Rhode Island; 1939, studied child development and family life for 6 months at the Merrill-Palmer School, Detroit; 1939-1941, studied child development at the University of Michigan, Ann Arbor, earning a master's degree in

1941; 1949-1951, attended the three year course at the Institute for Psychoanalysis, Chicago, graduating in 1951 with a diploma in psychoanalytic child care.

CAREER: 1928, assistant instructor of nursing arts, and then head nurse in a private ward, Michael Reese Hospital School of Nursing, Chicago; 1930-1931, supervisor of a private pavilion, Michael Reese Hospital; 1931-1933, supervisor of Sarah Morris Children's Hospital, a branch of Michael Reese Hospital; 1936-1939, under the auspices of the Rockefeller Foundation, served as instructor and supervisor of pediatric nursing, Peiping Union Medical College School of Nursing, China; 1940, in a sabbatical year, she travelled, first to Kolar, India, where she spent a month working with the former superintendent of Michael Reese, who then became superintendent at Ellen T. Cowen Memorial Hospital in Kolar; from Kolar, she went to northern India, then through Iraq and Syria to Italy, and back to Michigan; 1941-1942, instructor in pediatric nursing, University of Michigan; 1942-1946, assistant professor of pediatric nursing at Yale University, New Haven, Connecticut, and assistant director in charge of pediatric nursing, New Haven Hospital; 1946-1959, professor of pediatric nursing, University of Chicago; 1959-1963, research for the Rockefeller Foundation; 1963-1970, professor of pediatric nursing, University of Wisconsin, Madison; retired in 1970, and then travelled (especially to perinatal and pediatric meetings, often summering in Maine and New York State where she lived with friends in resort areas), maintained a massive correspondence, helped students and former students with theses, and wrote articles. In her retirement, she was an active volunteer worker for a Madison nursery school, for the Madison Art Museum, and for Bethel Lutheran Church Day Care Center, Madison, Wisconsin.

CONTRIBUTIONS: Florence Blake's greatest contributions were in pediatric nursing. While teaching pediatric nursing at Yale and serving as assistant director of pediatric nursing at New Haven Hospital, she became chairperson of a committee established by the National League of Nursing Education committee to plan an advanced course in pediatric nursing. An opportunity to create such a course for graduate nurses at the University of Chicago attracted her to Chicago in 1946. At that time, there was only one other graduate course in pediatric nursing in the country. Furthermore, the Children's Hospital in Chicago had never been used for students at the baccalaureate or master's level. In 1959, when the University of Chicago closed its nursing program, a Rockefeller Foundation grant enabled her to study children with operable cardiac defects, resulting in an important publication on pediatric nursing published by the Children's Bureau in 1964. When she accepted a position as professor of pediatric nursing at the University of Wisconsin-

Madison School of Nursing. The master's program in pediatric nursing admitted its first students in 1964

In addition to her role of developer of graduate nursing programs and advanced programs in pediatric nursing, her textbooks (*Essentials of Pediatrics* and *The Child, His Parents, and the Nurse*) were major forces in shaping pediatric nursing practice in hospitals and pediatric nursing courses in schools of nursing. Some of her innovations in pediatric nursing practice included developing ways nurses could use play with children to familiarize them with the care they would receive, and she instituted clinical conferences and process recordings of interactions with parents. After her retirement in 1970, she maintained an active interest in the care of children and also worked with older adults in adult day-care; she was sensitive to the developmental needs of senior citizens. In 1958, the nursing education alumni of Columbia University's Teachers College gave her an award for distinguished achievements in nursing education. In June 1974, she received from the American Nurses' Association's division of maternal-child nursing practice an award for her contributions to maternal and child health nursing.

WRITINGS: *Essentials of Pediatrics* (1934 and five subsequent editions; *The Child, His Parents and the Nurse* (1954); *Essentials of Pediatric Nursing* (1963); *Open Heart Surgery -- A Study in Nursing Care* (1964); *Nursing Care of Children* (1970, 1976).

REFERENCES: *American Journal of Nursing* (April 1984), p. 550; correspondence with Carolyn Aradine, R.N., Ph.D.; *Historical Register of Yale University, 1937-1951* (1952); *Nursing Outlook* (November-December 1983), p. 342; corrspondence with Ruth E. Redmann, a friend and colleague of Florence Blake, Long Beach, California, May 29, 1987; Gwendolyn Safier, *Contemporary American Leaders in Nursing: An Oral History* (1977); unpublished memorial resolution of the faculty of the University of Wisconsin on the death of Emeritus Professor Florence G. Blake, University of Wisconsin archives, Madison; Edna Yost, *American Women of Nursing* (rev. ed., 1965).

JOELLEN WATSON HAWKINS

BLANCHFIELD, FLORENCE ABY (APRIL 1, 1884, Shepherdstown, West Virginia--May 12, 1971, Walter Reed General Hospital, Washington, D.C.). *Army nurse.* Daughter of Joseph Plunkett Blanchfield, stonemason and cutter, and Mary Lavinia (Anderson) Blanchfield, nurse. Never married. EDUCATION: 1889-1898, attended public school in Walnut Springs, Virginia; 1898-1899, attended Orando Institute, a private school in Orando, Virginia; May 31, 1906, graduted from the South Side Hospital Training School for Nurses, Pittsburgh, Pennsylvania; 1907, post-graduate study in Baltimore, Maryland, at Dr. Howard A. Kelly's Sanatorium and study of operating room management and techniques, Johns Hopkins Hospital, Baltimore; 1908, post-graduate pediatric nursing course, Children's Hospital, Pittsburgh; 1914-1915, secretarial course at Martin's Business College, Pittsburgh, Pennsylvania; 1920-1921, extension courses in business and public speaking, University of California, Berkeley; 1920-1921 and 1929-1930, correspondence course in English composition from Columbia University, New York City; later in life studied dressmaking and automobile mechanics.

CAREER: 1906, private duty nursing, Baltimore; 1907-1908, supervisor of the operating room, South Side Hospital, Pittsburgh; 1908-1909, supervisor of the operating rooms, Montefiore Hospital, Pittsburgh; 1909-1913, superintendent of the Suburban General Hospital, Bellevue, Pennsylvania; 1913, surgical nurse and anesthetist, Ancon Hospital, Panama Canal Zone; 1914-1915, emergency surgical nurse, United States Steel Corporation's mill, Bessemer, Pennsylvania; 1915-1917 and 1919-1920, superintendent of nurses and of the training school, Suburban Hospital, Pittsburgh; August 20, 1917, entered service as a reserve nurse with Base Hospital Number 27, University of Pittsburgh Medical School Unit; August-September 1917, surgical nurse, Base Hospital Number 27, stationed at Ellis Island, New York; October-November 1917, nurse, Base Hospital Number 27, stationed at Angers, France; December 1917-January 1919, acting chief nurse, Camp Hospital Number 15, Camp Coetquidan, France; May 1919-January 1920, relieved from active duty; January-March 1920, nurse, Army Nurse Corps (ANC), Letterman General Hospital, San Francisco; April-November 1920, stationed at Camp Custer, Battle Creek, Michigan; November 1920-October 1921, stationed at Fort Benjamin Harrison, Indiana; October 1921-May 1922, instructor and recreation director, Army School of Nursing, Letterman General Hospital; June 1922-October 1924, assistant chief nurse, Sternberg General Hospital, Philippines; October 1924-January 1925, chief nurse, Camp John Hay, Philippines; February-March 1925, acting recreational director, Letterman General Hospital; March 1925, assigned to Walter Reed General Hospital, Washington, D.C.; April-October 1925, special duty nursing (TDY Secretary of War); November 1925-June 1929, chief nurse, Fort McPherson, Georgia; June-August 1926, chief nurse, Fort McClellan, Alabama; June-November 1929, assigned to Walter Reed General Hospital; December 1929-January 1932, chief nurse, Jefferson Barracks, Missouri; February 1932-October 1934, chief nurse, Fort William McKinley, Philippines; October 1934-March 1935, chief nurse, Tientsin, China; July 1935-February 1939, assigned to the office of the superintendent, ANC, Washington, D.C.; February 1939-February 1943, first assistant to superintendent, ANC; February-May 1943, acting superintendent, ANC; June 1943-September 1947, superintendent, ANC (appointed chief, ANC, July 28, 1947).

CONTRIBUTIONS: Florence Blanchfield was one of the most influential nurses in military history, serving during World Wars I and II and taking a leadership role during World War II. Much of her long career in the ANC was devoted to obtaining full military rank for nurses, who had long been the unsung heroines of the many wars in which the United States had been involved. As superintendent of the ANC during World War II, she established at Fort Meade, Maryland (1943) the first basic training course for newly commissioned nurses; similar courses were subsequently established in each of the nine service commands. She believed that confidence in the military medical services would be enhanced if nurses were available near the front, and she arranged for nurses to be assigned to hospitals near the front lines so they would be available to provide surgical nursing care. Her belief was validated during the battle for Anzio beachhead, when soldiers reported that their courage was strengthened by the presence of nurses. She was responsible for the 57,000 nurses who made up the ANC and, through their work, for the nursing care of nearly eight million soldiers. She became known as the "little colonel," but all that was little about her was her stature. Her energy, understanding, and efficiency, her consideration for all the persons with whom she worked, and her analytical ability made her an especially competent superintendent.

The association between the Nursing Service of the American Red Cross and the ANC had been a close one from the beginning, and she believed that the association was critical to ensuring a supply of nurses to meet the need of the military under rapidly changing conditions. In fact, she believed that there should not be a draft of nurses, and she defended her position when military leaders asked the president to authorize the drafting of nurses into the armed forces. She also believed that military nursing would benefit from close cooperation with the American Nurses' Association. Her leadership and that collaboration, along with the hard work and support of Congresswoman Frances Payne Bolton, led in 1947 to the Army-Navy Nurse Act, granting permanent status and full commissions to nurses. She was the first woman to be commissioned in the regular army, receiving from General Dwight D. Eisenhower Assigned Army Service Number 1 at the rank of colonel (July 18, 1947).

Other innovations that began under her leadership included constructive service credit for experience in civilian nursing, compilation of a nursing procedures manual, an organized administrative structure for the corps, opportunity for advanced study in civilian institutions for members of the corps, and army hospital affiliations for seniors in the Cadet Nurse Corps. In 1943, she initiated public relations for military nursing through the creation of the Army Nurse Branch of Technical Information in the Surgeon General's Office, designed to inform the public about the work of army nurses and to foster recruitment of nurses for the ANC. An official song was adopted, an official ANC ring was issued, twenty-one issues of a magazine (*The Army Nurse*) were published beginning in January 1944, and the *Army Nurse Corps Songbook* was compiled, printed, and distributed.

The example of her mother, who also practiced nursing, along with her brother's illness and death, apparently influenced her choice of a career. Her two sisters were also nurses, and, in fact, her sister Ruth studied under her. Early nursing experiences after graduation helped her to focus on a career in the military. In 1913, she went to Ancon Hospital in the Panama Canal Zone for a six-month tour of duty as a civil service employee; she worked in the operating pavilion as an anesthetist and surgical nurse. Returning home, she was on one of the first ships to sail through the newly completed canal. Upon her return, she was appointed superintendent of nurses at Suburban Hospital in Pittsburgh, where she provided leadership for the development of the training school. She believed that every nursing school superintendent ought to possess an academic degree, and since she did not possess such credentials, after the training school was established, she indicated her intention of resigning in order to join the army as a military nurse during World War I. Hospital administrators protested her decision, and she agreed to take a leave of absence rather than to resign. In August 1917 she sailed for France with Base Hospital Number 27 (University of Pittsburgh unit), one of twenty-eight nurses for 1,300 patients. After completing her military service, she returned to Suburban Hospital but resigned to allow a nurse with a degree to assume the superintendent position. At this point, she re-enlisted in the military, working her way up to serve eventually as superintendent of army nurses during and immediately after World War II.

Throughout her career, she received numerous honors. On June 14, 1945, she received the Distinguished Service Medal of the U.S. Army, the twenty-fourth nurse and the twenty-fifth woman to receive it. She also received the World War I Victory Medal, the American Campaign Medal, the World War II Victory Medal, and the European African Middle East Campaign Medal. In 1951, she was honored with the Florence Nightingale Medal of the International Red Cross. On July 10, 1963, she was awarded the West Virginia Distinguished Service Medal. The U.S. Army Hospital at Fort Campbell, Kentucky, was named the Colonel Florence A. Blanchfield Army Community Hospital and dedicated on September 17, 1982. She received victory medals for her service in World Wars I and II, and in 1944 she received the American Campaign Service Medal; on January 19, 1945, she received the European Service Medal.

After retirement, through her activities as a member of the Retired Officers' Association, she continued to work for the ANC and for all women in the military. She also worked with Mary W. Standlee on a history of the ANC. She died of atherosclerotic heart disease in 1971 at Walter Reed General Hospital and was buried with full military honors in the Nurses' Section, Arlington National Cemetery, Virginia.

WRITINGS: Numerous articles on military nursing; manuscript on the history of the Army Nurse Corps, written with Mary W. Standlee.

REFERENCES: *American Journal of Nursing* (July 1945), p. 575; Edith A. Aynes, "Colonel Florence A. Blanchfield," *Nursing Outlook* (February, 1959), pp. 78-81 and *From Nightingale to Eagle, An Army Nurse's History* (1973); *Current Biography* (September 1943), pp. 5-6; Doris W. Egge, "A Concise Biography of Colonel Florence Aby Blanchfield, ANC," June 1974, document of the Center of Military History, Department of the Army, Washington, D.C.; *Notable American Women: The Modern Era*, pp. 83-85; Portia B. Kernodle, *The Red Cross Nurse in Action 1882-1948* (1949); unpublished biographical notes, Nursing Archives, Mugar Memorial Library, Boston University; *Who's Who in America*, vol. 24 (1946-1947), p. 213.

JOELLEN WATSON HAWKINS

BOWMAN, JOSEPHINE BEATRICE (December 19, 1881, Des Moines, Iowa-- ?). *Superintendent of the U.S. Navy Nurse Corps.* Daughter of Colonel M. T. V. Bowman, Civil War officer who served on the staff of General William T. Sherman, and Josephine (Webber) Bowman. EDUCATION: 1904, diploma, Medico-Chirurgical Hospital Training School for Nurses, Philadelphia (later known as the School of Nursing of the Hospitals of the Graduate School of Medicine, University of Pennsylvania). CAREER: 1904-1908, private duty nursing in Pennsylvania; 1908, served with the American Red Cross on disaster nursing duty, Hattiesburg, Mississippi, flood; 1908, appointed to the U.S. Navy Nurse Corps; 1911, chief nurse, Navy Nurse Corps; 1914, supervisor, American Red Cross Nurse Unit, Royal Naval Hospital, Portsmouth, England (able to serve while relieved from active service with the U.S. Navy for six months); 1915-1918, served at various naval stations, including on the first hospital ship and in the Orient; 1918-1920,

chief nurse, U.S. Naval Hospital, Great Lakes, Illinois; December 1, 1922-January 1, 1935, superintendent of the U.S. Navy Nurse Corps; 1935, retired.
CONTRIBUTIONS: Josephine Bowman was a pioneer in Navy nursing, when there was widespread opposition to women, including from doctors who were opposed to having women in the medical corps. During World War I, she showed foresight and ability in organizing care for large numbers of naval personnel at the Great Lakes Naval Hospital, when the population at that station rapidly expanded from a capacity of 2,000 to 50,000. During the 1918 influenza epidemic, she was responsible for efficiently equipping naval barracks to provide hospital care for more than 1,000 patients. She was the first chief nurse to do duty on the *U.S. Relief*, the first hospital ship expressly designed and constructed for that purpose. She aided in the commission of that ship and established the status of the nurse aboard ship, which became policy. Bowman was a member of the National Committee on American Red Cross Nursing Service, of the Advisory Committee of Nurses to the Medical Director and to the Medical Council of the U.S. Veterans' Bureau, of the American Public Health Association, and of the American Association for the Advancement of Science. From 1930 to 1932, she was chairperson of the Government Section, American Nurses' Association. From 1931 to 1934, she served as president of the Graduate Nurses' Association of the District of Columbia.
WRITINGS: Many articles in the *American Journal of Nursing*, including "The History and Development of the Navy Nurse Corps," (25: 356-360) and "Disability Bill for Army and Navy Nurses," (30: 1017).
REFERENCES: *American Journal of Nursing*, 24: 1122 and 35: 1122; *Josephine Beatrice Bowman*, National League of Nursing Education, prepared by members of the staff of the Navy Nurse Corps; "Mrs. Higbee Is Succeeded by Miss Bowman," *Trained Nurse and Hospital Review* (January 1923), p. 41.

ALICE HOWELL FRIEDMAN

BRECKINRIDGE, MARY (February 17, 1877, Memphis, Tennessee--May 15, 1965, Hyden, Kentucky). *Public health nurse; nurse-midwife; founder of the Frontier Nursing Service.* Daughter of Clifton Rodes Breckinridge, cotton planter, commission merchant, U.S. congressman from Arkansas, minister to Russia under President Grover Cleveland, and Katherine (Carson) Breckinridge, housewife and mother. Married to Henry Ruffner Morrison, 1904 (died 1906); Richard Ryan Thompson, 1912 (divorced 1920). Children: son Breckinridge, born 1914 (died 1918) and daughter

Mary, born prematurely 1916 (died within six hours of birth). EDUCATION: From the age of six, daily lessons with German governesses; at age thirteen in Russia, tutored by French governess; 1896-1898, attended Rosemont-Dezaley School, Lausanne, Switzerland; 1898-1899, sent to Low and Heywood School, Stamford, Connecticut; 1907-1910, St. Luke's Hospital School of Nursing, New York City (graduated in 1910); 1921, postgraduate course in public health nursing, Teachers College, Columbia University, New York City; 1923, certified midwife, British Hospital for Mothers and Babies, Woolwich, London; 1924, post-graduate course at York Road General Lying-in Hospital, London. CAREER: 1910, after graduating from St. Luke's Hospital School of Nursing, returned home to care for her mother; 1912-1914, taught French and hygiene at Crescent College and Conservatory for Young Women, Eureka Springs, Arkansas; between 1914 and 1918, retired from teaching and nursing to bear her children and to care for her son; June 1918, worked under a three-month contract with the Children's Bureau to gather information about the nation's children and then as a public health nurse during the influenza epidemic in Washington, D.C., and then with the Boston Instructive District Nursing Association, 1918, while awaiting assignment to France; 1918-1921, volunteer with the American Committee for Devastated France, where she organized a disaster relief and a special program for children and pregnant women; 1920, during a leave in England, met English midwives and visited district nursing centers; 1925, organized the Kentucky Committee for Mothers and Babies, Leslie County, Kentucky, which in 1928 developed into the Frontier Nursing Service (FNS); to her death in 1965, served as director of the FNS and editor of its bulletin; 1939, founded the Frontier Graduate School of Midwifery, with Dorothy Farrar Buck serving as the first dean until her death in 1949.

CONTRIBUTIONS: Mary Breckinridge's most important contribution to nursing was as a pioneer in nurse-midwifery and in bringing modern nursing to the rural environment. She was founder of the Frontier Nursing Service (FNS) in 1928. During her forty years as director, the FNS grew from one clinic to five outpost centers, with administrative headquarters at Wendover, Kentucky, and a hospital, serving 1,000 square miles. She also founded the Frontier Graduate School of Midwifery (1939), which helped establish the role of educated nurse-midwife. The school was one of the first of its kind in the United States, graduating 285 nurse-midwives during Breckinridge's lifetime.

Her career in nursing was, in her own words, not the dream of girlhood but the result of her realization that she was not fitted to be of service to anyone. After the death of her first husband, reflecting upon her life and struck by her lack of ability to help a child with typhoid fever, she decided to enter nurses' training in order to be of help to children. The years from 1921 to 1924 were spent in preparation in public health, psychology, statistics, and biology at Teachers College (New York City), where M. Adelaide Nutting (q.v.) was her professor and friend, and in England where she trained as a midwife and became the first American certified as an English midwife. She decided to settle in Kentucky, where she had spent summers at the home of her great-aunt, Mrs. James Lees, from whose estate came some of the money used to found the FNS.

In Kentucky, she collected information about the lay midwives providing service in Leslie, Knott, and Owsley counties, and she gathered support for the establishment of a nursing service for mothers and children. On May 28, 1925, the Kentucky Committee for Mothers and Babies was launched. In 1926, the Big House in Wendover was completed, and it still serves as FNS headquarters. Hyden Hospital and Health Center was completed in 1928, and between 1927 and 1930, five outposts for the FNS were built. In 1928, the name was changed to the Frontier Nursing Service.

In the first years of service, the FNS nurses demonstrated a decrease in maternal and infant mortality and morbidity in Leslie County. Breckinridge was adamant about keeping precise records, and these, along with the survey of all families in Leslie County, provide information about unreported births and deaths for the fifteen years prior to the founding of the FNS, and serve to demonstrate the effectiveness of the service. In addition, the FNS accumulated the only extant set of obstetrical data on a native rural population in the United States, numbering 9,000 cases by 1951. The *Quarterly Bulletin* of the FNS commenced in June 1925 in response to a request by the original committee for printed reports of the progress of work.

Throughout her life, Mary played a major role in organizing branch committees and enlisting the aid of prominent citizens all over the country, raising money to support her work in Kentucky. From her experience in France, she brought the idea of a Courier Service, staffed by young women nineteen and older, who spend six weeks to several months caring for the horses (and now the jeeps) that transport nurses and other health care providers to families along the mountain creeks and performing a multitude of tasks to assist the nurses. Many couriers continued to serve the FNS for years or even for their lifetimes as members of the committees. In October 1928, the American Association of Nurse-Midwives started in Kentucky, with the sixteen charter members all staff of the FNS.

Breckinridge received many honors during her lifetime. In September 1962, she and her staff were honored with the first of what

was to become a series of Mary Breckinridge Days, with a parade led by the guest of honor, speeches, and a luncheon. The ten-thousandth baby delivered by the service was commemorated by a park named after Mary Breckinridge, on the middle fork of the Kentucky River. In 1982, she was elected to the American Nurses' Association Hall of Fame.
WRITINGS: *Wide Neighborhoods* (1952); articles in the *FNS Quarterly Bulletin* (1925-1965); "The Nurse-Midwife--a Pioneer," *American Journal of Public Health* (November 1927); "Is Birth Control the Answer?" *Harper's* (July 1931); numerous reports on the work of the FNS.
REFERENCES: Mary Breckinridge, "An Adventure in Midwifery," *Survey Graphic* (October 1, 1926), reprinted in *Frontier Nursing Service Quarterly Bulletin* (Winter 1985), pp. 18-25; "The Nurse-Midwife--a Pioneer," *American Journal of Public Health* (November 1927), pp. 1147-1151, "Is Birth Control the Answer?" *Harper's* (July 1931), pp. 157-163, and *Wide Neighborhoods* (1952); Nancy Dammann, *A Social History of the FNS* (1982); Bertha S. Dodge, *The Story of Nursing* (1954); Robin McKown, *Heroic Nurses* (1966); *Notable American Women*, 4: 103-105; *National League of Nursing Education Biographical Sketches, 1937-1940* (1940); Ernest Poole, *Nurses on Horseback* (1941).

JOELLEN WATSON HAWKINS

BRINTON, MARY WILLIAMS (c. July 27, 1895, Bala, Pennsylvania--?). *Missionary nurse.* Married Clarence C. Brinton, June 20, 1936. EDUCATION: Graduate of Miss Irwin's School, Philadelphia; 1914, enrolled in YMCA class for trained attendents, which was affiliated with St. Mary's Hospital for Children, Philadelphia; 1917-1920, attended Presbyterian Hospital School of Nursing, Philadelphia, graduating in 1920; postgraduate studies in anesthesia at Howard Hospital, Philadelphia, in administration at Philadelphia General Hospital, and laboratory training at Memorial Hospital, Roxborough, Pennsylvania; also had post-graduate training at the Deaver Clinic and Lankenau Hospital. CAREER: 1920, on the staff of the Visiting Nurse Society, Philadelphia; nurse in the accident ward, Presbyterian Hospital, Philadelphia; industrial nurse, Philadelphia Electric Company; nurse at the Grenfell Mission, Labrador; June 1927, nurse at the Grenfell Mission Hospital, on the island of Battle Harbor, Newfoundland, and at the Grenfell Mission, St. Anthony, Newfoundland; mission nurse in Wrangell, Skagway, Cordova, and Telegraph Creek, Alaska, and at Hudson Stuck Memorial Hospital (Fort Yukon, Alaska); assistant supervisor of maternity, Chestnut Hill Hospital, Wissahickon Valley, Pennsylvania; to 1935, service with the Piper Clinic, University

Hospital, Philadelphia; during World War II, volunteer, Pennsylvania Hospital, Philadelphia.
CONTRIBUTIONS: Although her career was cut short by marriage, Mary Brinton was a pioneer in nursing in Newfoundland and in Alaska. Her first missionary experience was in the Grenfell Mission, Labrador, where she did private duty nursing for six months and then joined the staff of the Grenfell Mission Hospital on the island of Battle Harbor. The history of the Grenfell Mission Hospitals began in 1889 when Dr. Wilfred Thomason Grenfell engaged in medical missionary work for the National Mission to Deep-Sea Fishermen. Over the years, he established four hospitals in Newfoundland and one in Labrador, providing medical and nursing care to natives, including Indians and Eskimo. Brinton began her missionary work in the Grenfell Mission in Labrador, and then she went to Grenfell Mission, St. Anthony, Newfoundland, doing similar work. Experience in Philadelphia, first as a visiting nurse, then in the accident ward of Presbyterian Hospital, and finally as an industrial nurse with a utility company helped to prepare her for the accident cases she saw while working in Newfoundland and later in Alaska.

After her first tour of duty as a missionary nurse, she travelled through Spruce Brook and Quebec, and then returned home to Philadelphia for a respite. But nursing in the far north country was in her blood, and she went to Wrangell in southeastern Alaska and spent four months there working as a nurse in a small hospital. From there she went to Skagway and eventually to Fort Yukon, where she worked for a time in another small hospital. She also did private duty nursing, nursing an artist in Cordova, and a trapper at Telegraph Creek who had been injured in a hunting accident. Returning once more to Wrangell, she set out for home through Ketchikan and Seattle, where she took the train east, stopping at Rochester, Minnesota, to visit the Mayo Clinic at the invitation of Dr. William Mayo, whom she had met in Wrangell.

She stopped in Chicago also, calling on Dr. Joseph Bolivar DeLee, the pioneering obstetrician who in 1899 had founded the Chicago Lying-in Hospital. Back in Philadelphia, after some post-graduate study and a period as supervisor of the maternity ward of Chestnut Hill Hospital, she was asked by Dr. Edmund B. Piper to be his office nurse and to administer anesthesia to his obstetrical patients. Her work was interrupted by appendicitis in 1935; following surgery, she sailed to Europe for a period of recuperation. While there she visited St. Bartholomew's Hospital in London and hospitals in Copenhagen, Norway, and Paris (including the American Hospital at Neuilly). Then she travelled to Vienna on the *Orient Express* and visited hospitals there. Finally she travelled to Salzburg, returning to the United States late in that same year.

In the winter of 1936, on her way to Guatemala to continue her missionary work, she met on the ship the man who was to become her husband. They were married a few months later, in June 1936, ending Brinton's formal nursing career. Coming from a family of privilege and money and marrying into one, she did not need to work, but she did volunteer to serve on hospital committees. As World War II began, her summer home in Prouts Neck, Maine, became a dispensary. In the winter of 1939, she returned to Philadelphia and was elected president of the Presbyterian Hospital Alumnae Association; in 1945, she was present at the twenty-fifth anniversary reunion of the class of 1920.
WRITINGS: *My Cap and My Cape* (1950).
REFERENCES: Mary W. Brinton, *My Cap and My Cape* (1950); Lavinia L. Dock, *A History of Nursing*, vol. 4 (1912); Bertha S. Dodge, *The Story of Nursing* (1950).

JOELLEN WATSON HAWKINS

BROWN, AMY FRANCES (c. 1910--December 1984). *Author.* EDUCATION: 1930, Bachelor of Education degree and second major in English, Western Illinois State Teacher's College, Macomb, Illinois; 1932-1933, graduate studies in English, University of Iowa, Iowa City; 1936, graduated from State University of Iowa School of Nursing, Ames, Iowa; 1937-1938, graduate studies in public health nursing, University of Kentucky; 1940, master of nursing degree, Western Reserve University, Cleveland, Ohio; 1955, Ph.D., University of Chicago. CAREER: Taught in a rural school for several years before entering nursing; May-October 1936, staff nurse, Lutheran Hospital, Fort Dodge, Iowa; 1936-1938, instructor, Good Samaritan Hospital, Lexington, Kentucky; 1940-1943, instructor of pharmacology and medical and psychiatric nursing, Vanderbilt University School of Nursing, Nashville, Tennessee; 1943-1944, clinical instructor and supervisor of medical nursing, Medical College of Virginia School of Nursing, Richmond, Virginia; 1944-1945, director of nursing education, Kentucky State Board of Nurse Examiners; 1945-1947, assistant professor of nursing, Francis Payne Bolton School of Nursing, Western Reserve University; 1948-1955, assistant and associate professor of medical nursing, State University of Iowa College of Nursing; 1955-1956, associate professor of nursing, Loyola University, Chicago; 1956-1957 and 1958-1959, instructor of medical nursing and special in-service program, Moline Public Hospital, Moline, Illinois; 1960, visiting professor, Nazareth College, Louisville, Kentucky; visiting consultant, St. Joseph Hospital School of Nursing, Lexington, Kentucky.

CONTRIBUTIONS: Through her writings, Amy Frances Brown influenced generations of nursing students. For many years, in issue after issue of the *American Journal of Nursing*, the many editions of her books were reviewed, or she was reviewing a colleague's book. She was eminently suited for her career as an educator and as an author, as her first degree was in education with a special diploma in English. She was inducted into the American Academy of Nursing in 1976.
WRITINGS: *Clinical Instruction* (1949); *Medical Nursing* (3d ed., 1957); *Research in Nursing* (1958); *Medical and Surgical Nursing* (1959); *Medical and Surgical Nursing II* (1959); *Curriculum Development* (1960); also wrote many articles, some of a clinical nature, such as "Teaching Drugs and Solutions," *American Journal of Nursing* (May 1939), pp. 509-512; also wrote articles to teach nurses about writing and speaking, such as "Guided Practice in Speech," *American Journal of Nursing* (April 1940), pp. 431-434 and "Learning to Write Effectively," *American Journal of Nursing* (November 1940), pp. 1256-1260.
REFERENCES: *American Journal of Nursing* (April 1940), p. 415, (March 1942), p. 297, (August 1943), p. 777, (December 1944), p. 1184, (November 1945), p. 966, and (November 1955), p. 1320; material from the nursing archives, Spalding University School of Nursing and Health Sciences, Louisville, Kentucky.

LORETTA P. HIGGINS

BROWNE, HELEN E. (February 3, 1911, Bury St. Edmonds, England--January 20, 1987, Milford, Pennsylvania). *Nurse-midwife.* Daughter of Phil Browne, gentleman farmer, and Agnes Browne. Never married.
EDUCATION: Graduated from Ipswich High School, Ipswich, Suffolk, England; 1931-1934, attended St. Bartholomew's Hospital School of Nursing, London, England, graduating in 1934; 1934-1935, one-year course in midwifery, British Hospital for Mothers and Babies, Woolwich, London. CAREER: 1935-1938, private nurse-midwifery practice, England; July 28, 1938-c. 1942, district nurse-midwife, then supervisor, then 1947-1965, assistant director, and 1965-1975, director, Frontier Nursing Service, Wendover, Kentucky.
CONTRIBUTIONS: Helen Browne was a pioneer in the establishment of nurse-midwifery service and in the demonstration of what nurses are capable of doing in a rural community. Born and educated in England, at the invitation of Mary Breckinridge (q.v.) she came to the United States as a young nurse-midwife. Breckinridge had contacted the British Hospital for Mothers and Babies to request a nurse-midwife who would be willing to work in Kentucky, and Helen Browne responded. During

her early years at Frontier Nursing Service (FNS), she was a district nurse-midwife, first at Red Bird-Flat Creek Clinic. During World War II, she was appointed supervisor of Hyden Hospital, Hyden, Kentucky, and following the war, in 1947, she became assistant director of FNS. When Breckinridge died in 1965, Browne was unanimously elected director (May 18) and served in that position until her retirement in 1975. Under her dedicated leadership, Mary Breckinridge Hospital was built, the name of the school was changed to the Frontier School of Midwifery and Family Nursing, and the curriculum was expanded to combine family nursing and nurse-midwifery in an integrated program. Because she believed that nurse-midwives should speak with one voice, she worked for the merger of the FNS-based American Association of Midwives with the American College of Nurse-Midwifery, to become the American College of Nurse-Midwives. Known as Brownie to all who knew her at the Frontier Nursing Service, she was remembered for her patience, her caring, her foresight, and for her ability to raise funds necessary to expand the services and programs of the FNS. After her retirement in 1975, she moved to Milford, Pennsylvania, but continued to serve the FNS as a volunteer speaker and fund-raiser, and as a member of its board of governors.

Over the course of her career, she received several important honors in recognition of her contributions to the field. She received a distinguished service award from Berea College, Berea, Kentucky, and in 1964, she was appointed an officer of the Most Excellent Order of the British Empire (OBE). In 1976, following her retirement, she received an honorary doctorate in nursing from Eastern Kentucky University, Richmond, Kentucky, and was appointed by Queen Elizabeth II a commander of the OBE. In 1987, a memorial fund was established in her honor to restore Wendover, the home of the FNS.

REFERENCES: *Boston Globe* (January 22, 1987), p. 73; *Frontier Nursing Service Quarterly Bulletin* (Winter 1987), pp. 1-4; remarks of Jane Leigh Powell at the memorial service held April 10, 1987, published in the *Frontier Nursing Service Quarterly Bulletin* (Spring 1987), pp. 9-12.

JOELLEN WATSON HAWKINS

BUNGE, HELEN LATHROP (October 11, 1906, LaCrosse, Wisconsin--April 12, 1979, Madison, Wisconsin). *Nurse-educator; researcher.* Daughter of George W. and Sarah (Wheeler) Bunge. Her great-grandfather was professor of chemistry and natural history at the University of Wisconsin. Never married. EDUCATION: 1924-1926, attended Connecticut College for Women, New London, Connecticut;

1928, A.B., University of Wisconsin, Madison; 1930, certificate of graduate nurse, University of Wisconsin; 1936, M.A., Teachers College, Columbia University, New York City; 1940-1942, graduate study in the doctoral program, Teachers College, Columbia University (she deferred writing her dissertation in order to accept a position teaching at the Frances Payne Bolton School of Nursing, Western Reserve University, Cleveland, Ohio); 1950, Ed.D., Teachers College, Columbia University.
CAREER: 1930-1931, head nurse, Wisconsin General Hospital, Madison, Wisconsin; 1931-1940, instructor and assistant to the director of the University of Wisconsin School of Nursing; 1940-1942, assistantship, division of nursing education, Teachers College, Columbia University; 1943-1946, assistant professor, Frances Payne Bolton School of Nursing, Western Reserve University, Cleveland, Ohio; 1946-1953, professor and dean, Frances Payne Bolton School of Nursing; 1953-1959, executive officer, Institute of Research and Service in Nursing Education, Teachers College, Columbia University; 1959-1967, director of the Nursing School, associate dean of the Medical School, and professor of nursing, University of Wisconsin, Madison; 1967-1969, dean, University of Wisconsin School of Nursing.
CONTRIBUTIONS: Helen Bunge was on the cutting edge of nursing education throughout her career. Probably her greatest contribution to nursing, however, was in promoting nursing research. In 1947 she chaired the committee on research of the American Association of Collegiate Schools of Nursing, and it recognized the need to publish the increasing number of research projects in nursing. As a result of the work of her committee, the first journal devoted to nursing research was created; Bunge served as the editor of *Nursing Research* for its first five years. She continued as chairperson of the editorial advisory board and as a member of the journal's review panel for five more years.

Not only was she influential in promoting the publication of studies in nursing research, she was an active researcher who substantially added to the professional literature of her field. She served as a consultant and/or co-author of many studies about nursing education. These included a study of nursing education in the state of Washington, which according to Mary M. Roberts (q.v.) was "especially notable for its emphasis on methods for improving inter-professional relationships." That clearly reflected her focus on the need to promote multidisciplinary education and practice. In recognition of this, in 1967, President Lyndon Johnson invited her to the signing of the bill which was intended to establish a "Partnership for Health" (House bill 6418). She was a member of the first U.S. Public Health Service nursing research study section, which evaluated applications for grants in nursing research. In addition, she wrote and spoke extensively, both nationally and internationally, about research in nursing. She was the executive officer of the first institute of research and service in nursing education, funded by a five-year, $100,000 grant from the Rockefeller Foundation and located at Teachers College.

Although her experience as a nurse-educator began in 1931 when she became an instructor at the University of Wisconsin School of Nursing, she was not involved in administration until the hectic period of World War II. In 1943, she became coordinator of Western Reserve University's basic program, which had a large number of undergraduates seeking the first degree in nursing. Eventually the bachelor's degree was to become a requirement for entrance to the program, but during the war years Bunge was responsible for administering the earlier type of program. Although Bunge was only an assistant professor, she took on many administrative responsibilities when the dean, Marion Howell (q.v.), became heavily involved in national defense activities regarding the procurement of nurses for the war effort. When Howell resigned due to illness, Bunge was appointed to succeed her as dean (1946).

At that time, Bunge emphasized the need for a well-prepared faculty in order for the university to compete with other universities establishing high-quality nursing programs at the baccalaureate level. She stressed the importance of experience in the field in order to maintain high standards for clinical courses. She suggested joint appointments for the faculty between the university and regional social service agencies, which would enable the professors to keep up to date in clinical areas and which would provide the students with good role models. She was well liked by students and faculty alike, all of whom appreciated her sense of humor. She was admired by the local community as well as the university community, and upon her resignation from the deanship, the *Cleveland News* published an editorial tribute. She also received a letter of commendation from Frances Payne Bolton, the U.S. congresswoman from Ohio, and a congratulatory letter from the governor of Ohio.

During the 1950s, Bunge had been sought to head up the nursing program of her alma mater, the University of Wisconsin. Since she believed that the future of nursing education was in public higher education and since her family and friends urged her to return home to Wisconsin, she accepted the position in 1959. There had been a delay in her acceptance of this position, for she believed that certain issues needed to be resolved before she assumed the leadership of the Wisconsin nursing program. Although the undergraduate nursing school at Wisconsin had started in 1924, due to competition with the hospital-based diploma nursing programs which graduated students after a shorter period of study, the university's nursing school had only a small number of students. It clearly was not going to be able to support itself on the basis of tuition and fees of the students, and as a result Bunge insisted on receiving a commitment for sufficient financial support to enable her to put the program on a firm footing. In addition, she envisioned the development of a top-flight graduate nursing program, which would certainly require extensive financial support. She did not envision financial support coming from research grants, at least not at the outset, as she insisted on waiting for properly prepared faculty before she would begin writing grant applications.

Another issue was that of autonomy. At that time, the school of nursing was administratively placed within the medical school complex. She did not consider nursing as coming under the control of the medical faculty, and she placed a high priority on interpreting nursing to the university administration. Before taking up her position as dean, therefore, Bunge did a study of nursing and nursing education in Wisconsin. Even with an extensive understanding of the state of nursing and nursing education in the area, she found it difficult to deal with the administrative situation at the university. She had to work, for instance, with four different deans of the medical school, a new university president, a vice-president, the first chancellor at the Milwaukee branch (who also opened a nursing program), and several other layers of administration. Her energy, patience, her strong University of Wisconsin background, and her own distinguished achievements all helped her not only to survive but to accomplish a great deal.

The graduate nursing program began in 1964, approximately five years after her arrival on campus. Over the course of her tenure as dean, she increased undergraduate enrollment, obtained federal funds to support graduate programs in pediatric and psychiatric nursing, secured federal grants for institutional research, faculty research and development, and equal opportunity grants for minorities, and she developed a new baccalaureate curriculum. Although she worked for many years to secure a new building for the Nursing School, this was not achieved until after her death. One of her proudest accomplishments, however, was when in 1967 the school became autonomous, as one of the ten separate schools on the Madison campus.

She was a member of many committees of the American Nurses' Association, the National League of Nursing Education (NLNE), and the Association of Collegiate Schools of Nursing. She was member of the influential subcommittee of the NLNE which revised *A Curriculum Guide for Schools of Nursing* (1937). She also served as president of the Wisconsin League for Nursing, chairperson of the committee on chronic illness and nursing homes, a member of the citizens' advisory committee on community mental health resources, a member of the nursing advisory committee for the development of regional medical programs, a member of the subcommittee on health manpower, and a board member of the Wisconsin division of the American Cancer Society. She was on the national advisory committees for the American Red Cross and the Veterans Administration, and she served on the executive committee of the Florence Nightingale International Foundation.

Throughout her career, she received numerous awards in recognition of her service, beginning in 1928 when she was elected to Phi Beta Kappa. In 1940 she received the Isabel Hampton Robb Fellowship at Columbia University's Teachers College. In 1967, she received the Achievement Award in Research and Scholarship presented by the Nursing Education Alumni Association of Teachers College. Two years later, in 1969, when she retired as dean of the nursing school, she received several awards, including the distinguished service award presented by the University of Wisconsin Alumni Association, the M. Adelaide Nutting Award of the National League for Nursing, and the University of Wisconsin School of Nursing Alumni established in her honor, the Helen L. Bunge Award. When she left Western Reserve University, a similar award was established in her honor, also known as the Helen Lathrop Bunge Award (1970). In 1984, she was elected to the American Nurses' Association Nursing Hall of Fame.

WRITINGS: Many journal articles particularly about nursing research, including "Changing the Basic Curriculum at the Frances Payne Bolton School of Nursing, Western Reserve University," Ed.D. dissertation, Columbia University, 1949; J. A. Curran and H. L. Bunge, *A Study of Nursing Care and Nursing Education in Washington* (1951); H. L. Bunge et al, *A Study of Nursing Education in Wisconsin* (1955, mimeographed publication of Columbia University Teachers College Institute of Research and Service in Nursing Education); "Is Research the Answer?: An Interview with Helen L. Bunge," *Nursing World* (July 1958), pp. 18-20; "The First Decade of Nursing Research," *Nursing Research* (1962), pp. 132-137; "Research in Nursing: Is There a Need?" *International Nursing Review* (1969), pp. 33-37.

REFERENCES: Margene O. Faddis, *The History of the Frances Payne Bolton School of Nursing* (1948); Marie Farrell, "Helen L. Bunge: An Idealist and a Realist," *Nursing Research* (1962), p. 139; Hortense Hilbert, "Five Years of Leadership," *Nursing Research* (October 1957), p. 51; Lucille E. Notter, "Helen Bunge, First Editor of Nursing Research," *Nursing Research* (August 1970), p. 291; Mary M. Roberts, *American Nursing* (1954), p. 525: Louise C. Smith, *Helen L. Bunge: Nurse, Teacher, Scholar* (1970); *Who's Who of American Women* (1968-1969).

ALICE HOWELL FRIEDMAN

BURGESS, ELIZABETH CHAMBERLAIN (November 2, 1877, Bath, Maine--July 22, 1949, New York City). *Educator and expert in legislative issues.* Daughter of George Henry Burgess and Marcia Hill (Woodbury) Burgess. Never married. EDUCATION: Attended the Misses Orton and Nichols private school in New Haven, Connecticut, graduating in 1895; 1901-1904, attended Roosevelt Hospital School of Nursing, New York City, graduating in 1904; 1910-1912, attended Teachers College, Columbia University, New York City, 1912, received diploma in teaching and administering schools of nursing; 1923, B.S. from Teachers College; 1925, M.A. from Teachers College. CAREER: 1904, operating room nurse at French Hospital, New York City; 1905-1906, private duty nursing, New York City; 1906-1910, assistant superintendent of nurses, Roosevelt Hospital, New York City; 1910-1912, part-time teaching at Bellevue and St. Luke's training schools for nurses, New York City; 1912-1916, superintendent of nurses and director of school of nursing, Michael Reese Hospital, Chicago; 1916-1920, inspector of nursing training schools for New York State Department of Education; during World War I, took leave from Department of Education to serve as assistant inspector of nursing services in the Office of the Surgeon General of the U.S. Army; 1920-1922, secretary of the New York State Board of Nurse Examiners; 1922-1947, instructor, assistant professor, associate professor, and professor, Teachers College, Columbia University; became ill soon after her retirement and died at Roosevelt Hospital, where, many years earlier, her career had begun.

CONTRIBUTIONS: Elizabeth Burgess' major contribution to nursing history came as a result of her participation in two major studies of American nursing. The first, *Nursing and Nursing Education in the United States: A Report of the Committee for the Study of Nursing Education* (1923), commonly known as the Goldmark Report, made ten recommendations to improve nursing education, most of which were startling for their time. The second study was completed by the Committee on the Grading of Nursing Schools (1926-1934), a group consisting of representatives of seven organizations as well as members at large. She was one of two representatives from the National League of Nursing Education (NLNE), and she played a major role during the eight years of the committee's existence. The committee began by completing surveys which determined the current status of the nursing profession (the educational level of applicants to nursing schools), distribution of nurses, and information on faculty and curricula at the various schools. The third and last publication to come out of this committee had a profound impact on nursing education and set the stage for the future external accreditation of schools of nursing. Rather significantly, her work on those two studies grew from an earlier survey she had made as part of her responsibilities during World War I. During that time, she assisted Annie Goodrich (q.v.) in making a national survey of nursing in military hospitals and in organizing the Army School of Nursing.

In addition to her work on the two most important committees in nursing history of the 1920s and 1930s, she played major roles in various professional organizations on the state and national levels, in addition to being active in her alumnae association. She served as president of District 13 of the New York State Nurses' Association as well as on the board of directors. Her most important contributions, however, were made as a leader in the NLNE (now the National League for Nursing). She was president for four years (1929-1933) and a member of the board of directors for many years. She was a member of the Committee to Study Administration in Schools of Nursing, chair of a joint American Nurses' Association and League Committee on Legislation, and chair of the membership committee of the Association of Collegiate Schools of Nursing. Finally, she shared her knowledge with countless students whom she taught at Teachers College over the twenty-five-year period from 1922 to her retirement in 1947.

WRITINGS: Many articles in the *American Journal of Nursing*.

REFERENCES: *American Journal of Nursing* (July 1928), p. 714, (December 1934), pp. 1183-1184 and (September 1949), p. adv. 25; Elizabeth C. Burgess, *National League of Nursing Education Biographical Sketches* (1940); Cordelia W. Kelly, *Dimensions of Professional Nursing* (1962); Isabel M. Stewart, "Elizabeth Chamberlain Burgess," *American Journal of Nursing* (August 1958), pp. 1101-1105; *Who Was Who in America*, vol. 2 (1950).

LORETTA P. HIGGINS

BUTLER, IDA FATIO (1868 or 1869, Watertown, New York {Madison Barracks}--March 11, 1949, West Hartford, Connecticut). *Red Cross nurse.* Her mother died when she was very young, and she was raised by her grandfather, Dr. John Butler, superintendent of the Hartford Retreat. Never married. EDUCATION: Educated in private schools in Hartford and Berlin, Connecticut; August 1901, graduated from the Hartford Hospital School of Nursing. CAREER: September 1901-March 1902, head nurse of a gynecological ward, University of Pennsylvania Hospital, Philadelphia; April 1902-January 1916, head nurse, Hartford Hospital; 1916-1918, supervisor and guide to probationers, director of the nursing residence, Hartford Hospital; March 1918-November 15, 1938, Red Cross service; 1918, chief nurse at Children's Hospital, Hopital Violet, Lyons, France; 1918-1919, supervisor of a Washington, D.C., home for convalescent victims of the flu epidemic; 1919, fifteen-week lecture tour on Red Cross nursing activities, delivering over 190 lectures in ninety-five cities and towns; 1919-1920, director of the nurses' division of the Foreign and Insular Division; 1920-1936, assistant director of the Red Cross Nursing Service; 1936-1938, director, Red Cross Nursing Service; 1938, retired.

CONTRIBUTIONS: Ida Butler devoted the major portion of her career to service in the American Red Cross. She was one of the earliest members of the American Red Cross Nursing Service, having joined shortly after graduation and possessing badge number 248. Before her call to active service, she helped recruit nurses for wartime service, and she taught Red Cross classes when she was not on duty at the Hartford Hospital. During World War I, she was called to active service for the Red Cross and was assigned to foreign service in January 1918. She sailed on March 6, 1918, and assumed the position of chief nurse at the children's hospital, Hopital Violet, Lyons, France. She helped to organize a second children's hospital, Hopital Holtzman, and remained until October of that year when she returned to the United States to recruit other nurses for Red Cross service. She began a fifteen-week speaking tour on Red Cross nursing activities, visiting ninety-five towns and delivering 190 scheduled speeches to Chautauqua circuit audiences. In June 1920, she was made the assistant director of the Red Cross Nursing Service, and upon the death of Clara Noyes (q.v.) in June 1936, she assumed the role of director, being formally appointed to the post on October 21, 1936. She was active in recruitment of nurses for the Red Cross throughout her career, including for relief work following the 1927 Mississippi River flood and the 1937 Ohio-Mississippi river flood.

As director of the Red Cross Nursing Service, she was known as a devoted, courageous, and fair leader. She was known for her wise judgment, her ability to achieve results, and her selfless devotion to the Red Cross and to the nursing profession. Her cooperation and contributions to the analysis of all the nursing functions of the Red Cross led to reorganization of those services. As director, she was a member of the board of directors of the American Nurses' Association, to which she devoted time and energy for the cause of the profession. She was president of the D.C. Graduate Nurses Association (1921-1922), and she also served as secretary of the National Committee on Red Cross Nursing Service.

After her retirement in 1938, she served as temporary secretary of the Nursing Council on National Defense (November 1940-1944), was chairperson of the Connecticut State Defense Council (1940), and chaired the Connecticut State Nurses Council on National Defense (during World War II). She also continued her Red Cross work and her work with professional organizations; at the ages of seventy and seventy-two, she directed all arrangements for the biennial nursing conventions jointly sponsored by the American Nurses' Association, the National League of Nursing Education, and the National Organization of Public Health Nurses.

In 1937, she was awarded the Florence Nightingale Medal by the International Red Cross Committee of Geneva. She also received the French Reconnaissance Medal from the French government for her service during World War I and the Connecticut Distinguished Service Medal for her service in World War II.

WRITINGS: Numerous unpublished reports, speeches, and letters; articles in professional journals including "Lyons Revisited," *American Journal of Nursing* (November 1937), pp. 1219-1221.

REFERENCES: *American Journal of Nursing* (November 1938), pp. 1278-1279 and (May 1949); Ida F. Butler, typed curriculum vitae, 1936, Nursing Archives, Mugar Memorial Library, Boston University; Ida F. Butler, "Lyons Revisited," *American Journal of Nursing* (November 1937), pp. 1219-1221; Portia B. Kernodle, *The Red Cross Nurse in Action, 1882-1948* (1949); Meta Rutter Pennock, *Makers of Nursing History* (1940), p. 67; *Red Cross Courier* (December 1936), p. 22 and (April 1939), pp. 22-23; Julie C. Stimson, "Ida F. Butler," *National League of Nursing Education Biographical Sketches 1937-1940* (1940); *Trained Nurse and Hospital Review* (January 1937), pp. 19-20.

JOELLEN WATSON HAWKINS

C

CABANISS, SADIE HEATH (October 8, 1863, Petersburg, Virginia--July 11, 1921, Richmond, Virginia). *Virginia's pioneer nurse.* Daughter of Charles J. Cabaniss, attorney, and Virginia R. (Heath) Cabaniss. Never married. EDUCATION: 1874, graduated from St. Timothy's School, Catonsville, Maryland; 1893, graduated from Johns Hopkins School of Nursing, Baltimore, Maryland. CAREER: Governess in a private home in Virginia; taught at Mt. Psgah Academy, a private school in Culpeper, Virginia; 1893, night supervisor at Johns Hopkins Hospital; 1895-1900, supervisor of operating room nurses, Old Dominion Hospital, Richmond, Virginia; c. 1900-1910, director, Nurses' Settlement of Richmond, Virginia; 1909, public health nurse, Hanover County, Virginia; c. 1914, served with the North Carolina State Health Department; 1915-?, director, nurses' settlement of St. Augustine, Florida.

CONTRIBUTIONS: Sadie Cabaniss was a pioneer nurse in Virginia, known as the first rural nurse in that state. After graduating from Johns Hopkins School of Nursing, where she came under the influence of Isabel Hampton (q.v.) and M. Adelaide Nutting (q.v.), she was recommended to take charge of the operating room of Richmond's Old Dominion Hospital, then administered by the Sisters of Mercy. During her first two years there, Cabaniss organized the work of the operating room and worked in several other nursing capacities. She was so successful in demonstrating the value of a well-organized nursing service that she was asked to begin training other members of the nursing staff. Between 1895 and 1900, she developed and directed the training school for nurses at the Old Dominion Hospital. This was the first nurse-training school in Virginia which followed the Nightingale method of nursing education. The Nightingale method provided for supervision by a professional nurse, affiliation with a quality hospital which would provide a variety of clinical experiences, and the hospital and school would be separately administered. She recognized that the graduate nurses needed evidence of their competence, and as a result she created a system whereby graduates received certificates to testify to their education; the first diplomas were signed by the faculty of the Medical College of Virginia, which had a close affiliation with the Old Dominion Hospital.

Cabaniss led the various training schools in Virginia to organize their graduates into alumnae associations, and these later came together to form the Graduate Nurses' Association of Virginia. She was elected as its first president and held that position for the first five years of the association's existence. The association, having the proper credentials, became part of the Associated Alumnae of the United States and Canada, the forerunner of the American Nurses' Association. Cabaniss served the Associated Alumnae as its vice president, and through her influence, the tenth annual convention was held in Richmond, in 1907. She was anxious to have the convention in a southern city, as the South had so little exposure to modern trends in hospital or nursing care that the convention would play a major role in introducing rural and small town nurses to the developing movement to advance the profession. The first work of the Graduate Nurses' Association of Virginia, when she was president, was to frame a law to regulate the practice of nursing in the commonwealth. When the law was passed in 1903, Virginia became one of the first three states to require registration of nurses. Cabaniss was then appointed to serve on the first board of examiners in Virginia, serving as its chairperson for nine years. In addition to her work in organizing a professional school for nurses and fighting for the establishment of a nurse-registration act, Cabaniss worked to upgrade the quality of training of attendants. In Richmond, most attendants worked in the City Home, where the care was under the direction of other patients or from paupers who were untrained and often intoxicated and unable to provide even the basic nursing services required. When smallpox took the life of an untrained attendant, the city was then ready to follow Cabaniss' advice and change the system of nursing service by having at least one trained nurse present at all times.

From that position, Cabaniss became aware of the needs of patients after discharge from the hospital, and as a result she organized the Nurses' Settlement of Richmond, which was similar to Lillian Wald's (q.v.) Henry Street Settlement, in New York City. The Nurses' Settlement of Richmond provided follow-up nursing care for patients in their homes, a service that had never been available to the sick poor of the city. Her work in public health nursing made her aware of the seriousness of tuberculosis as a communicable disease, and she helped create dispensaries for tubercular patients of the Richmond area who could not be accommodated through the local hospitals.

Two memorials were established in honor of the contributions that Cabaniss made to the history of public health nursing and nursing education in the state of Virginia. The chair of nursing education at the University of Virginia was named in her honor, after the first steps were taken in that direction in the spring of 1923 by the Graduate Nurses' Association of Virginia. Fifty thousand dollars was raised by the association and presented to the University of Virginia to establish the Cabaniss chair. In addition, in September 1928, the Cabaniss Memorial School of Nursing Education at the University of Virginia was opened. To raise the funds, *Signal Fires*, a masque of service with the pageant of the lives of Florence Nightingale and Sadie Cabaniss, was presented.

During the Spanish-American War, Cabaniss helped to control epidemics of measles and typhoid fever among the soldiers. During World War I, she worked as a public health nurse in the shipyards of Savannah, Georgia.

REFERENCES: *American Journal of Nursing* (January 1927), pp. 33-35; Louise Burleigh, "The Florence Nightingale Play Competition," *American Journal of Nursing* (December 1921), pp. 40-41; Nannie J. Minor, "A Pioneer Nurse in Virginia," paper read before the Graduate Nurses' Association of Virginia (1923), located in the Virginia Nurses' Association Collection, Special Collection Archives, Tompkins-McCaw Library, Virginia Commonwealth University, Richmond, Virginia; Anne F. Parsons, "Sadie Heath Cabaniss: Virginia's Pioneer Nurse," located in the Virginia Nurses' Association Collection, Special Collection Archives, Tompkins-McCaw Library, Virginia Commonwealth University, Richmond, Virginia (copies of the Minor and Parsons speeches are in the Sophia Palmer Collection, Nursing Archives, Mugar Memorial Library, Boston University).

ALICE HOWELL FRIEDMAN

CAMP, HARRIET. See **LOUNSBERY, HARRIET (CAMP).**

CANNON, IDA MAUD (June 29, 1877, Milwaukee Wisconsin--July 7, 1960, Watertown, Massachusetts). *Public health nurse; pioneer in medical social service.* Daughter of Colbert Hanchett Cannon, official of the Great Northern Railroad, and Sarah Wilma (Denio) Cannon, schoolteacher who died when Ida was four years old. Never married. EDUCATION: 1896, graduated from St. Paul High School, St. Paul, Minnesota; 1896-1898, attended City and County Hospital Training School for Nursing, St. Paul, graduating in 1898; 1900-1901, took courses in sociology at the University of Minnesota, Minneapolis; 1906-1907, attended Boston School for Social Workers (later Simmons College School of Social Work). CAREER: 1898-1900, director, hospital at state school for the feeble-minded, Fairbault, Minnesota; 1903-1906, visiting nurse, St. Paul Associated Charities; 1906, volunteer in hospital social service at Massachusetts General Hospital, Boston; 1907-1945, full-time social worker and, 1907-1945, head social worker and chief of the Social Service Department, Massachusetts General Hospital; director of the medical social work curriculum at the Boston School of Social Work and lecturer at Boston University, Boston College, and New York schools of social work, as well as holding the adjunct position with the Boston School.

CONTRIBUTIONS: Although Ida Cannon is best known as the founder of medical social work rather than as a nurse, it was her nursing background and career that sparked her interest in social welfare. Indeed, her unique combination of skills and knowledge enabled her to pioneer in medical social work. Influenced by an article in *Harper's Bazaar* written by Isabel Hampton Robb (q.v.), she entered a training school for nursing. Her work from 1898 to 1900 as organizer and director of the hospital at the state school for the feeble-minded at Fairbault, Minnesota, helped make her aware of the social needs of hospital patients. She had to give up that position due to temporary blindness caused by formaldehyde she used to fumigate the rooms, and during her time off she studied sociology and psychology at the University of Minnesota. While there, she heard a speech by Jane Addams, which incited in her an interest in social work. This interest was nurtured during her work as a visiting nurse among the poor of St. Paul from 1903 to 1906 and during her work as an organizer of a summer camp for the tubercular children of Minneapolis in 1905.

In the autumn of 1906, she moved to Cambridge, Massachusetts, to live with her brother and to attend the Boston School for Social Workers. She became a volunteer in the newly established (1905) hospital social service unit at Massachusetts General Hospital, which was administered by Dr. Richard Clarke Cabot, physician to out-patients. She first heard Dr. Cabot speak at the Massachusetts State Conference of Social Work in Worcester and was interested in his idea of social service within hospitals. Little did she know that she would spend the rest of her professional life working with Dr. Cabot. In 1907, after a summer visiting London and Paris hospitals, she joined the staff at Massachusetts General and in that same year was made head worker of social service, a post she held until her retirement in 1945. In 1915, the post was renamed chief of social service. She and Cabot worked together on the evolution of both the social service department and the role of the medical social worker. Until 1914 when ward work was officially recognized, the social service department remained out-patient work and an unofficial service;

on October 17, 1919, it was officially incorporated into the hospital organization. Not only did she bear a large part of the burden of organizing and running the social service department at Massachusetts General, but she shared with Dr. Cabot the task of selling the department to other members of the staff and to the board. Loosely connected with the hospital at its inception, for the first fourteen years of its existence, the social service department was responsible for even the financing of its work. Cannon characterized some of the work of her early years as not unlike scenes in *Alice in Wonderland*: the unreality of physicians prescribing a vacation, a job, or a set of teeth to persons for whom even the basics of existence were beyond reach.

Cannon's energy was not singularly directed toward the creation and operation of the social service department, however. The teaching function of the department was initiated in 1912. She held an adjunct position with the Boston School of Social Work and until 1925 was director of that school's special medical social work curriculum. Medical students and nursing students in the Nurse Training School of Massachusetts General were also accommodated with rotations through the social service department.

A leader in social work practice and education, Cannon was also a leader in its evolution as a profession. During her career, she served as an officer and on major committees concerned with the development of social work. She was one of the leaders in the formation of the American Association of Hospital Social Workers (later the American Association of Medical Social Workers), its vice-president from 1918 to 1919, and its president from 1920 to 1927. She was on the executive council and the training committee, and in 1926 she chaired the committee on relations between hospitals and communities. In 1920, she served on a committee of the American Hospital Association undertaking a survey of hospital social work and in 1923 was on that association's committee on training for hospital social work. From 1930 to 1931, she was a member of the national committee in the Department of Immigration and Foreign Communities of the International Institute. She was a delegate to the White House Conference on Child Health and Protection in 1930 and 1931 and chaired a subcommittee on medical social service. During 1932 she was president of the Massachusetts Conference on Social Work and a delegate to the International Conference of Social Work in Frankfurt. Four years later, in 1936, she was again a delegate to the International Conference, which was held in London. During 1938-1939, she was vice-president of the National Conference of Social Work.

She served her state and region in various capacities. On January 12, 1925, she was appointed consultant for the Unitarian Social Service Council. For 1937 and 1938, she was a member of the board of directors of the Massachusetts Mental Hygiene Society, and in 1938 she was a member of the board of directors of the Community Federation of Boston. During the same time, 1937-1939, she was on the committee on management of the International Institute of the YWCA of Boston and on the executive committee of the Boston Health League. For the Massachusetts State Department of Health, she served on the advisory committee on medical social service (1940-1945). She also served on the advisory committee for the Massachusetts Department of Public Welfare (1942). A resident of Cambridge, she served on its Board of Public Welfare and as a trustee of the Cambridge City Hospital and of Tewksbury State Hospital and Infirmary.

She was never too busy to serve as a lecturer and as a consultant to other hospitals seeking to emulate Massachusetts General. She was active in initiating the development of social work in hospitals in Belgium, Denmark, England, France, and Germany. She was also a prolific writer, turning out two books, one of which (*Social Work in Hospitals*) was the authoritative text for many of the early years of the profession. Her department gained some notice in 1942 for its work in caring for victims and families of the Cocoanut Grove (night-club) fire. In the *Annals of Surgery* for June 1943, she wrote an article describing the activities of the social service department during and after that disaster.

Following her resignation in 1945, she retired to the Cambridge home she shared with her sister and brother, and in addition to continuing to write, she enjoyed her hobbies of astronomy and bookbinding. She was a member of the committee for the fiftieth anniversary celebration of the social service department, held October 20-22, 1955. Two years later, in 1957, she suffered a stroke and was confined to a nursing home in Watertown until she died in 1960. She was honored with memorial services at First Church in Harvard Square, Cambridge.

While alive and after her death, she received a great deal of recognition for her pioneering service to humanity. She received two honorary degrees, a doctor of humanities from the University of New Hampshire (1937) and a doctor of science from Boston University (1950). In 1959, she received both the Lemuel Shattuck Award by the Massachusetts Public Health Association and honorary membership in England's Institute of Almoners. The Ida M. Cannon award of the Massachusetts Social Service Department was named in her honor. In 1960, she was posthumously awarded a citation and commemorative medal at a reunion dinner of the Social Service Department. A memorial fund at the hospital was established by friends in 1961. Her portrait hangs in the Cabot Room of Massachusetts General Hospital.

WRITINGS: *Social Work in Hospitals* (1913, rev. ed., 1923); *On the Social Frontier of Medicine* (1952); numerous articles in professional journals, including "Changes in Hospital Care through Social Service," *Trained Nurse and Hospital Review* (April 1938) and "Some Social Aspects of Syphilis," *American Journal of Nursing* (May 1938); many volumes of unpublished reports, letters, and diaries, located in the Social Service Department Archives, Massachusetts General Hospital, Boston.
REFERENCES: *Annual Reports of the Social Service Department*, Massachusetts General Hospital; *Boston Herald*, July 9, 1960; Ida M. Cannon Papers, Social Service Department Archives, Massachusetts General Hospital (personal papers, letters, diaries, bibliography, typed biography by Mary K. Taylor); Ida M. Cannon, "Changes in Hospital Care through Social Service," *Trained Nurse and Hospital Review* (April 1938), pp. 364-368, *Social Work in Hospitals* (1913, rev. ed., 1923), and *On the Social Frontier of Medicine* (1952); *Dictionary of American Biography*, supplement 6: 133-135; Nathaniel W. Faxon, *The Massachusetts General Hospital 1935-1955* (1959); *Massachusetts General Hospital News* (December 1960); *Notable American Women*, pp. 97-98; Roy Lubove, *The Professional Altruist: The Emergence of Social Work as a Career, 1880-1930* (1965); Meta Rutter Pennock, ed., *Makers of Nursing History* (1928), pp. 60-61 and (1940), pp. 98-99.

JOELLEN WATSON HAWKINS

CARR, ADA M. (Parish of Kenilworth, County of Warwick, England--June 28, 1951, Baltimore, Maryland). *Public health nurse.* Never married. EDUCATION: Attended school in the Convent of the Sacred Heart, Canada; 1893, graduated from Johns Hopkins Hospital School of Nursing, Baltimore, Maryland. CAREER: 1893-1901, head nurse, then assistant superintendent of nurses, Johns Hopkins Hospital School of Nursing; 1902-1903, superintendent of nurses, Newport Hospital, Newport, Rhode Island; 1908-1912, superintendent, Baltimore Visiting Nurse Association; 1913-1916, head of the department of education, Instructive District Nursing Association, Boston; 1916-1918, district nurse, Instructive Visiting Nurse Association, Providence, Rhode Island; 1918-1922, consulting editor, *Public Health Nursing*, Cleveland, Ohio; 1923-1930, editor, *The Public Health Nurse*, New York City.
CONTRIBUTIONS: Ada Carr was a leader in both institutional and community nursing. She was in the forefront of the public health nursing movement, and active with the National Organization for Public Health Nursing (NOPHN) when it was organized in 1912. She is best remembered for the "high level" of *The Public Health Nurse*, a magazine

which she edited for seven years. Prior to that, she had been a consultant to *Public Health Nursing*, a predecessor of *The Public Health Nurse*. She also was a prolific writer of articles about public health nursing, and at one time she wrote all the book reviews for *The Public Health Nurse*. She was also remembered by the staff of the NOPHN as the one who urged the preservation of the records of that association. Her suggestion was followed, with the result that NOPHN materials are in an archives at the New York City office of the National League for Nursing. Within the field of public health nursing, Carr raised the critical question as to whether "the education and instructive features of visiting nursing" should be "given such importance as to make skilled nursing only a secondary consideration." The debate which followed this question continued for many years to separate the ideology of the official (state, city, or county) public health nurse from the visiting nurse and the private agency nurse.

Another significant contribution of Carr was that she may have been the first nurse to conduct post-graduate studies in public health nursing. She realized that the typical hospital training program of the time did not prepare a nurse to care for patients in their homes and community. As head of the department of education of the Boston Instructive Visiting Nurse Association, she was responsible for developing and teaching such courses, which were necessary for hospital-trained nurses who had little or no experience outside the hospital setting. The certificate program in public health nursing at Simmons College, Boston, was a direct outgrowth of this work with the visiting nurse association.

When she assumed her position with the Baltimore Visiting Nurse Association, there was only one nurse caring for patients in their homes. When she left the association after almost five years, six were doing that work. While superintendent of nurses at Newport Hospital, in Newport, Rhode Island, she increased the educational program from two to three years, very much in line with the philosophy she came to accept when she studied at Johns Hopkins under the tutelage of M. Adelaide Nutting (q.v.). It was also when Carr was superintendent of nurses at the Newport Hospital that she began her lasting friendship with Mary Sewall Gardner (q.v.), who also went on to be an outstanding leader in the field of public health nursing.

WRITINGS: *The Early History of the Hospital and the Training School* (1909); "Reading Lists on Organization, Administration, and Development of Public Health Nursing" (1920), M. Adelaide Nutting Historical Nursing Collection, Columbia University Teachers College Library, New York City; "William H. Welch and Nursing," *International Nursing Review* (1950); numerous articles in *The Public Health Nurse*.

REFERENCES: *American Journal of Nursing* (1951); Howard S. Brown, *History of Newport Hospital* (1976); Lavinia Dock and Isabel Stewart, *A*

Short History of Nursing (1931); M. Louise Fitzpatrick, *The National Organization for Public Health Nursing, 1912-1952* (1975); Janet Herrich, "Historical Perspectives on Public Health Nursing," *Nursing Outlook* (November-December 1983), pp. 317-320; *The Public Health Nurse* (1951); Winifred Rand, "Ada M. Carr," biographical sketch published by the National League of Nursing Education (n.d.).

ALICE HOWELL FRIEDMAN

CHRISTY, TERESA ELIZABETH (March 31, 1927, Brooklyn, New York--April 1982). *Historian of Nursing*. Daughter of James P. Christy and Charlotte (Pardy) Christy. Never married. EDUCATION: 1949, B.S., Manhattanville College of the Sacred Heart, Purchase, New York; 1957, M.S., DePaul University, Chicago, Illinois; 1968, Ed.D., Teachers College, Columbia University, New York City. CAREER: 1947-1948, operating room nurse, Halloran Veterans Administration Hospital, Staten Island, New York; 1949-1950, labor and delivery room nurse, French Hospital, New York City; 1950-1960, instructor of nursing arts, St. Joseph's Hospital, Joliet, Illinois; 1960-1964, assistant professor of nursing, Molloy College, Rockville Center, New York, serving as chairperson of the department of nursing, 1963-1964; 1966-1967, lecturer, Teachers College, Columbia University, and 1968-1970, assistant professor; 1970-1974, associate professor of nursing, Adelphi University, Garden City, New York; 1974-1975, associate professor, and 1975-1982, professor of nursing, University of Iowa, Iowa City, Iowa.

CONTRIBUTIONS: Teresa Christy was best known for her writings, particularly for her "Portrait of a Leader" series in *Nursing Outlook* (1969-1975). These articles presented new information about nursing leaders of the twentieth century and provide historians of nursing with a wealth of information which is not available without a great deal of detective work in primary sources. Her series included articles on Lavinia Dock (q.v.), Annie Goodrich (q.v.), M. Adelaide Nutting (q.v.), Sophia Palmer (q.v.), Isabel Hampton Robb (q.v.), Isabel Maitland Stewart, (q.v.), and Lillian D. Wald (q.v.). She was concerned that "in current feminist writings, the work of the great leaders in nursing has been overlooked," and she set out to research and write about the "lives of great American nurses who were intelligent, industrious, dedicated visionaries--people whom nurses of the present could emulate." Nine of her articles were included in *Pages from Nursing History* (1984), a collection of original articles from the *American Journal of Nursing*, *Nursing Outlook*, and *Nursing Research*. Her contribution represented one-third of the essays in the book, indicating the extent of her work as compared with others in her field.

Christy is also remembered for her scholarly work, *Cornerstone for Nursing Education* (1969), which was based upon her doctoral dissertation. It was a significant contribution to the literature of the profession, for it documents the work of the nursing division of Columbia University's Teachers College and its influence on the development of nursing education. She was a popular speaker and a participant in numerous programs and conferences. She gave dozens of lectures on nursing history to audiences from coast to coast and in that way helped to renew an awareness of the history of nursing and to instill in others an appreciation for the importance of studying nursing history. She also influenced a large number of students, for she taught at five universities, including the University of Iowa, where she was a full professor at the time of her death in 1982. She served as director of Adelphi University's graduate program in nursing. In 1977, she served as chairperson of the American Nurses' Association hall of fame committee, which was responsible for nominating persons for induction in the association's nursing hall of fame.

She received a number of honors in recognition of her contributions to her profession. In 1976, she received the centennial scholar award of Johns Hopkins University and the alumnae achievement award of Columbia University's Teachers College nursing education alumnae association. In 1977, she received the Sigma Theta Tau founder's award for research in the history of nursing. In 1978, she received the University of Iowa college of nursing outstanding teacher award and in that same year was named as a fellow of the American Academy of Nursing.

WRITINGS: *Cornerstone for Nursing Education: A History of the Division of Nursing Education at Teachers College, Columbia University, 1899-1947* (1969); numerous articles in nursing journals, including "Portrait of a Leader" series in *Nursing Outlook* (January, March, June, and October 1969, March and August 1970, and December 1975).

REFERENCES: *American Journal of Nursing* (1970), p. 1976, and (1982), p. 862; *Contemporary Authors* (vols. 73-76, pub. 1978), pp. 120-121; M. Louise Fitzpatrick, "Portrait of a Leader: Teresa E. Christy," *Society of Nursing History Gazette* (1982), pp. 1-2.

ALICE HOWELL FRIEDMAN

CLAYTON, S{ARAH} LILLIAN (1876, Sassafras, Maryland--May 2, 1930, Philadelphia). *Nurse; educator, administrator.* Never married.

EDUCATION: 1893-1894, nursing student, Children's Hospital, Philadelphia; 1896, received diploma, Philadelphia General Hospital School of Nursing; 1900-1902, special training for missionary work at the Baptist Institute of Christian Workers, Philadelphia; 1910-1911, completed hospital economics course, Teachers College, Columbia University, New York City; 1912, post-graduate study at the University of Minnesota.
CAREER: 1896-1899, night supervisor, Philadelphia General Hospital; 1899-1900, private duty nursing; 1902-1907, assistant superintendent, Miami Valley Hospital, Dayton, Ohio; 1911, superintendent of nurses, Minneapolis City Hospital, Minneapolis, Minnesota; 1914, first educational director, Illinois Training School of Nurses, Chicago; 1915-1930, superintendent of nurses, Philadelphia General Hospital, and director of nursing, Philadelphia Department of Health bureau of hospitals; 1922, instructor (summer session), Teachers College, Columbia University.
CONTRIBUTIONS: The Boxer Rebellion caused Lillian Clayton to abandon her plans to become a missionary nurse in China, and after five years of private duty nursing, she turned to hospital administration and nursing education, fields to which she contributed a great deal over the course of her career. She was innovative in her style of nursing administration and avant-garde in her willingness to use the results of experimentation and studies in both hospital administration and nursing education. For instance, while serving as superintendent of nurses at the Philadelphia General Hospital, she made a comparative study of the staffing of similar institutions to determine the staff levels needed for good nursing service. Then she worked diligently to reach these at "Old Blockley," as the hospital was known. She created the Women's Advisory Council to secure public support for the Philadelphia General Hospital and to involve influential women in the crusade to improve patient care as well as the living and working conditions of nurses. She was a leader in the movement to employ general duty nurses for patient care rather than total reliance upon students for this service.

As a leader in nursing education, she was a major force behind the movement to give student nurses formal preparation before they were expected to care for patients. Her ideas for pre-clinical nursing courses continue to be followed, especially in diploma schools, hospital-based nursing programs which are unaffiliated with colleges or universities. She was among the first to recognize the need to include the social and health aspects of nursing in the basic curriculum. She expanded the clinical experiences for students beyond the pre-clinical course, seeking out-of-hospital experiences such as could be developed through affiliations with visiting nurse associations. She always emphasized the need to prepare students for the realities of patient care. She was interested in the individual student and frequently had informal conferences with them. She was one of the first nurse-educators to advocate student governance in an attempt to democratize nursing education. She was interested in the development of character within the student. Her classes in ethics, innovative for that time, encouraged discussion about the ethical issues of the day. Her interest in professional ethics can be seen from the fact that she served on the Committee for the Formation of a Code of Ethics for Nurses (1926).

In addition to her contributions to hospital administration and nursing education, she was an active member of various professional organizations. She served on numerous committees that influenced the direction of nursing and nursing education. She was elected president of the National League of Nursing Education in 1917 and served for three years. During World War I, she was a member of the Committee on Nursing of the Council of National Defense, and she helped to organize the participation of civilian hospitals in the affiliations of students from the Army School of Nursing. She also served in other important capacities: as a member of the board of the Harmon Associates (which provided retirement planning for nurses), as a member of the local and national committees of the Red Cross Nursing Service, and as a member of the board of directors of the International Council for Nurses. She was president of the American Journal of Nursing Company. She was appointed to the Pennsylvania Board of Nurse Examiners and served as chairman for five years.

She was elected president (1926-1930) of the American Nurses' Association (ANA). She led the association as it grew from a membership of 47,000 to 100,000. She encouraged the association to consider and plan for the needs of both the individual nurse and for nurses as a group. During her term in office, she was an advocate of a program for financial planning for nurses in their retirement; she urged greater publicity for the profession and was outspoken in her belief that the public needed to know more about nursing. She was an early spokesman for research in nursing, telling the delegates to the 1928 convention of the ANA that "we are not truly a profession until we have research to our credit."

She received various awards in recognition of her accomplishments. She was the first recipient of the Walter Burns Saunders Medal for "distinguished service in the cause of nursing," receiving the award for her work as an "educator, administrator, humanitarian." A memorial tablet was placed in the lobby of the newly built administration building of the Philadelphia General Hospital in 1928 to recognize her "extraordinary devotion and constructive service." The class of 1929 placed a bronze table in the nurses' home of the Miami Valley Hospital, Dayton, Ohio, in honor of Clayton and Ella Crandall (q.v.), a former superintendent, and a fountain was dedicated to the two "who had set standards of nursing in a city where there had been no school of nursing before." Clayton died one month before the completion of her term as president of ANA. A tribute to her was read by Annie Goodrich (q.v.) at the 1930 convention of the ANA, and she received a posthumous honorary degree (master of science in nursing education) from Teachers College, Columbia University. Beginning in 1947, scholarship awards at the Philadelphia General Hospital nursing school were given in her name.

WRITINGS: Many articles published in the *American Journal of Nursing*, including "Affiliation for Schools with Public Health Nursing Associations," (1924), p. 1140; "Forms of Government in Schools," (1926), p. 872; "Place of Teaching Supervision in Educational Programs" (1923), p. 479, "Problems of Administration" (1930), p. 417, and "Standardization of Nursing Techniques" (1927), p. 939; also contributed to *Modern Hospital* a number of articles on clinical experiences for students.

REFERENCES: *American Journal of Nursing* (1924), p. 388; L. Flanagan, *One Strong Voice: A Story of the American Nursing Association* (1976); Mary M. Roberts, *American Nursing: History and Interpretation* (1954), pp. 650-651, and "S. Lillian Clayton, 1876-1930," *American Journal of Nursing* (1954), pp. 1360-1363; unpublished biography in History of Nursing Collection, Teachers College, Columbia University.

ALICE HOWELL FRIEDMAN

COLLINS, CHARITY E. (March 21, 1882, possibly in Atlanta, Georgia--?). *Public health nurse; school nurse.* At some time married to a Mr. Miles. EDUCATION: Completed the eighth grade and three years of high school at Spelman Seminary, Atlanta, Georgia; October 1, 1903, entered the nurse-training school of MacVicar Hospital, associated with Atlanta Baptist Female Seminary, Atlanta, Georgia, (which evolved into Spelman College), graduating on November 16, 1906. CAREER: 1906-1911, private duty nurse; 1911-c. 1930, public school nurse, Atlanta, Georgia; 1918, U.S. Public Health Service during the influenza epidemic.

CONTRIBUTIONS: Charity Collins was one of the earliest public school nurses in the country and perhaps the first black nurse in such a position. In 1911, she was appointed public school nurse by the city of Atlanta, which then had nine schools and over 4,000 children; by 1929, there were fourteen schools and 20,000 children, with the number of public health nurses growing to five. She was the first black nurse appointed by the Atlanta Department of Health. During her long years of service, an infant welfare center was established to provide well-child care, oral hygiene programs for students were organized, along with prenatal clinics for black women. Parent-teacher associations were established in the schools, and a great deal of attention was given to health education. Collins was credited for having much to do with the establishment of these examples of community work and with the close cooperation between physicians and parents that characterized health care for mothers and children in Atlanta early in this century.

It is probable that Collins lived out her career as a school and public health nurse in Atlanta. We know from one account of her life that she was a school nurse for at least nineteen years in Atlanta. She received a certificate from the U.S. Public Health Service, signed by Surgeon-General Rupert Blue, in recognition of her service during the 1918 influenza epidemic. On October 12, 1919, the name of Charity Collins came before the Georgia State Board of Examiners of Nurses as one of the applicants for registration without examination; her application was approved, and she was issued certificate number 1,054.

REFERENCES: Mary Elizabeth Carnegie, *The Path We Tread: Blacks in Nursing 1854-1984* (1986); Lavinia L. Dock, ed., *A History of Nursing*, vol. 3 (1912); official minutes and unpublished records, Georgia State Board of Examiners of Nurses, Atlanta; Adah B. Thoms, *Pathfinders: A History of the Progress of Colored Graduate Nurses* (1929).

JOELLEN WATSON HAWKINS

COOKE, GENEVIEVE (1869, Dutch Flat, California--January 28, 1928). *Editor and organizer.* Parents were pioneers who crossed the country in a covered wagon before she was born. EDUCATION: Attended common schools; 1887-1888, studied nursing at California Women's Hospital, San Francisco, graduating in 1888; 1900-1901, studied anatomy and dissection, Cooper Medical College, San Francisco (now Stanford University Medical School); 1901, studied physical training at Harvard University summer school, Cambridge, Massachusetts; attended the lateral curvature clinic, Children's Hospital, Boston; 1903, completed course in massage taught by Dr. Douglas Graham of Boston. CAREER: 1888-1900 private duty nurse, San Francisco; visiting instructor in massage, Children's Hospital, Lane (now Stanford), St. Francis, and University of California hospitals, San Francisco; instructor of corrective exercises at Miss Mabie's gymnasium and in her own office; founder, editor, and business manager for nine years of *Pacific Coast Nursing Journal.*

CONTRIBUTIONS: Genevieve Cooke's major contribution was as founder and business manager of the *Pacific Coast Nursing Journal*, the organ of the California State Nurses' Association. She apparently was influenced in her career choices as a result of her attendance at the International Congress of Nurses in Buffalo, New York, in 1901, where she met numerous leaders of nursing organizations and became aware of the importance of journals in the development of professionalism. She was a charter member of the California State Nurses' Association, and she urged the other members to approve a proposal for the association to publish a journal. Beginning as the *Journal of the California State Nurses' Association* and published out of her apartment, that same year it was renamed *The Nurses' Journal of the Pacific Coast.* Managing to rescue the *Journal*'s bank book, check book, subscription list, and advertising contracts from the devastation caused by the April 1906 San Francisco earthquake, she relocated the *Journal*'s office and published the issue after the earthquake only six weeks late. In 1912, she persuaded the board of directors of the California State Nurses' Association to change the publication's name to *The Pacific Coast Journal of Nursing.* As editor of that publication, she worked for an eight-hour day for nurses and for nurse registration. She was known for her sense of professional ethics, refusing to sacrifice her principles even at the expense of loss of advertising revenue for the *Journal.*

In addition to her work in publishing the *Journal*, she was active in professional associations on the local, state, national, and international levels. For many years she was a member of the council of the California State Nurses' Association; she was secretary for one term and twice the president of the San Francisco County Nurses' Association. As a delegate from the California State Nurses' Association at the national convention in Detroit in May 1906, she began a long and important career with the American Nurses' Association. In 1907, she attended the International Congress of Nurses in Paris, and she was elected first vice-president of the American Nurses' Association, a position she was reelected to in 1908 and 1909. From 1910 to 1912, she served an elected position as a member of the board of directors of the American Journal of Nursing Company. She served as president of the American Nurses' Association from 1913 to 1915. She was ill for many of the last years of her life.

WRITINGS: "Nurse Views on Aid for San Francisco," *American Journal of Nursing* (August 1906), pp. 823-825; "Nurses as Specialists in Mechanotherapy," *The Nurses' Journal of the Pacific Coast* (April 1907), pp. 158-159; "Inception of Our Journal," *Pacific Coast Journal of Nursing* (May 1915), pp. 209-210.

REFERENCES: Daisy Caroline Bridges, *A History of the International Council of Nurses: 1899-1964* (1967); Lyndia Flanagan, *One Strong Voice* (1976); Theresa Earles McCarthy and S. Gotea Dozier, "Genevieve Cooke," *American Journal of Nursing* (March 1928), pp. 146-147; "Our Professional Editors: Miss Genevieve Cooke," *British Journal of Nursing*

(January 27, 1906), p. 72; "Who's Who in the Nursing World: Genevieve Cooke, R.N.," *American Journal of Nursing* (July 1923), p. 852.

LORETTA P. HIGGINS

CRANDALL, ELLA PHILLIPS (September 16, 1871, Wellsville, New York--October 24, 1938, New York City). *Public health nursing leader.* Daughter of Herbert A. Crandall, manufacturer, and Alice (Phillips) Crandall, seamstress. Never married. EDUCATION: Attended public schools in Dayton, Ohio; 1890, graduated from high school; 1897, graduated from "Old Blockley," the Philadelphia General Hospital; 1909, took a post-graduate course at New York School of Philanthropy (later New York School of Social Work), New York City. CAREER: 1899-1909, superintendent, Deaconess Home and Hospital, Dayton, Ohio (later Miami Valley Hospital), and first director of the hospital's school of nursing; 1909-1910, supervisor, Henry Street Visiting Nurse Service, New York City; 1910-1912, instructor in public health nursing, Teachers College, Columbia University (she helped develop courses in district nursing and health protection and continued as a lecturer until 1919); 1912-1920, executive secretary, National Organization for Public Health Nursing; 1921-1922, director of the Maternity Center Association's committee to study community organization for self-support for health work for women and young children, New York City; 1922, director of the New York Association for Improving the Condition of the Poor's bureau of educational nursing, New York City; 1922-1925, associate director, American Child Health Association; 1925-1938, executive secretary of the Payne Fund.

CONTRIBUTIONS: Ella Crandall was one of the founders of the National Organization for Public Health Nursing, having served as a member of the special commission established by the American Nurses' Association and the Society of Superintendents of Training Schools to study efforts to deal with disease, filth, and poverty in slums and small towns. In 1911, she suggested that the American Red Cross undertake the provision of nursing service to rural areas, and in 1912 the Red Cross Rural Nursing Service was established, made possible through the use of the relatively inexpensive and dependable Ford automobile. In June 1912, she took office as the organization's first executive secretary, and later in that year with a trip to the southern states she began her travels to visit nurses in the field. In March 1913, she served at the Dayton, Ohio, flood, in charge of fifty nurses doing sanitary inspections. In 1915, she travelled 82,021 miles and gave eighty-three public addresses across the United States. To promote the importance of public health nursing, she visited chambers of commerce, industrialists, and civic clubs. To observe their work in public health, she visited individual nurses and directors of visiting nurse services.

During World War I (1917-1918), she served in Washington, D.C., as executive secretary for the three committees on nursing of the Council of National Defense, the General Committee on Nursing, the Subcommittee on Public Health Nursing of the Committee on Hygiene and Sanitation, and the Committee on Home Nursing. She also served on a subcommittee (first meeting, September 20, 1918) to develop programs for civilian hospitals to work with the Army School of Nursing to train nurses for army service. In 1918, yet another committee demanded her time, its objective to prepare a campaign to encourage nurses to enroll for service in the American Red Cross. On December 9, 1919, a resolution to recognize army nurses with rank was presented by the National Committee on Red Cross Nursing to the Central Committee of the American Red Cross; Crandall had helped draft that document and was one of its co-signers. Apparently Crandall had some difference in philosophy with Clara Noyes (q.v.) during the latter's tenure as director of the Red Cross Nursing Service. There is some evidence that Crandall felt that the Red Cross had taken advantage of the services of the National Organization for Public Health Nursing. Whatever occurred, the result was Crandall's resignation from the organization in 1920, and indeed, her eventual decision to leave nursing.

Early in her career she and her friend S. Lillian Clayton (q.v.) started the school of nursing of Miami Valley Hospital, Dayton, Ohio, creating from an old deaconess hospital a modern institution. She served as a member of the executive committee of the Society of Superintendents of Training Schools in 1908-1909 and as president of the Ohio State Association for Graduate Nurses. She also was a member of the board of directors of the American Nurses' Association (1913-1916, 1918-1920) and on the American Red Cross committee on nursing (1916-1918). Her career ended as executive secretary of the Payne Fund, founded by Mrs. Chester Bolton (Frances Payne Bolton), a Cleveland philanthropist who later was a congresswoman. The fund was created to support research in education, as well as experimental projects directed at educating youth for peace. With the Payne Fund, Crandall became particularly interested in a study of the magazine-reading habits of young people. A sudden and swift illness with pneumonia took her life in 1938, and she died in Roosevelt Hospital in New York City.

WRITINGS: Numerous articles for nursing journals, almost all on public health nursing.

REFERENCES: *American Journal of Nursing* (October 1920), pp. 3-4, (November 1922), p. 129, (December 1938), pp. 1406-1409; Annie M.

Brainard, *The Evolution of Public Health Nursing* (1922); Lavinia Dock et al., *History of American Red Cross Nursing* (1922); M. Louise Fitzpatrick, *The National Organization for Public Health Nursing, 1912-1952* (1975); Mary Sewall Gardner, "Twenty-five Years Ago," *The Public Health Nurse* (March 1937), pp. 141-144, and *Public Health Nursing* (1916); National League of Nursing Education, *Leaders of American Nursing* (1924); *Notable American Women*, pp. 398-399; Mary M. Roberts, *American Nursing: History and Interpretation* (1954); *The Public Health Nurse* (October 1920), pp. 553-555, and (December 1938), pp. 726-727; *The Trained Nurse and Hospital Review* (November 1938), pp. 410-411; unpublished papers, M. Adelaide Nutting Historical Nursing Collections, Teachers College, Columbia University (microfiche 2436).

JOELLEN WATSON HAWKINS

CUMMING, KATE (c. 1833, Edinburgh, Scotland--June 5, 1909, Birmingham, Alabama). *Civil War nurse.* Never married. CAREER: April 7, 1862 left Mobile, Alabama, to begin work nursing the sick and wounded of the Confederate Army, returning to Mobile on May 27, 1865. CONTRIBUTIONS: Kate Cumming served as a Civil War nurse, being twenty-eight years-old when the war began. As a refined lady in the Southern tradition, she volunteered for service with the Confederate Army. Her family was opposed to her decision, although her father eventually gave her his blessing. Many of the women who volunteered with her and who provided nursing service after the Battle of Shiloh returned home after a short time. Cumming persisted, however. She was not a trained nurse; she learned by doing. Although in 1860 an American edition of Florence Nightingale's *Notes on Nursing: What It Is, and What It Is Not* was published, the medical establishment was not ready for a large number of nurses to serve with the military. The Northern authorities accepted the role of nurses before the Confederate leaders recognized the need to do so. As a result, it was not until September 1862 that Confederate nurses were granted official status. When that happened, Cumming became a matron whose duties included not only caring for the ill and wounded but also responsibility for the domestic services of the hospital, including supervision of food and laundry services. Because the military hospitals were mobile units, the nurses moved with them. During her three years of service, she travelled to sites scattered about Alabama and Georgia. After the Battle of Shiloh, the sick and wounded Confederate soldiers were moved to Corinth, Mississippi, where the Tishomingo Hotel was used as a hospital.

Cumming was matron of this hospital, which was so overcrowded that Ella K. Newsom (q.v.) wrote that "every yard of space on the floors, as well as all the beds, bunks and cots were covered with the mangled forms of dying and dead soldiers."

Second only to her loyal and dedicated service to the Confederate soldiers was the publication of her journal soon after the war's end. Although she apologized that dates and places might not be exact, she painted a detailed picture of the conditions under which medical and nursing care were provided, as well as excellent descriptions of that care. In addition, she told poignant stories of the lives of the soldiers, as well as of the doctors and nurses. Hers was a record of the war not dimmed by years of delay before writing. In her journal she did more than describe her daily activities; she also articulated a philosophy and analyzed the problems that she encountered in nursing the soldiers. For example, she discussed prejudice against women, the unprofessional behavior of some women, and the incompetence of those in charge of transporting the soldiers. Although a loyal Southerner, she criticized when it was justified. She lamented that more Southern women were not involved in nursing the wounded or in helping to provide for supplies for the military hospitals.

WRITINGS: *The Journal of a Confederate Nurse* (ed. Richard Barksdale Harwell, 1959), originally published as *A Journal of Hospital Life in the Confederate Army of Tennessee from the Battle of Shiloh to the End of the War: With Sketches of Life and Character and Brief Notices of Current Events during that Period* (1866); *Gleanings from Southland* (1895), an abridged version of her first book.

REFERENCES: H. H. Cunningham, *Doctors in Gray: The Confederate Medical Service* (1958); Bertha S. Dodge, *The Story of Nursing* (1954); Richard Barksdale Harwell, ed., *The Journal of a Confederate Nurse* (1959).

LORETTA P. HIGGINS

CUSHMAN, EMMA D. (Missouri--December 31, 1930, Cairo, Egypt). *Missionary nurse.* Descendant of Robert Cushman, who chartered the *Mayflower.* Never married. EDUCATION: 1892, graduated from Paterson General Hospital, Paterson, New Jersey; post-graduate studies in the care of women and in pharmacy. CAREER: Schoolteacher, New York State; 1892-1899, superintendent of Scarritt Hospital, Kansas City, Missouri (operated a missionary training school in Konia, Turkey); 1900-1930, member of the medical staff of the American Board of Foreign Missions.

CONTRIBUTIONS: Emma Cushman devoted most of her career to foreign service under the auspices of the American Board of Foreign Missions. When a call came to Scarritt Hospital for a missionary nurse to serve in Konia, Cushman volunteered. Embarking in 1900, her first assignment was at the American Hospital in Konia, at that time, almost entirely populated by Muslims, with a small percentage of Greeks and Armenians. The nurses, however, were all Greek and Armenian. In 1908, she organized a training school there to provide for the education of nurses so desperately needed in the Middle East. Because there were no nursing textbooks written in Arabic or Armenian, she translated various texts for use in the school.

She provided nursing care during the Balkan Wars, returning afterward to Konia. When foreigners were ordered to leave Turkey, she refused to desert her post. In most difficult surroundings, she continued to provide nursing care for tens of thousands of war victims, including British soldiers who were prisoners of war, Roman Catholic priests and nuns, refugees from various parts of Turkey, and Armenians who sought refuge from genocide at the hands of the Turks. During this time, Konia was closed to outsiders. Cushman was to a great extent the only individual representing the interests and principles of the Allied nations, and she was given the title of acting consul of the allied and neutral nations. Forty-six racial or national groups were represented in this central prison camp.

In 1922, she cared for refugees who fled when Turkish forces counter-attacked and took control of Smyrna. Cushman at one time oversaw a 4,000-bed trachoma hospital at Istanbul and a 1,000-bed orphanage near there. When 22,000 Christian children were evacuated from Anatolia, she accompanied them to Corinth, Greece, and worked in the 2,500-student orphanage school until her services were no longer needed. She trained the children in skills needed for life: farming, artisan crafts, and housekeeping. Her work was completed in Corinth during the late 1920s, and she retired to a small house built for her by some of the orphan children in the village of St. Theodore, near the Corinthian canal. Her nearly thirty years of living in the Mediterranean area left her ill and suffering from both the climate and the lack of hygiene. In December 1930, the American Board of Foreign Missions sent her to Egypt so she could spend Christmas among the orphans from Armenia who had found refuge there and who were sponsored by the Near East Foundation. While in Egypt, she died of malaria and anemia on December 31, 1930.

During the course of her career, she received numerous citations in recognition of her humanitarian work. These included the (French) Cross of the Legion of Honor for her work with French prisoners and the highest civilian decoration accorded by Greece, the Gold Cross of the

Redeemer; she received the blessing of the Greek patriarch in Constantinople. In the statements which accompanied the awards, she was characterized as a nurse, almoner, administrator, priest, financier, and statesman.

REFERENCES: *American Journal of Nursing* (April 1930), pp. 417-418; Lavinia L. Dock and Isabel M. Stewart, *A Short History of Nursing* (4th ed., 1938); William T. Ellis, *Bible Lands To-Day* (1927); Minnie Goodnow, *Nursing History* (7th ed., 1943); Paterson General Hospital, *Centennial Publication* (1971), p. 29.

JOELLEN WATSON HAWKINS

D

DAKIN, FLORENCE (May 29, 1869, Brooklyn, New York--?). *Nurse-administrator.* Daughter of George W. V. Dakin and Anna Maria (Olcott) Dakin. Never married. EDUCATION: Graduate of Brooklyn Heights Seminary, Brooklyn, New York; attended Hollins Institute, Roanoke, Virginia; 1902, graduated from New York Hospital School of Nursing, New York City. CAREER: 1902, superintendent, Fannie Paddock Hospital, Tacoma, Washington; instructor of nurses and supervisor of ward management, City and County Hospital, San Francisco; assistant in the commissary department, New York Hospital, New York City; assistant superintendent of nurses, Paterson General Hospital, Paterson, New Jersey; instructor, Middletown Hospital and School for Trained Attendants, Middletown, Ohio; 1925-1938, inspector of nurses' training schools, State of New Jersey.

CONTRIBUTIONS: Florence Dakin was well known as a teacher of trained attendants and as author of *Simplified Nursing* (1925), a book which evolved from her own experience in teaching attendants. The book was especially practical for the training of home nurses, trained attendants, and nursing housekeepers. In the first half of this century, hospital housekeeping was a responsibility assigned to many departments of nursing service, and there were no textbooks or teaching materials for training the auxiliary workers in the hospital setting. Textbooks focused on the training of the professional nurse, and there was clearly a need for guidance in the preparation of what were to become nurses' aides and other auxiliary personnel. Florence Dakin's experience as a nurse who served as assistant in the commissary and as supervisor of ward management provided her with insight into the economics of hospital management and with material which she used in her book. The book was not used in formal educational programs; rather, professional nurses who were placed in the position of training aides and other auxiliary workers could rely upon the book for information and guidance as to the roles of various personnel, and techniques which could be used in providing the needed education.

WRITINGS: *Simplified Nursing* (1925).
REFERENCES: Meta Rutter Pennock, *Makers of Nursing History* (1940); *Who's Who in American Women* (1958), p. 302.

ALICE HOWELL FRIEDMAN

DAMER, ANNIE (1858, Stratford, Ontario, Canada--August 9, 1915, New York City). *Public health nurse; leader in the American Nurses' Association.* Never married. EDUCATION: 1885, graduated from Bellevue Hospital Training School, New York City. CAREER: 1885-1893, private duty nursing for a young girl; 1893-1898, nurse-investigator for the Charity Association of Buffalo, New York; 1898-c. 1901, nurse in charge of the dispensary for tubercular patients, Bellevue Hospital; 1901-c. 1911, took charge of Echo Hill Farm, Yorktown Heights, New York, the home for convalescent children established under the auspices of Lillian Wald (q.v.) and her Nurses' Settlement on Henry Street.

CONTRIBUTIONS: Annie Damer made two significant contributions during her active career, which was cut short by her illness and untimely death; she was instrumental in establishing tuberculosis nursing in New York and was a leader in a number of professional organizations. As the nurse in charge of the dispensary for tubercular patients at Bellevue Hospital, she organized the work of visiting nurses who went out to teach dispensary patients how to protect themselves and others from tuberculosis. At that time, there was a tent pavilion connected with Bellevue for care of tubercular cases. Patients were warmly covered in bed while nurses worked in cold approximating that of the outdoors. Following this position, Damer took charge of the home for convalescent children under the auspices of Lillian Wald and her Nurses' Settlement on Henry Street. The home was called Echo Hill Farm and was located at Yorktown Heights, New York. The farm consisted of seventy-eight acres for which Damer was responsible, along with the children needing special care.

During her years in Buffalo, Damer began her activities with nursing organizations. From 1900 to 1901, she was president of the Buffalo Nurses' Association and extended the invitation for the International Council of Nurses to meet there in September 1901. She chaired the arrangements committee for that third international congress. A member of the first Board of Nurse Examiners in New York State, she later became its president. She served as president of the New York State Nurses' Association for several terms. In 1901, she was elected second president of the Associated Alumnae (later the American Nurses'

Association), serving until 1902; she was elected again in 1905 and served two terms until 1909. She was also president of the board of directors of the *American Journal of Nursing.* Actively interested in the work of the Red Cross, in 1904 she served on a committee of Associated Alumnae to study affiliation of that organization with the American Red Cross. In April 1908, she was asked to serve on the Red Cross Nursing Service committee and in that same year, she served on a subcommittee of the Standing Committee on Education of the Society of Superintendents of Training Schools for Nurses to prepare an outline for class work in home nursing, for use by the Red Cross and other organizations. Her loyalty to her alma mater led her to become president of the Bellevue Alumnae Association. She also was a member of the Board of Women Managers of the Pan-American Exposition in Buffalo, and she represented the interests of the nursing profession.

In 1911, exhausted from her work at Echo Hill Farm and from her work on numerous important committees, she took time off to travel to England. The trip, however, was far from a vacation; she met with a number of British nurses and devoted time to learning about the practice of district nursing and tuberculosis treatment in British sanatoriums. An accident forced her to retire from active nursing work, but she continued to be interested in the affairs of the profession until her death. Her last years, however, were spent as an invalid, and she could no longer participate in organizational work. In 1914, she was honored for her contributions to the profession by being awarded honorary membership in the American Nurses' Association.

WRITINGS: Many published and unpublished speeches and papers; her presidential addresses to the Associated Alumnae were published in convention reports, *American Journal of Nursing* (1901-1902, 1905-1909).

REFERENCES: *American Journal of Nursing* (September 1915), p. 1077, (October 1915), pp. 74-75; Daisy Caroline Bridges, *A History of the International Council of Nurses, 1899-1964: The First 65 Years* (1967); *British Journal of Nursing* (July 8, 1911), p. 24; Lavinia L. Dock, Sarah E. Pickett, Clara D. Noyes, Fannie F. Clement, Elizabeth G. Fox, and Anna R. Van Meter, *History of American Red Cross Nursing* (1922); Lucy B. Fisher, "Miss Annie Damer, President of Associated Alumnae," *Nurses' Journal of the Pacific Coast* (April 1907), pp. 150-154; Lyndia Flanagan, *One Strong Voice: The Story of the American Nurses' Association* (1976); *Pacific Coast Journal of Nursing* (October 1915), p. 423.

JOELLEN WATSON HAWKINS

DARCHE, LOUISE (August 20, 1852, Lampton Mills, near Toronto, Canada--June 1899, London, England). *Educator.* Never married. EDUCATION: 1883-1885, attended Bellevue Hospital Training School for Nurses, New York City, graduating in 1885. CAREER: 1870, principal of a school at St. Catharine's, Ontario; c. 1886-1888, private duty nursing, including nursing for the son of a Chicago millionaire; January 1, 1888-February 1, 1898, superintendent of Training School for Nurses, Charity Hospital, Blackwell's Island, New York City; spent six months with her sister in Canada after her resignation; travelled in Europe; a few months prior to her forty-seventh birthday, she died in an English nursing home run by her good friend, Diana Kimber (q.v.).

CONTRIBUTIONS: Louise Darche devoted her later professional life, even to the point of sacrificing it, to improving the school of nursing at Charity Hospital on Blackwell's Island, New York City. Standing in her way was a powerful and corrupt political machine that treated her badly. The state of nursing and patient care at the hospital were in such a disorganized and incompetent state when she began her work that it was difficult to recruit well-qualified applicants who were interested in enrolling in the training school. One of her improvements was to take charge of the training of the male nurses, who had not received a formal education or proper supervision. By the end of her tenure, she was responsible for more than one hundred nurses and an average daily census of 800 patients. She developed a plan for a City Department of Nursing, and she worked toward its establishment.

Darche also helped her colleagues in nursing education by clarifying puzzling issues that beset the relatively new profession. For example, much discussion hinged on Florence Nightingale's rules for schools of nursing and their adaptation in the United States. Other questions involved the purpose of nurses' training: was its emphasis to be service or education? She supported the extension of the training programs from one to two years, so the second-year students could become head nurses and act as teachers for the first-year students. As one of the speakers at the 1893 meeting at the Chicago World's Fair, where the National League of Nursing Education was conceived, she argued that it was crucial for nurses to unite in favor of improved standards for the profession. She was supported in the plan to establish a publication which would be the official organ of the national association of nurses. She was the first secretary of the American Society of Superintendents of Training Schools for Nurses, which was established at that 1893 meeting and which was to become the National League for Nursing.

In 1916, the graduates of the City Hospital School of Nursing, as the Blackwell's Island school came to be called, established a scholarship

fund to be known as the Darche and Kimber Scholarship fund to commemorate the work of these two women who played major roles in the early history of the school and in the early history of the nursing profession. Darche was also one of a few nurses to be chosen by the Matrons' Council of Great Britain and Ireland as honorary members of that organization.
WRITINGS: "Improved Methods of Nursing," *Lend a Hand* (August 1895), pp. 122-125; several of her speeches were published in reports of nursing organizations.
REFERENCES; *American Journal of Nursing* (October 1919), p. 40; Jane E. Mottus, *New York Nightingales* (1981); M. Adelaide Nutting Collection, Teachers College, Columbia University, New York City; National League of Nursing Education, *Early Leaders of American Nursing Calendar* (1922); *The Nursing Record & Hospital World* (March 19, 1898), p. 233 and (June 10, 1899), pp. 456-458.

LORETTA P. HIGGINS

DAVIS, FRANCES REED {ELLIOTT} (April 28, 1882, Shelby, North Carolina--May 2, 1965, Mount Clemens, Michigan). *Public health nurse; nurse-educator.* Daughter of Darryl Elliott and Emma Elliott. Married William A. Davis, December 24, 1921. EDUCATION: 1907, completed normal school training at Knoxville College, Knoxville, Tennessee; 1913, received diploma from Freedmen's School of Nursing, Washington, D.C.; 1916, completed community health nursing course (as designated by the town and country nursing service of the American Red Cross), Teachers College, Columbia University, New York City; 1929-1930, attended Teachers College on a Julius Rosenwald Scholarship but was unable to complete the course due to ill health and deaths in the family. CAREER: 1907, taught school in Henderson, North Carolina; 1913, private duty nursing, Washington, D.C.; 1914, supervisor of nurses, Provident Hospital, Baltimore, Maryland; summers of 1916 and 1920, camp nurse for a community-based camp for needy mothers and young children, Washington, D.C.; 1916, staff nurse, Henry Street Settlement, New York City; 1917, staff nurse, American Red Cross, Jackson, Tennessee; early 1918, visiting nurse, American Red Cross, Chattanooga, Tennessee; 1918, director of nurses, John A. Andrew Memorial Hospital, Tuskegee, Alabama; 1919, director of nursing, Dunbar Memorial Hospital, Detroit, Michigan; 1920, staff, Detroit Visiting Nurse Association; 1922, staff, Detroit Health Department; 1923, superintendent of nurses and director of nurses' training, Dunbar Memorial Hospital; 1927, staff nurse, Child Welfare Division, Detroit Health Department; 1935, Detroit Visiting Nurse

Association; 1938, director, community nursing service, Inkster, Michigan; 1944, staff nurse, Eloise Hospital and Infirmary, Inkster, Michigan.

CONTRIBUTIONS: Frances (Elliott) Davis was the first Black nurse to be enrolled officially by the Red Cross Nursing Service and designated as its first black nurse by presentation of Red Cross nursing pin number 1A. She had read with admiration of the pioneer work the Red Cross was doing in rural areas and decided to become a Red Cross nurse in the rural South. Although meeting the Red Cross qualifications of high scholastic standing, graduating from a three-year nursing program, and having a course in public health nursing at Columbia University, with clinical experience with the Henry Street Settlement, she did not automatically receive her Red Cross pin as did all other town and country Red Cross nurses. She wrote about this to Mary S. Gardner (q.v.), director of the Bureau of Public Health Nursing and president of the National Organization for Public Health Nursing. On July 6, 1918, she received congratulations from Gardner for the honor of "being the first colored nurse to be enrolled in the Red Cross." She was to be honored at the 1965 National Red Cross convention in Detroit, but her death came a few days before the event. In all her positions, she insisted upon quality education and employment for black nurses. One way was through her active membership in many nursing organizations, including Freedmen's Hospital Alumnae Association, the National Association of Colored Graduate Nurses, the American Red Cross, the National League of Nursing Education, the Detroit District and Michigan State Nurses' Association, and the American Nurses' Association.

From 1923 to 1927, she served as director of the training school of Detroit's Dunbar Hospital, and in that capacity she organized the first training school for black nurses in the state of Michigan and graduated the first class of black nurses who took the state board examinations and were admitted to practice in the state.

She was a skillful and educated nurse who loved to take care of people, and she took leaves from many of her positions to nurse her friends and members of her family. She lived through two world wars, the Great Depression, the influenza epidemic, and labor unrest in the automobile industry, and as a community leader she tried to relieve the distress that these situations brought to families, especially to mothers and their children. She organized loan closets and commissaries to relieve the need for clothes and food among the unemployed, and she developed nursery schools to provide day-care for children whose mothers were called to work in war industries. During the Depression, she organized youth projects, so her town (Inkster, Michigan) would qualify for National Youth Administration funds and so young people could be gainfully employed. Following her example, many young women became nurses.

REFERENCES: Mary Elizabeth Carnegie, *The Path We Tread: Blacks in Nursing, 1854-1984* (1986); *Notable American Women*, pp. 180-182; Jean Maddern Pitrone, *Trailblazer: Negro Nurse in the American Red Cross* (1969); Adah B. Thoms, *Pathfinders: A History of the Progress of Colored Graduate Nurses* (1929).

ALICE HOWELL FRIEDMAN

DAVIS, MARY E. P. (c. December 1840, New Brunswick, Canada--June 9, 1924, Norwood, Massachusetts). *Pioneer nurse; administrator; journalist.* Daughter of Captain John Davis and Charlotte (McFarland) Davis. Never married. EDUCATION: 1878, one of the first graduates of the Boston Training School for Nurses (later the Massachusetts General Hospital School for Nurses) (the school, one of the three Nightingale schools in the United States, had opened five years earlier; Linda Richards (q.v.) was the director of nurses while Davis was a student). CAREER: 1878-1879, graduate nurse, Massachusetts General Hospital, Boston; c. 1889-1899, superintendent of the hospital and nurses' training school at the University of Pennsylvania, Philadelphia; superintendent of nurses at the Washington Training School for Nurses (later known as Capitol City School), Washington, D.C.; superintendent at the Boston Insane Hospital, Dorchester, Massachusetts; first registrar of the Central Directory for nurses, Boston; corresponding secretary of the Massachusetts State Nurses' Association.

CONTRIBUTIONS: Mary Davis was a pioneer in the founding of the *American Journal of Nursing*, the first journal to be owned and managed exclusively by nurses. She served as its business manager from 1900 until 1909. As leader of a stock company beginning in 1899, she was able to provide a sound financial base for the new magazine. She interviewed publishers, arranged for typesetting and printing, and secured nearly 600 subscriptions which helped make it financially possible for the *Journal* to begin. The first issue was ready for October 1900. Although it was not the first nursing journal, it is the one that survives today.

Davis was one of the eighteen superintendents of nurses who in 1893 founded the American Society of Superintendents of Training Schools for Nurses (now the National League for Nursing), the first national nursing organization in the United States. She was a member of the influential committee of that organization which outlined the goals, specified the qualifications of its members, and described the duties of its officers. The society accepted the work of the committee and its emphasis on the plan to establish a uniform standard of education for all nurses as necessary for the development of the profession.

Her principal executive position was that of superintendent of the University of Pennsylvania Hospital. During her ten years in that position, the hospital was reorganized and enlarged, and the first three-year course for nurses at that hospital was established. While superintendent, Davis gave the presidential address of the third annual convention of the Society of Superintendents of Training Schools for Nurses. Once again she spoke out strongly in favor of improved nursing education, and she advocated a universal standard of training. She also outlined the characteristics and qualifications needed in a superintendent of nurses, explaining that if the superintendents were not qualified as nurses as well as teachers, they could not provide their pupils with a suitable education. To help superintendents and others to prepare for such responsibilities, she was a strong advocate of an advanced course to meet this need, and the leadership of the society was proposing that such a course be established at Teachers College of Columbia University. The course on hospital economics began in October 1899 with two students enrolled; Davis was one of those who examined applicants for entrance to the course.

She was also interested in the pre-nursing educational programs, and she was a leader of those who around 1900 saw the need for preparatory courses for prospective nursing students. She argued in favor of increased educational standards, and in order to accomplish that goal, she believed that it was necessary for beginning students to be adequately prepared academically for a rigorous nursing program. She argued that the preparatory program should be within a technical school rather than organized by the hospital or training school. She reasoned that because of their physical constraints as well as the inadequate academic preparation of nursing staff members, most hospitals were not capable of providing pre-nursing training.

With her classmate Sophia Palmer (q.v.), and with John Simmons of Boston, she envisioned having such a course offered through the newly organized Simmons College. Simmons had left his fortune to establish in Boston a college for "utilitarian education for girls where they could learn art, science, and industry." The proposed project did not come to fruition, and plans in other states for "central" schools were equally unsuccessful in those days. Although outwardly sympathetic toward the goal of improved education, superintendents of training schools would not allow the "probationers" to be away from the hospital for this formative year. To do so would have meant the loss of their labor, mainly in their housework responsibilities.

Davis' attitudes on the formative education of nurses were very progressive, as indicated in her writings and speeches. She wanted students to understand what they were doing for patients and why they were doing it. She insisted that for the students, "the mind should not get separated from the body." She said the goal was to teach the student to reach wisdom, which is "to know yourself." She recognized the need for what today is called stress management, and wanted nurses to be taught how to reduce tensions and relax.

In 1895 she, along with her classmate Sophia Palmer, rallied other classmates and graduates of the Boston Training School to form an alumnae association, which came into existence on February 14 of that year. That organization remains in existence as the Massachusetts General Hospital School of Nursing Alumnae Association. The members were among those who in 1897 joined with nine other alumnae associations to found the Nurses Associated Alumnae of the United States and Canada (which became the American Nurses' Association). Davis was a moving force in the founding (1903) of the Massachusetts State Nurses' Association (MSNA), and she was the second president of that association (1911-1913). She was the first chairperson of the legislative committee of the MSNA and served during the years when the association submitted legislation for nurse registration, which was finally enacted into law in 1910. She also developed the Suffolk County (Massachusetts) Central Directory which was to help graduate nurses obtain employment, but which differed from others in operation in Massachusetts at that time, in that this one was controlled and operated by the nursing profession.

When the library of the Massachusetts General Hospital School of Nursing was enlarged and refurbished in 1940, it was renamed the Palmer-Davis Library in recognition of the two graduates, Sophia Palmer (q.v.) and Mary E. P. Davis, who were pioneers in the nursing profession. In 1982, at the annual convention of the American Nurses' Association, Davis was inducted in the association's Hall of Fame. She met the criteria for induction in that she contributed to the health history of the United States. It was recognized that her work toward producing the journal made the publication a "powerful, co-ordinating force within the profession."

WRITINGS: Many journal articles; among those in the early *American Journal of Nursing* are "What We Are Overlooking of Fundamental Importance in the Training of the Modern Nurse" (1907), p. 764, and "Preparatory Work for Nurses" (1903), p. 256.

REFERENCES: *American Journal of Nursing* (October 1924), pp. 811-812; American Nurses' Association, *Nursing Hall of Fame* (1982), p. 6; Teresa Christy, *Cornerstone for Nursing Education* (1969); Mary Ellen Doona, "Nursing Revisited: Palmer, Davis and Simmons," *The*

Massachusetts Nurse (March 1984); Mary Ellen Doona, "The Cause is Just," *The Massachusetts Nurse* (July 1982), pp. 4-6; Massachusetts Nurses' Association, *Landmarks in Nursing: A Centennial Review* (1976), p. 6; National League for Nursing Education, *Some Leaders of American Nursing* (1923); Sylvia Perkins, *A Centennial Review 1873-1973, of the Massachusetts General Hospital School of Nursing* (1975); town of Norwood, death certificate (1924).

ALICE HOWELL FRIEDMAN

DEANE, ELIZABETH M. (1854, possibly in New Jersey--July 21, 1913, Hoboken, New Jersey). *Missionary nurse to Alaska.* Never married. EDUCATION: 1895-1897, attended the New York Training School for Deaconesses, New York City, graduating in 1897. CAREER: 1897-1911, deaconess in Alaska; 1911-1912, nursing work in Graniteville, South Carolina.

CONTRIBUTIONS: As one of the earliest graduates of the New York Training School for Deaconesses, Elizabeth Deane was the first deaconess who served in the territory of Alaska, leaving immediately after she was "set apart" by Bishop Whipple as a deaconess under the Protestant Episcopal church of the United States (May 27, 1897). Her first assignment was at Circle City, where she served alone for five years (1897-1902), providing nursing care to native Alaskans. When the first church hospital in the interior of Alaska was built, Grace Hospital, she was placed in charge of it. Later she served at Valdez, Ketchikan, and Chena. The long hours, hard work, and exposure to cold and disease forced her in the autumn of 1911 to return to the United States to recuperate. After her return to the United States, for a year she helped Deaconess Sands at Graniteville, South Carolina. She hoped to be able to return to Alaska, but her health and strength did not return, and she was provided a retirement allowance by the Board of Missions.

REFERENCES: Unpublished material from the Deaconess History Project, Episcopal Women's History Project, New York City; Minnie Goodnow, *Nursing History* (7th ed., 1943); New York Training School for Deaconesses, *Alumnae Bulletin* (October 1913); *The Spirit of the Missions* (September 1913), p. 587.

JOELLEN WATSON HAWKINS

DELANO, JANE ARMINDA (March 12, 1862, Townsend, Schuyler County, New York--April 15, 1919, Savenay Hospital, France). *Red Cross* *nurse; army nurse.* Daughter of George Delano, farmer and Civil War soldier, and Mary Ann (Wright) Delano, homemaker. Never married. EDUCATION: Attended Cook Academy, a Baptist boarding school, Montour Falls, New York; 1884-1886, Bellevue Hospital School of Nursing, New York City, graduating January 1887; 1896, attended classes at the University of Buffalo Medical School, Buffalo, New York; 1898, attended New York School of Civics and Philanthropy (later New York School of Social Work); 1907, studied in New York City. CAREER: Taught for two years in a district school in her own community; 1887, private duty nurse to New York City Mayor Abram S. Hewitt; 1887, superintendent of nurses, Sandhills Emergency Center, Jacksonville, Florida; 1888, visiting nurse in mining camp, Copper Queen Mining Co., Brisbee, Arizona; 1888-1890, in private practice; 1891-1896, assistant superintendent (some sources say superintendent) of nurses, University Hospital School of Nursing, Philadelphia; 1897-1900, in private practice; 1900-1902, director of the Girls House of Refuge, Randall's Island, New York; 1902-1907, director, Bellevue Hospital School of Nursing, also superintendent of Mills Training School for male nurses; 1907-1908, cared for her aged mother until she died; 1909-1912, superintendent of the Army Nurse Corps; 1909-1919, chairperson of the National Committee on Red Cross Nursing Services for the American Red Cross; 1909, member of the War Relief Board of the Red Cross; 1908-1911, president of the board of directors, *American Journal of Nursing*; 1909-1912, president of the American Nurses' Association; 1912, resigned from the Army Nurse Corps to devote full time to the Red Cross; 1918, director of the department of nursing of the American Red Cross when that department was created; January 1919, went to France for a last tour of inspection and died there in April.

CONTRIBUTIONS: Jane Delano's greatest contribution was her organization of nursing within the American Red Cross (ARC). She developed a system with the American Nurses' Association (ANA) to secure and evaluate the credentials of nurses to enroll in the ARC and by 1911, 1,300 nurses were enrolled. Under her influence, the Red Cross Nursing Corps became the Army Nurse Reserve.

An important demonstration of the fieldwork of the nurses she recruited into the ARC occurred in the Ohio Valley floods of March 1913. She helped to develop volunteer nurses' aide auxiliary corps for the ARC after expressing considerable opposition to lay nurses in the Red Cross. With Isabel McIsaac (q.v.), she developed the *American Red Cross Textbook on Elementary Hygiene and Home Care of the Sick* (1913).

She engineered a supply of over 21,000 professional nurses for World War I. As of November 15, 1918, there were 21,344 nurses on duty in the Army Nurse Corps. The total number of American graduate nurses who served in World War I was 26,868, of whom 19,877 were enrolled through the ARC. Her work to provide Red Cross nurses for World War I was made more difficult due to rumors that Red Cross nurses in Europe had been raped, had become pregnant, had contracted venereal diseases, and had been mutilated in battle. During the war, she had a much-recorded confrontation with Annie Goodrich (q.v.) concerning creation of an Army School of Nursing, which Delano opposed. True to her commitment to the United States, however, when the school was created, she spent the remainder of her life recruiting students.

In May 1912, she served as a delegate to the Ninth International Red Cross Conference in Washington, D.C., and was on the program as well. In 1912, the Red Cross Town and Country Nursing Service was established; she had a part in its creation, although she was not directly involved. She designed the cap in 1911 and the cape for Red Cross nurses, the latter first worn in 1914. In January 1911, she began writing the Red Cross Department of the *American Journal of Nursing {AJN}*, a practice that continued for some thirty years. Undoubtedly, as president of the board of *AJN*, Delano had something to do with the continuation of that section. At her death, she left money and the royalties from the text to support Delano Red Cross Nurses to serve in remote areas. The first nurse, Stella Fuller, was assigned to Alaska.

Early experiences in nursing prepared Delano for her leadership role in the Red Cross. As a student at Bellevue, she was singled out for her unusual capabilities, and Mrs. William Preston Griffin, president of the training school committee, predicted that of all the nurses in the school, she would render the most distinguished service to humanity. During her work in Florida at the Sandhills Emergency Center (Hospital), she experienced the yellow fever epidemic of 1888. She was referred to as the Florence Nightingale of America for her memorable work there. Legend has it that she suggested the use of protective screens, although the role of the insect vector in spreading the disease was not yet understood. She was also a pioneer when she served as nurse for the Copper Queen Mining Company in 1888, called there to care for miners stricken with typhoid fever.

As director of the School of Nursing at Bellevue (1902-1907), she introduced some revolutionary reforms; she insisted that students be referred to as the "nurses" instead of the "girls," instituted dietary changes, made certain that students had time off, and encouraged social activities and cultural opportunities such as attending the opera. While still at Bellevue, in 1903, she discussed with her friend Mary A. Clarke the thought of entering Red Cross work. Both the November 4, 1902, fireworks disaster on Madison Avenue, New York City, and the June

1904 burning of the steamer *General Slocum* in the East River helped to confirm her belief in the need for services for handling emergencies.

In 1910, she was appointed by President William Howard Taft to the position of superintendent of the Army Nurse Corps. She surveyed army hospitals throughout the West and in the Philippines, and she was commissioned by the ARC to visit Japan to study Red Cross conditions there. Also in 1910 the National Committee on Red Cross Nursing Service held its first meeting (on January 20), ratifying the appointment of Delano as chairperson. She set up her Red Cross office in her home while continuing her army work in the State, War, and Navy Building until her resignation from the army in 1912 (her letter of resignation is dated March 11, 1912). On January 2, 1919, she sailed for France for a final tour of inspection of the hospitals where her Red Cross nurses were serving. On February 10, she arrived at Savenay ill with mastoiditis. Although she underwent several operations, she never recovered and died in Base Hospital Number 69 on April 15, 1919. It was reported that her last words were: "My work, my work, I must get back to my work." Her body was temporarily interred in the American military cemetery at Savenay. Seventeen months later, she was buried with military honors in Arlington National Cemetery, and May 7, 1919 was declared a national memorial day for Jane Delano. The Distinguished Service Medal of the United States and Distinguished Service Medal of the American Red Cross were awarded posthumously; the nurses' residence at the Army Medical Center, Washington, D.C., was named for her; a sculpture memorializing her and 296 other Red Cross nurses who died during World War I was placed in the garden of Washington, D.C., headquarters of the Red Cross, unveiled in 1934. In 1982, she was elected to the American Nurses' Association Hall of Fame.

WRITINGS: *American Red Cross Textbook on Elementary Hygiene and Home Care of the Sick*, with Isabel McIsaac (1913); circular about surgical dressings, 1915.

REFERENCES: *American Journal of Nursing* (April 1912), p. 548, and (June 1919), pp. 688-700; American Red Cross, *Jane Delano, Innovator in Nursing* (pamphlet, 1972); *British Journal of Nursing* (May 24, 1919), p. 355; Gladys Bonner Clappison, *Vassar's Rainbow Division* (1918); Mary A. Clarke, *Memories of Jane A. Delano* (1934); Major Joel Andrew Delano, comp., *The Genealogy, History, and Alliances of the American House of Delano, 1621-1899* (1899); *Dictionary of American Biography* V: 218-219; Lavinia L. Dock, Sarah E. Pickett, Clara D. Noyes, Fannie F. Clement, Elizabeth G. Fox, and Anna R. Van Meter, *History of American Red Cross Nursing* (1922); Lyndia Flanagan, *One Strong Voice: The Story of the American Nurses' Association* (1976); Patrick F. Gilbo, *The American Red Cross: The First Century* (1981); Mary E. Gladwin, *The Red Cross and Jane Arminda Delano* (1931); Annie Warburton Goodrich, *The Social and Ethical Significance of Nursing* (1932); *National Cyclopedia of American Biography*, XIX: 131-32; *Notable American Women*, pp. 456-457; *Pacific Coast Journal of Nursing* (May 1919), pp. 266-268; Meta Rutter Pennock, ed., *Makers of Nursing History* (1928); Mary M. Roberts, *American Nursing: History and Interpretation* (1954).

JOELLEN WATSON HAWKINS

DEMING, DOROTHY (June 8, 1893, New Haven, Connecticut--January 22, 1972, Winter Park, Florida). *Public health nurse; author.* Daughter of Clarence Deming and Mary Bryan (Whiting) Deming. EDUCATION: 1914, B.A., Vassar College, Poughkeepsie, New York; c. 1914, post-graduate studies, Yale University, New Haven, Connecticut; 1920, graduated from Presbyterian Hospital School of Nursing, New York City. CAREER: 1920, private duty nursing; 1921, staff nurse, New Haven Visiting Nurse Association, New Haven, Connecticut; 1922-1923, supervisor, Harlem Center and field director, Manhattan branch of the Henry Street Settlement, New York City (also served briefly as acting director of the Henry Street Settlement); c. 1924, director, Holyoke Visiting Nurse Association, Holyoke, Massachusetts; 1927, editor, *Public Health Nursing*, and assistant to the director, National Organization for Public Health Nursing, New York City; 1935-1942, general director, National Organization for Public Health Nursing; 1942-1952, member of the technical staff, American Public Health Association, New York City.
CONTRIBUTIONS: Dorothy Deming's main contributions came through her extensive work with the National Organization for Public Health Nursing (NOPHN). Beginning in 1927 and continuing for the next twenty-five years she served the organization during a most difficult time in its history: that of the Great Depression, World War II, and the immediate postwar era. During her tenure with the organization, its services expanded to all parts of the country, including consultation in orthopedics and industrial nursing. A consultative staff of ten became available for appraisals, studies, and other services upon request of local or state agencies. This was especially significant, as the need for public health nursing services reached a total of 6,000 agencies nationwide. During the same time, town, city, county, and state agencies became involved in public health nursing, and professional consultation was especially helpful for agencies which had to explain their work to non-professional administrators or legislators. As a result of her extensive public health nursing background, with the New Haven Visiting Nurse Association, the Holyoke Visiting Nurse Association, and the Henry Street

Visiting Nurse Association, she was recruited by the American Public Health Association to assist with the preparation of examinations required for the merit systems of personnel management employed by governmental agencies. Social security grants required the establishment of a merit system in the hope of reducing political interference from state or local politicians and to enable official agencies to document the qualifications of the members of their staffs. Eventually, forty states utilized the examinations developed through this program.

In addition to her work for the NOPHN, Dorothy Deming was also a well-known author. She wrote a series of "Penny Marsh" books for teenage readers, hoping that her books would convince high school girls that a college and nursing career would enable them to enter a worthwhile profession which would not only be self-satisfying but benefit society. She completed most of the work required for a Ph.D. from Yale University, but she did not finish her dissertation, which was eventually published as part of the Connecticut tercentenary celebration of 1955 (*The Settlement of Connecticut Towns*). She also wrote a book on practical nursing based on an extensive study of the field, which demonstrated her personal belief that the nursing profession had to re-evaluate its relationship with practical nurses who also were involved in the delivery of health-care services. Prior to her book, *The Practical Nurse: A Comprehensive Study* (1947), little had been written on the subject.

WRITINGS: *Penny Marsh, Public Health Nurse* (1938); *Penny Marsh, Supervisor of Public Health Nurses* (1939); *Penny Marsh Finds Adventure in Public Health Nursing* (1940); *Ginger Lee, War Nurse* (1942); *The Practical Nurse: A Comprehensive Study* (1947); *The Settlement of Connecticut Towns* (1955); many articles in professional journals.

REFERENCES: *Trained Nurse and Hospital Review* (1941), p. 372; *Current Biography* (1943), pp. 167-168; Ella E. McNeil, *A History of the Public Health Nursing Section, American Public Health Association, 1922-1972* (1972), pp. 8, 10; *National League of Nursing Education Biographical Sketches* (n.d.); Mary M. Roberts, *American Nursing: History and Interpretation* (1954); information from the Vassar College alumni office.

ALICE HOWELL FRIEDMAN

DENSFORD, KATHARINE. SEE **DREVES, KATHARINE {DENSFORD}**.

DEUTSCH, NAOMI (November 5, 1890, Brno, Czechoslovakia--November 26, 1983, New Orleans, Louisiana). *Public health nurse.* Daughter of Gotthard Deutsch and Hermine (Bacher) Deutsch, who migrated to the United States in 1891 and settled in Ohio. Never married. EDUCATION: 1908, graduated from Walnut Hills High School, Cincinnati, Ohio; 1912, graduated from Jewish Hospital School of Nursing, Cincinnati; 1916-1917 and 1919-1921, attended Teachers College, Columbia University, New York City, receiving B.S. degree in 1921. CAREER: 1912-1918, public health nurse, Visiting Nurse Association of Cincinnati, and public health nurse, Irene Kauffman Settlement, Pittsburgh, Pennsylvania; 1918-1925, public health nurse and field director, Henry Street Visiting Nurse Service, New York City; October 1925-1933, director, Visiting Nurse Association, San Francisco; fall 1933-1935, lecturer and then assistant professor of public health nursing, University of California, Berkeley; 1936-1943, director, public health nursing unit, Federal Children's Bureau, Washington, D.C.; March 1, 1943-1945, principal nursing consultant, Pan American Sanitary Bureau, Panama; 1945-1946, research associate in nursing education, Teachers College, Columbia University; 1946-1950, instructor in nursing education, Teachers College, Columbia University.

CONTRIBUTIONS: Naomi Deutsch was a leader in the organization of public health nursing and responsible for organizing and directing the public health nursing unit of the Federal Children's Bureau, Washington, D.C. After her first positions in Cincinnati and at a settlement house in Pittsburgh, she worked with Lillian Wald (q.v.) at Henry Street Settlement in New York City. After working at Henry Street for seven years (1918-1925) and after earning her bachelor's degree (1921), Deutsch was invited to organize and direct the Visiting Nurse Association (VNA) of San Francisco. She directed the association from 1925 to 1933 and during those years also taught a class in public health nursing. It was a natural transition for her to be appointed instructor and then assistant professor of public health nursing at Berkeley and to continue as a consultant to the VNA. Before leaving California to accept a federal position with the Children's Bureau, she was honored by the California League of Nursing Education and the California State Nurses' Association.

Since Lillian Wald was instrumental in the creation of the Children's Bureau, it is likely that she had a role in the selection of Deutsch to serve as director of its public health nursing unit. Funding of increased activities of the bureau was made possible through the Social Security Act of 1935, and as a result of this support the unit was established in 1936, with Deutsch as its first director. During World War II, she represented the Children's Bureau on the Nursing Council on National Defense. In 1943 she resigned from the Children's Bureau to take a position with the Pan American Sanitary Bureau. She was headquartered in Panama where she worked with Dr. John R. Murdock in the development of health programs in the Caribbean and Central America. After her retirement from the Pan American Sanitary Bureau, she returned to the United States and settled in New York City, where she taught at Teachers College until 1951 or 1952. In the 1960s she moved to New Orleans to live with her sister. She was involved in volunteer activities with civic organizations, notably the League of Women Voters, and with Planned Parenthood. She continued to be interested in the evolution and development of public health nursing until the end of her life.

Deutsch's activities were not limited to her professional positions. While in California, she served as president of the California State Organization for Public Health Nursing (1933-1935). She was also a member of the board of directors of the California State Nurses' Association. In the 1940s, she served as chairperson of the joint committee on inter-American nursing of the American Nurses' Association, the National League of Nursing Education, and the National Organization for Public Health Nursing. She was an active member of the latter two groups, serving on the board of directors, and she was a member of the governing council of the American Public Health Association, the American Association of Social Workers, and the National Council of Social Work. While in California, she served as president of the California State Conference of Social Work.

WRITINGS: Numerous articles in professional journals.

REFERENCES: *American Journal of Nursing* (January 1941), p. 94, (August 1941), p. 934, and (April 1943), p. 402; Max Binheim, ed., *Women of the West* (1928 ed.); M. Louise Fitzpatrick, *The National Organization for Public Health Nursing, 1912-1952* (1975); Durwood Howes, ed., *American Women, 1935-1940: A Composite Biographical Dictionary* (1941), I: 228; information provided by L. Edward Lashman, nephew of Naomi Deutsch; unpublished materials, Nursing Archives, Mugar Memorial Library, Boston University; *Pacific Coast Nursing Journal* (September 1934), p. 487 and (January 1936), pp. 34-35; Mary M. Roberts, *American Nursing: History and Interpretation* (1954); officer's record, November 28, 1945 and supplemental page (last entry 1950), in Teachers College, Columbia University, New York City; unpublished materials, records of the Visiting Nurse Association of San Francisco.

JOELLEN WATSON HAWKINS

DEWITT KATHARINE (June 11, 1867, Troy, New York--December 3, 1963, Poughkeepsie, New York). *Editor; leader in private duty nursing.* Daughter of Rev. Abner DeWitt, a Presbyterian minister, and Mary Eliza (Hastings) DeWitt. Never married. EDUCATION: Attended Troy Seminary, Troy, New York; 1887, graduate of Mt. Holyoke Seminary, South Hadley, Massachusetts; 1891, graduated from Illinois Training School for Nurses, Chicago; post-graduate studies in obstetrics, Illinois Training School. CAREER: 1887-1888, schoolteacher; 1891-1907, private duty nursing in Illinois, Massachusetts, North Carolina, Ohio, and other states; 1907-1920, assistant editor, 1920-1921, acting editor, 1921-1922, co-editor, and 1922-December 31, 1932, managing editor, *American Journal of Nursing*.

CONTRIBUTIONS: Katharine DeWitt made two major contributions to the nursing profession. Her first was to provide much-needed leadership in the field of private duty nursing, helping to raise it from a domestic role to the practice of a profession. Although many of the early training schools established registries for their alumnae, as did DeWitt's alma mater, they often had little control over what duties were expected of their graduates in addition to providing nursing care for patients. Often, the private duty nurse was expected to cook, wash dishes, clean the house, and do the laundry. DeWitt helped private duty nurses to see their roles as professionals through her prolific writing on the subject and through her activities in professional organizations.

A teacher by nature, DeWitt as a student demonstrated her abilities by showing the famous obstetrician Dr. Joseph B. DeLee, then an intern, how to ascultate the fetus. While working primarily with Dr. DeLee in the early 1900s, she taught private duty nursing to the senior class at the Illinois Training School for Nurses. DeWitt had followed in her mother's footsteps by graduating from Mt. Holyoke Seminary, but her teaching career took another direction. Perhaps she was influenced to study nursing by the experiences she had when as a senior she assisted in the Mt. Holyoke dispensary.

She believed that the nurse must teach hygiene and preventive medicine, and at the first session ever held on private duty nursing (at the 1910 meeting of the Nurses' Associated Alumnae, later to become the American Nurses' Association), she served as chairperson and stressed the role of the private duty nurse in the prevention of disease and in the improvement of personal hygiene of the patient. Since the vast majority of graduates were working as private duty nurses, Sophia Palmer (q.v.), editor of the *American Journal of Nursing*, recognized that the *Journal* had to include articles and editorials related to the problems of the private duty nurse, and she asked DeWitt to serve as an assistant editor. For a number of years, DeWitt wrote articles and editorials about private duty nursing and encouraged other nurses engaged in the same work to write about the nursing care of their patients. In 1913, she published *Private Duty Nursing*, revising it for a second edition in 1917.

Her editorial position at the *Journal* enabled DeWitt to make her second major contribution to the profession: communicating what nurses do through editorials and articles. Interestingly, DeWitt had contributed to the first issue of the *American Journal of Nursing* (October 1900) an article on "Specialties in Nursing," and before her formal appointment as assistant editor had assisted Sophia Palmer with her correspondence when Palmer visited Chicago. Since the *Journal*'s editorial offices for the first twelve years of its existence were in Palmer's home in Rochester, New York, DeWitt had to move to Rochester to join the *Journal*'s editorial staff, which for a number of years consisted of Palmer and DeWitt. DeWitt edited the private duty section, as well as assuming other editorial responsibilities. Since the editorial staff was so small, she and Palmer had to participate in every phase of the publication process, including writing articles and editorials, editing the various sections of the *Journal*, and proofreading. When the Red Cross Nursing Department was established in 1907, DeWitt was its editor, and as a result in 1918 she was called upon to aid the National Committee on Red Cross Nursing Service in a nationwide publicity campaign to recruit nurses for military service.

When Palmer died suddenly, DeWitt assumed the editorship of the *Journal* for more than a year, until Mary Roberts (q.v.) joined her. When Roberts became editor in 1923 and was installed in the new offices in New York City, Katharine remained in Rochester, New York, where she served as managing editor until the two offices were combined in 1929. As managing editor, she assumed responsibility for the business operations of the *Journal*.

During her busy years assisting Palmer, DeWitt also spent countless hours in service to professional organizations. Beginning early in her career when she was a private duty nurse, she became an active member of her alumnae association and served as its president. Her literary talents were already apparent in the reports she produced for the association, reports often written in a closet after her patient had been settled for the night. As secretary of the Associated Alumnae for eight years, she helped to facilitate establishment of its national headquarters, its reorganization during the years from 1916 to 1922, the great convention in 1916, establishment of an office of interstate secretary in 1917, and the publicity campaign during World War I. She also played a role in the creation of the American Nurses' Memorial in 1921 and the establishment of the Isabel McIsaac (q.v.) Loan Fund in 1917. For both that fund and the Robb Memorial Fund, she served as secretary, continuing well past her retirement in the case of the Robb Memorial Fund.

After her retirement from the *Journal* in 1932, she went abroad for a year and then established her home in Poughkeepsie, New York. On the occasion of her retirement, the New York State Nurses' Association paid tribute to her at its thirty-first meeting, held October 4, 1932, at Lake Placid. The association presented her with an inscription of over 4,000 names of nurses who subscribed to the *Journal*. In the many years left to her, she continued to write articles for the *Journal* and other professional magazines and to devote time to her church and to caring for the needs of others. She also served as acting president of District 12, New York State Nurses' Association, on its board of directors, and on committees, and as a board member of the Poughkeepsie Visiting Nurse Association. In 1954 she was honored by the House of Delegates of the American Nurses' Association with its first "Honorary Recognition."

WRITINGS: *Private Duty Nursing* (1913, 1917); countless articles in professional journals.

REFERENCES: American Journal of Nursing, *The Story of the American Journal of Nursing* (1940); *American Journal of Nursing* (March 1906), p. 348, (November 1931), p. 1147, (December 1932), pp. 1233-1237, and (October 1950), pp. 590-597; Joseph B. DeLee, "Katharine DeWitt--Student Nurse, and Private Duty Nurse," *American Journal of Nursing* (September 1932), pp. 963-966; Lavinia L. Dock, Sarah E. Pickett, Clara D. Noyes, Fannie F. Clement, Elizabeth G. Fox, and Anna R. Van Meter, *History of American Red Cross Nursing* (1922); Helen W. Munson, *The Story of the National League of Nursing Education* (1934); National League of Nursing Education, *Biographical Sketches* (1923); *Nursing Outlook* (January 1964), p. 62; *Poughkeepsie Journal*, December 3, 1963; Mary M. Roberts, "The Private Duty Nurse Who Became 'Recording Angel,'" *American Journal of Nursing* (March 1955), pp. 306-308.

JOELLEN WATSON HAWKINS

DIX, DOROTHEA LYNDE (April 4, 1802, Hamden, Maine--July 17, 1887, Trenton, New Jersey). *Crusader for the mentally ill and imprisoned; superintendent of Civil War nurses.* Daughter of Joseph Dix, itinerant Methodist minister, and Mary (Bigelow) Dix, homemaker and invalid. Never married. EDUCATION: Attended local school in Hamden, Maine; 1814-1816, attended school in Boston; 1819, returned to Boston where she attended school and public lectures, and studied privately and in the libraries of the city. CAREER: 1816, at the age of fourteen, opened a school for small children, Worcester, Massachusetts, and 1816-1819, taught there; 1821-1826, conducted a "dame school" for young girls at her grandmother's estate, the Dix mansion; also taught poor children in the barn, and taught at the Fowler Monitorial School; 1826-1831, ill much of the time, wintering with relatives, spending summers (as well as the winter of 1830-1831) as a governess for William Ellery Channing's family on Narragansett Bay, Portsmouth, Rhode Island, and at St. Croix, Virgin Islands; 1831-1836, ran a combined day and boarding school at Boston which was well known, especially among Unitarians; suffering from a nervous collapse, sailed for Europe on April 22, 1836, and spent eighteen months recuperating at Liverpool, England; autumn of 1837, returned to the United States, spent several years ill and unable to work; 1841-1842, outraged by conditions at the Middlesex House of Correction, East Cambridge, Massachusetts, launched a campaign for improvement and began an eighteen-month survey of every jail, almshouse, and house of correction in the state; 1842-1854, continued her campaign on behalf of the mentally ill in many states, as well as in two Canadian provinces; September 1854-September 1856, travel in Europe, investigating prison and asylum conditions; September 1856-1861, resumed her work on behalf of the insane; 1861-1866, superintendent of Union Army nurses; 1866-1881, continued to expose prison and asylum conditions, raised funds for orphans' homes, disaster victims, public drinking fountains in Boston, and so forth; 1881-1885, retirement at the Trenton State Hospital, New Jersey; buried in Mt. Auburn Cemetery, Cambridge, Massachusetts.

CONTRIBUTIONS: Dorothea Dix's greatest contribution was her tireless work on behalf of the mentally ill and the imprisoned. Her influence and work, however, extended far beyond the places she personally visited; her work inspired the creation of hospitals as far away as Japan, and she is acknowledged as one of the most important impetus for reform in the treatment of the mentally ill. Her work began on March 28, 1841, when she was asked to teach Sunday school at the Middlesex House of Correction, and she found among the drunks and prisoners some insane women forced to endure inhuman conditions. Seeking the help of reformers Samuel Gridley Howe, Horace Mann, Charles Sumner, Rev. Robert C. Waterton, and Dr. William Ellery Channing, she succeeded in securing better quarters for the women. In that year, 1841, she launched a survey of every jail, almshouse, and house of correction in Massachusetts, completing her work by the end of December 1842. In January 1843, Dr. Howe presented the report to the legislature, resulting in increased support for the newly opened asylum at Worcester.

Having succeeded in Massachusetts, Dix turned her attention to neighboring states. In state after state, her reports served to direct public attention to the need for state mental hospitals, with her first success being Trenton State Hospital, New Jersey, the first hospital built with public funds as a direct result of her work. By the spring of 1848, she had travelled over 60,000 miles and visited over 9,000 insane, epileptic, and retarded persons in prisons across the country. When her work began, there were 13 mental hospitals in the United States; by 1880 there were 123. She had a direct role in founding or enlarging 32 state mental hospitals here and abroad and in establishing St. Elizabeth's Hospital, the federal hospital for the insane in Washington, D.C. (then known as the Hospital for the Insane of the Army and Navy). She was the inspiring force for numerous other hospitals. By 1870, six hospitals had honored her by hanging her portrait in a prominent location, and Dixmont Hospital, in Pennsylvania, was named for her.

In 1848, she began a crusade on behalf of a proposal which if implemented would have raised a tremendous amount of money to provide adequate care of the insane. Her proposal would have established a public land trust, known as the five-million-acre bill (later raised to 12,225,000 acres), to be sold on behalf of the indigent insane. After she lobbied for six years, Congress finally passed the bill in 1854, but President Franklin Pierce vetoed it, undoubtedly breaking her heart in the process. Almost immediately after the veto, she took ill and spent much of the next seven years in semi-retirement, trying to recuperate.

In 1861, she was appointed superintendent of U.S. Army nurses, but the overwhelming nature of the task made her seem disorganized and, to some, inept. She believed that nurses should be "plain looking women," and she refused to accept women who were over the age of thirty, as well as nuns and members of other religious sisterhoods. In spite of her peculiar beliefs which prevented many women from serving as Civil War nurses, her contributions during the Civil War were significant. She helped to set up and staff infirmaries in the Washington, D.C., area, and she performed valuable service, especially on behalf of the sick and wounded. She sent instructions to volunteer sewing societies, helped to stockpile medical supplies, issued a call for canned fruit to prevent scurvy, and engaged in numerous activities that seemed to direct her attention in too many directions. In October 1863, the secretary of war issued an order authorizing the surgeon-general to appoint nurses and stating that nurses were to be subordinate to medical officers. This undermined her authority and indicated the controversy that plagued her tenure in the position. In January 1867, General William Tecumseh Sherman presented her with a stand of flags made especially for her, as recognition of her important service during the Civil War.

Her contributions would not be complete without acknowledging her reputation as a teacher and as a writer. Her book, *Conversations on*

Common Things, an elementary science text first published in 1824, passed through sixty editions by 1869. She had great personal sympathy for women's rights, peace, temperance, and public education, but she was not active in these causes, choosing to devote her life to improving conditions among the mentally ill. Upon her death, Dr. Charles H. Nichols of Bloomingdale Asylum, New York City, wrote: "Thus has died and been laid to rest, in the most quiet, unostentatious way, the most useful and distinguished woman America has yet produced." On July 4, 1899, Dorothea Dix Park in her birthplace, Hamden, Maine, was dedicated to her memory. The U.S. Postal Service issued a one-cent stamp in her honor, and in 1976 she was elected to the American Nurses' Association Hall of Fame.

WRITINGS: *Conversations on Common Things* (1824); *Hymns for Children* (1825); *Evening Hours* (1825); *Meditations for Private Hours* (1828); *Garland of Flora* (1829); *American Moral Tales for Young Persons* (1832); *Remarks on Prisons and Prison Discipline in the U.S.* (1845); *Letter to Convicts in the Western State Penitentiary of Pennsylvania* (1848).

REFERENCES: *American Journal of Nursing* (December 1949), p. 743; Albert Deutsch, *The Mentally Ill in America* (2d ed., 1949); Phebe A. Hanaford, *Daughter of America* (1883); Mary A. Gardner Holland, *Our Army Nurses* (1897); *Journal of Education* (March 28, 1901), p. 53; Joan Marlow, *The Great Women* (1979); Helen E. Marshall, *Dorothea Dix* (1937); *National Cyclopedia of American Biography*, III: 438-439; *Notable American Women*, pp. 486-89; Meta Rutter Pennock, ed., *Makers of Nursing History* (1928); Francis Tiffany, *Life of Dorothea Dix* (1890); Dorothy Clarke Wilson, *Stranger and Traveler* (1975).

JOELLEN WATSON HAWKINS

DOCK, LAVINIA LLOYD (February 26, 1858, Harrisburg, Pennsylvania--April 17, 1956, Chambersburg, Pennsylvania). *Nurse-educator; author.* Daughter of Gilliard Dock and Lavinia Lloyd (Bombaugh) Dock, landowners through inheritance. Never married. EDUCATION: 1884-1886, attended Bellevue Hospital Training School for Nurses, New York City, graduating in 1886. CAREER: Visiting nurse with the Women's Mission of the New York City Mission and Tract Society; visiting nurse for a ladies' charitable society, Norwich, Connecticut; 1888, head nurse in a ward under the direction of Jane Delano (q.v.), a Bellevue classmate, during the yellow fever epidemic in Jacksonville, Florida; 1889, assisted during the Johnstown, Pennsylvania, flood; 1889, night supervisor at Bellevue Hospital; 1890-1893, assistant superintendent of nurses at the newly constructed Johns Hopkins Hospital, Baltimore, Maryland; 1893-1895, superintendent of the Illinois Training School, Cook County Hospital, Chicago; 1896-1915, resided at the Henry Street Settlement house, New York City, providing services to poor immigrants; 1915-1922, worked for women's rights and continued as foreign department editor of the *American Journal of Nursing*; 1922, moved to a country home outside Fayetteville, Pennsylvania, where she lived with her four sisters; died at the age of ninety-eight not long after breaking her hip in a fall.

CONTRIBUTIONS: Lavinia Dock played major roles in the early development of the American Nurses' Association, as well as being an author and historian and an advocate of social welfare and women's rights legislation. Her work as an organizer in the nursing profession began in 1893 when she became secretary of the American Society of Superintendents of Training Schools for Nurses (later the American Nurses' Association). She was involved in the *American Journal of Nursing* as a contributor to the first issue, for which she wrote a classic article entitled "What We May Expect from the Law." She was a proponent of registration for nurses and became one of the first registered nurses in New York State. For over twenty years she was editor of the foreign department of the *American Journal of Nursing*. As a pacifist, she allowed no mention of World War I in the articles published under that department. That her interests were global was also demonstrated in her involvement with the International Council of Nurses (ICN), as a founder, as author of the preamble to its constitution, and as secretary from 1899 to 1922. She was so convinced of the important work being done by the ICN that she donated the royalties from the third and fourth volumes of *A History of Nursing* to the organization. In 1922, she was honored by the ICN, when she was presented with a scroll in recognition of her contributions to that organization. Twenty-five years later, at the age of eighty-nine, she was a guest of honor at the Atlantic City convention of the ICN (1947).

She was a prolific author. Her best-known books are the series on the history of nursing co-authored with M. Adelaide Nutting (q.v.) and a short version co-authored with Isabel Stewart (q.v.). However, her first book, *Materia Medica for Nurses*, was very likely the most helpful to practicing nurses. She was proud of the project and wrote that she had conceived the idea and carried it through to completion without collaboration. Since her publisher doubted that the book could be a financial success and apparently would not publish it without subsidy, her father provided money for the initial printing. It sold upwards of 100,000 copies, however, and it made history as the first pharmacology book for nurses. It included many "recipes" for disguising the unpleasant taste of medications being prescribed at the time. In 1911, she published *Hygiene and Morality*, a brave act since at that time venereal diseases were not discussed at all, even to the extent that many physicians did not inform nurses that their patients were infected with venereal diseases.

Although she held important positions as an educator and training school superintendent during her first ten years in nursing, she faced her biggest challenges as a member of the staff at the Henry Street Settlement (1896-1915). In order to communicate with her patients, largely the immigrant poor, she studied languages and apparently became fluent enough to be able to understand not only their immediate need but the reasons for their immediate needs. Largely as a result of her daily contact with the immigrant poor, she began to develop, clarify, and articulate her beliefs about war, politics, and poverty. She became involved in larger social issues and began to move to the left in her political beliefs. She saw the relationship between the broad issues facing women and those of the nursing profession, believing that unless women had the vote, legislators would be unwilling to listen to the demands of a profession which consisted almost exclusively of women. As a result, she became a strong supporter of women's suffrage and in the process went far beyond the more conservative beliefs of many American women of the time. Her militant support of women's rights at times created a rift between her and her nursing colleagues, as well as her colleagues in social welfare work. That can be seen from the fact that after almost twenty years at Henry Street, she left in 1915 when her association with the National Woman's party caused a rift between her and other members of the staff.

In addition to her nursing practice, her organizational work, her publications, and her work for women's rights, she was a better-than-average pianist and artist. She might be described as a visionary and as a Renaissance woman.

WRITINGS: *Materia Medica for Nurses* (1890); *Short Papers on Nursing Subjects* (1900); *Hygiene and Morality* (1911); *A History of Nursing* (in four volumes, 1907, 1912, 1935), vols. I and II co-authored with M. Adelaide Nutting; *The History of American Red Cross Nursing*, with others, (1922); *A Short History of Nursing*, with Isabel M. Stewart (1938); countless articles in various journals.

REFERENCES: *American Journal of Nursing* (February 1922), p. 349, (May 1923), pp. 660-661, (February 1959), p. 195, and (June 1956), p. 712; *British Journal of Nursing* (April 1, 1922), p. 197, and (January 1926), p. 6; Teresa E. Christy, "Portrait of a Leader: Lavinia Lloyd Dock," *Nursing Outlook* (June 1969), pp. 72-75; *Dictionary of American Biography*, supp. 6, pp. 166-167; Janet Wilson James, *A Lavinia Dock Reader* (1985); *National League for Nursing Education Calendar* (1922);

Notable American Women, IV; *New York Times*, April 18, 1956; *Nursing Outlook* (May 1956), pp. 298-299, and (January 1977), pp. 22-26; Mary M. Roberts, "Lavinia Lloyd Dock," *American Journal of Nursing* (June 1956), p. 727, and "Lavinia Lloyd Dock-Nurse, Feminist, Internationalist," *American Journal of Nursing* (February 1956), pp. 176-179.

LORETTA P. HIGGINS

DOLAN, MARGARET {BAGGETT} (March 17, 1914, Livingston, North Carolina--February 27, 1974, Chapel Hill, North Carolina). *Public health nurse; educator.* Daughter of John Robert Baggett and Allene (Keeter) Baggett. Married Charles E. Dolan, June 3, 1941. EDUCATION: 1932, A.A., Anderson College, Anderson, South Carolina; 1935, graduated from Georgetown University School of Nursing, Washington, D.C.; 1944, B.S., University of North Carolina, Chapel Hill; 1953, M.A., Teachers College, Columbia University, New York City. CAREER: 1935-1936, staff nurse, Instructive Visiting Nurse Society, Washington, D.C.; 1936-1941, epidemiology nurse, U.S. Public Health Service; 1941-1943, nursing supervisor, Greensboro (North Carolina) City Health Department; 1945-1946, tuberulosis nurse-consultant, U.S. Public Health Service; 1947-1950, supervisor and special consultant, Baltimore County Health Department, Towson, Maryland; 1950-1959, associate professor, University of North Carolina, Chapel Hill; 1959-1973, professor and head of the department of public health, University of North Carolina; 1973, professor emeritus.

CONTRIBUTIONS: Margaret Dolan was recognized as a national leader in public health nursing. She served as president (1962-1964) of the American Nurses' Association (ANA), the National Health Council (1969-1971), and the American Public Health Association (1972-1973). She was only the second nurse in the history of the American Public Health Association to be elected as its president. She also was president of the American Journal of Nursing Company (1960-1961). During her tenure as ANA president, the early stages of the debate on the role of nursing in the delivery of primary care became a major concern of the organization. The ANA house of delegates passed a resolution to the effect that the primary role of the professional nurse was as a clinical practitioner, and Dolan upheld this declaration in her capacity as the association's official representative. She was concerned that if the nurse were considered as an adjunct to the physician, as was the case for many years, the nurse would never achieve anything resembling professional respect. She urged the creation of a strong and united ANA which would serve the individual nurse and her patient. She stressed the need for nursing to seek its special realm of knowledge and authority, which builds upon a foundation of knowledge and skill. She believed that the profession had to progress in the area of nursing education and to bring it more into line with the changing world, which had begun to expect every professional to have a college education, rather than to be a graduate of a hospital nursing school which issued diplomas rather than college degrees.

She reminded her colleagues that education alone, important as it was, would not be sufficient to solve the problems of the profession, which were due to economic conditions as well as the need for a sense of professionalism. She felt that without a drastic change in the compensation provided to nurses, the profession would be unable to recruit the best-qualified students and fill the need for experienced and educated nurses. That would be more of a problem as time passed because qualified females would be able to enter other professions and fields due to advances in the women's rights movement and the successful drive for civil rights for all Americans. When large numbers of women could enter medicine, law, business, and other professions, the attraction of nursing would decrease, making it even more necessary to increase the compensation provided to trained nurses. She urged nurses to seek the support of other health groups, as well as civic, business, and professional groups which could work together to improve conditions in the profession.

Dolan promoted health legislation at both the state and national levels. She was frequently called upon as a consultant on public health for the U.S. Department of Health, Education, and Welfare, as well as for the Department of the Army. For more than twenty years, she appeared before congressional committees on behalf of the ANA, and represented the needs and interests of the profession. She also served on a number of government advisory boards, including the President's Committee on Health Resources (1962-1968) and the President's Committee on the Status of Women (1960-1964). She was a member of the Social Security Administration's health insurance benefits advisory council (1968-1972) and on the board of directors of the National Assembly on Social Policy and Development (1968-1972). She was a fellow of the American Public Health Association and served as a member of its governing council and executive board (1968-1972). She was an active member of the North Carolina branch of the tuberculosis association, and also served on committees of the national organization as well.

She received a number of honors in recognition of her service to the profession and to humanity. In 1964, she was given honorary membership in the ANA. In 1968, the ANA gave her its Pearl McIver (q.v.) Public Health Award. In 1970, she received from Duke University an honorary doctor of laws degree. In 1973, the year in which she

retired, she received an honorary doctor of science degree from the University of Illinois. In 1984, she was inducted into the ANA Hall of Fame.
WRITINGS: Many articles in nursing and public health journals.
REFERENCES: Lyndia Flanagan, *One Strong Voice: The Story of the American Nurses' Association* (1976), pp. 8, 299, 556-565; *Who Was Who in America*, 1974-1976 (1978).

ALICE HOWELL FRIEDMAN

DOMITILLA, SISTER MARY, O.S.F. (born Lillian DuRocher, September 11, 1889, Monroe, Michigan--February 17, 1955, Saint Marys Hospital, Rochester, Minnesota). Daughter of Secomb DuRocher and Josephine (LaFountain) DuRocher, farmers. *Hospital administrator; educator.* Never married. EDUCATION: 1915-1918, attended St. Marys School of Nursing, Rochester, Minnesota, graduating in 1918; 1918-1920, attended Teachers College, Columbia University, New York City, graduating in 1920 with a bachelor of science degree and a diploma in teaching and supervision; 1934-1935, post-graduate study, Teachers College, receiving a master of arts degree in 1935. CAREER: 1906-1909, taught school; 1910, entered convent of the Sisters of St. Francis, Rochester, Minnesota; 1912-1915, teacher, Sacred Heart High School, Waseca, Minnesota; 1920-1931, educational director and science instructor, St. Marys Hospital School of Nursing, Rochester, Minnesota; 1931-1934, director of St. Marys Hospital School of Nursing; 1935-1937, director of the division of nursing education, College of St. Teresa, Winona, Minnesota; 1937-1939, assistant superintendent, St. Marys Hospital; 1939-1949, administrator, St. Marys Hospital; 1950, appointed hospital consultant for the four institutions administered by the Sisters of Saint Francis; religious superior of the sisters at St. Marys Hospital.
CONTRIBUTIONS: Sister Mary Domitilla had a long and distinguished career in nursing, and although her professional life was spent in Minnesota, her influence was nationwide. In Minnesota, she assumed control of St. Marys Hospital in 1939, and under her leadership it was transformed from a small and informal organization to one that by 1941 had expanded to 850 beds and sixty bassinets. Although the hospital grew in size and services it provided, she insisted that it never lose its personal touch, for which many patients chose the Catholic hospital of the day. She instituted new business and accounting systems, centralized the dietary department (and in the process reduced the domestic duties expected of nurses), and began a home nursing service and a psychiatric department. In 1941, she founded the hospital paper, the *News Bulletin.*

Although administrative duties took most of her time, she maintained a keen interest in the nursing school, which supported a number of different educational programs ranging in length from one to four years. She improved the curriculum and strengthened the faculty of the nursing school, and she established post-graduate programs in operating room management and internships for graduate dietitians. Sister Mary had many interests outside nursing, especially enjoying the outdoors, books, art, and music. Because she believed in the importance of leisure activities, she encouraged students to devote their spare time to recreational activities. To that end, when she helped to plan a new nurses' residence in 1927, she included an auditorium, recreation rooms, and a swimming pool.

She served as president of the Minnesota State Board of Nurse Examiners and as a member of that board for seventeen years (1923-1940). She served on many committees of various national nursing organizations. From 1922 to 1932, she was on the committee on education of the National League of Nursing Education, from 1923 to 1930, she was a member of the committee on ethical standards, and from 1938 to 1941, she served on the committee on nursing tests. From 1928 to 1934, she served on the committee for grading nursing schools, the only religious involved in that important study. She also served on the council on education of the Catholic Hospital Association, the committee for revision of the curriculum in schools of nursing, the committee on state board problems, and the committee on graduate curricula of the Association of Collegiate Schools of Nursing. She was a clear and forceful speaker, and as a result her participation was sought at numerous national meetings and conferences. She also was the author of two outlines, one in pharmacology and the other in chemistry, which were used as teaching aids in nursing schools. She was a member of the editorial board of *Hospital Progress*. She was one of the first two Catholic sisters to be admitted to the department of nursing and health at Columbia University Teachers College, and when the program at Catholic University was being planned, she was asked for her ideas about what direction the school should take. At that time, there was a great deal of discussion about whether the school should offer programs which would be restricted to Catholic sisters, but Sister Mary strongly opposed that idea, and apparently her ideas were taken seriously; the program at Catholic University was opened to laypersons as well as members of religious orders. In 1940, she received the distinguished service cross of the Catholic Hospital Association of the United States and Canada, in recognition of the achievement of noteworthy results in Catholic hospital work.

WRITINGS: "Improved Method of Applying Hot Dressings," *American Journal of Nursing* (October 1923), pp. 12-13; "State Board Examinations: Objective Type and Essay Type Compared," *American Journal of Nursing* (June 1934), pp. 587-591; *Outline of Chemistry* (1931); *Outline of Materia Medica and Special Therapeutics* (1933).
REFERENCES: *American Journal of Nursing* (April 1934), pp. 361-362, (June 1939), p. 690, and (December 1940), p. 1413; Sister Mary Brigh, O.S.F., "Sister M. Domitilla, O.S.F.," *The Minnesota Registered Nurse* (June 1950), pp. 83-84; Sister M. Olivia Gowan, "Influence of Graduate Nurses in the Formative Years of a University School of Nursing," *Nursing Research* (Summer 1967), pp. 261-266; Nursing Archives (Boston University) *News Bulletin* (March 1955), pp. 1-3; M. Adelaide Nutting Collection, Teachers College, Columbia University, New York City (microfiche number 2439); materials from the archives of St. Marys Hospital, Rochester, Minnesota.

LORETTA P. HIGGINS

DRAPER, EDITH AUGUSTA (?--April 5, 1941, Oakville, Canada). *Nurse-administrator.* Never married. EDUCATION: 1884, graduated from Bellevue Hospital School of Nursing, New York City. CAREER: c. 1884-1886, private duty nursing, Rome, Italy; 1886-1888, 1888-1893, assistant superintendent of nurses, St. Luke's Hospital, Chicago; assistant and then superintendent of nurses, Illinois Training School, Chicago; 1893, superintendent of nurses, Royal Victoria Hospital, Montreal, Quebec, Canada; 1896, superintendent of nurses, Brookbend Hospital, Sidney, British Columbia; superintendent of nurses, Otisville Hospital, Otisville, New York.
CONTRIBUTIONS: Edith Draper was one of the early graduates who set a high standard for the nursing profession. Not only was she in a position of influence as superintendent of the Illinois Training School, of which Isabel Hampton (q.v.) had been the superintendent as late as 1886, but she was in charge of the nursing service at the Cook County Hospital, one of the largest in the country. She was one of the Bellevue graduates who was present at the organizational meeting of the Society of Superintendents of Training Schools of Nurses, held in New York City. She also was a contributor to the first volume of the *American Journal of Nursing*. Indeed, while superintendent of the Illinois Training School at Cook County Hospital, Chicago, she pointed out the need for the profession to have its own publication. She presented a paper, "The Necessity of an American Nurses' Association," at the first general meeting of American nurses, held in 1893 in Chicago at the International

Congress of Charities, Correction, and Philanthropy. Her paper was included in *Nursing of the Sick* (1893), a germinal publication in the professionalization of American nursing. This book, edited by Lillian A. Hampton and others, was the re-issue of part III of the proceedings of the conference. She spoke of the need for an association to provide professional and financial assistance, promote lectures, and encourage the creation of publications which would serve to provide information on nursing needs and to allow for the exchange of ideas among nurses in various cities and states. At that meeting, she expressed the theme of each of the speakers when she declared, "To advance we must unite!" a much-quoted statement. She was one of twelve members of the Committee for the Organization of a National Association of Nurses, which presented a specific proposal, including a constitution, at the fourth annual convention of the society in 1897.
WRITINGS: "The Value of General Reading for Private Duty Nursing," *American Journal of Nursing* (1900), p. 205; "Isabel Hampton Robb," *American Journal of Nursing* (1912), p. 126.
REFERENCES: *American Journal of Nursing* (1941), p. 632; Lyndia Flanagan, *One Strong Voice: The Story of the American Nurses' Association* (1976), pp. 4, 28-29, 35, 293, 642-645; Mary M. Roberts, *American Nursing: History and Interpretation* (1954), p. 41; Grace F. Schryver, *History of the Illinois Training School for Nurses* (1930), pp. 60 and 70; Isabel M. Stewart, *The Education of Nurses* (1943), p. 120.

ALICE HOWELL FRIEDMAN

DREVES, KATHERINE J. {DENSFORD} (December 7, 1890, Crothersville, Indiana--September 29, 1978, St. Paul, Minnesota). *Nurse-educator.* Daughter of Loving Garriott Densford and Mary Belle (Carr) Densford. Married Carl Arminius Dreves, August 8, 1959; no children.
EDUCATION: Attended Oxford College for Women, Oxford, Ohio (one year); 1914, A.B., Miami University, Oxford, Ohio; 1915, M.A., University of Chicago; 1918, graduated from Vassar College Training Camp for Nurses, Poughkeepsie, New York; 1920, graduated from University of Cincinnati (Ohio) College of Nursing; 1937, post-graduate studies, Teachers College, Columbia University, New York City.
CAREER: c. 1910, elementary school manual training teacher in an industrial school (home for delinquents); 1915-1916, high school teacher of Latin and German, Michigan; 1916-1918, high school teacher, Bismarck, North Dakota; 1920-1925, head nurse, Cincinnati General Hospital, then public health nurse, Hamilton County, Ohio; (during those same years, served as supervisor of nurses, Cincinnati Tuberculosis

Sanatorium, and instructor of tuberculosis and public health nursing, University of Cincinnati); 1925-1930, assistant dean and associate director, Cook County School of Nursing (formerly Illinois Training School for Nurses), Chicago; 1930-1959, dean, University of Minnesota School of Nursing, Minneapolis; 1959, retired and named professor emeritus, University of Minnesota School of Nursing.

CONTRIBUTIONS: For twenty-nine years, Katherine Densford was director of the oldest university nursing program in the United States, at the University of Minnesota. Her greatest achievement at Minnesota was to strengthen the nursing program by integrating it into the academic life of the university, thereby providing students a fully integrated academic experience which was unique for the 1930s and 1940s. During her tenure as dean (1930-1959), she was seen as a crusader who sought to transform the nursing student from a health-care provider at the university hospital to a student who was in the process of learning both the theory and practice of nursing care. Densford insisted that the educational needs of schools of nursing no longer be submerged by the needs of the hospital and that the educational needs of the student must be the paramount concern of the faculty and administrators.

In spite of the fact that she took over the program at Minnesota in 1930, the early years of the Great Depression, she was able to foster curriculum reform, attract a qualified faculty, and even see to the construction of a desperately needed nursing school building. Her innovative ideas for the financing of continuing education resulted in the enrollment of many midwestern graduates of hospital training programs, with many of them not only taking advanced courses but eventually earning their bachelor's degree. Densford was a staunch supporter of a master's program which would help prepare nurse-educators; she postponed the development of such a program until 1950, however, when the University of Minnesota had a well-prepared faculty able to serve as graduate-level professors.

Densford was the fourteenth president (1944-1948) of the American Nurses' Association (ANA). She was president during the period in which professional organizations were undergoing reorganization and when the nursing profession took decisive action on economic matters. She fought to open ANA membership to black nurses from the South as well as from the North, and she was an early advocate of national health insurance. During her term as president, the ANA established the professional credentials and personnel service to assist returning veterans in selecting future careers in nursing. Densford urged the expansion of the role of nursing services to meet the health needs of the American people and to protect and promote the welfare of the professional nurse. At various times in her career, she served as the

ANA parliamentarian, and she was a member of the National Association of Parliamentarians.

She served ten years (beginning in 1946) as second vice-president of the International Council of Nurses (ICN). Through that organization, she expressed her belief that nurses must have a genuine concern for service to others, as well as sense of responsibility toward their calling, and she insisted that both of these goals could be demonstrated through continued participation in world affairs. Her activities on behalf of the ICN and other nursing organizations took her around the world as her interest and influence in global health care grew stronger. She was the ICN observer at the 1945 conference on international organization which led to the establishment of the United Nations. In 1958, she served as special representative to the tenth anniversary special commemorative session of the World Health Assembly and the eleventh World Health Organization assembly which was held in Minneapolis.

Densford was president of the Minnesota Nurses' Association (1940-1944) and the Minnesota League for Nursing Education (1933-1935). She was national president of Sigma Theta Tau, the national nursing honor society, from 1936-1938. Known as an "organization woman," she was a member and a leader of a variety of prestigious organizations. In addition to the ones already mentioned, she served on the board of directors of the Illinois State Nurses' Association and the American Journal of Nursing Company and was chairperson of the Minnesota Nursing Council for War Service. She was a member of the Minnesota State Board of Health for six years and of the Governor's Commission on the Status of Women. In her retirement, she served as co-chairperson of the campaign to raise one million dollars for the American Nurses' Foundation.

Over the course of her career, she received a number of awards and honors in recognition of her ability and service. In 1914, she was inducted into Phi Beta Kappa during her senior year at Miami University. In 1945, she received an honorary doctor of science degree from Baylor University, and in 1950 she received a doctor of laws degree from Miami University. In 1984, she was elected to the ANA's Nursing Hall of Fame.

WRITINGS: *Ethics for the Modern Nurse* (co-author with Millard S. Everett, 1946); *Counselling Programs in Schools of Nursing* (co-author, 1946).

REFERENCES: Grace Bonner Clappison, *Vassar's Rainbow Division* (1918), pp. 203-205; Lyndia Flanagan, *One Strong Voice: The Story of the American Nurses' Association* (1976), pp. 491-502; Laurie K. Glass, "An Organization Woman: Katherine Densford Dreves, 1891-1978," newsletter of the American Association for the History of Nursing (Spring 1985), and "Raising a Million Dollars: Katharine Densford Dreves and the American Nurses' Foundation," *Journal of Nursing History* (November 1985), pp. 56-67; James Gray, *Education for Nursing: A History of the University of Minnesota School* (1960); Grace Fay Schryver, *A History of the Illinois Training School for Nurses, 1880-1929* (1930).

ALICE HOWELL FRIEDMAN

DROWN, LUCY LINCOLN (August 4, 1848, Providence, Rhode Island--June 21, 1934, Lakeport, New Hampshire). *Superintendent of nurses.* Daughter of Leonard and Mary (Lincoln) Drown. Never married. EDUCATION: Attended public and private schools in Rhode Island and New Hampshire; completed course, Salem Normal School, Massachusetts; 1884, diploma, Boston City Hospital School of Nursing. CAREER: For twelve years taught in the public schools on New Hampshire and Massachusetts; 1884-1885, assistant superintendent of nurses, Boston City Hospital; 1885-1910, superintendent of nurses, Boston City Hospital.
CONTRIBUTIONS: Lucy Drown served as superintendent of nurses at Boston City Hospital for twenty-five years, and during that time she trained many young women who subsequently became leaders of the nursing profession. Many of her students became superintendents of nursing programs, including Mary Riddle (q.v.), the first president of the Massachusetts Nurses' Association and the first chairman of the Massachusetts Board of Registration in Nursing. Drown was described as a "gentlewoman of the old school, whose stern New England conscience demanded more of herself than of any other . . . whose organization assumed the precision of a geometrical figure, whose leadership was forceful and compelling, whose example pointed the way to industry, loyalty, and righteousness." Lavinia Dock (q.v.) considered her "as a pioneer not only in training school organization and in a more thorough profession instruction, but also in the development of private duty; in school associations, state, and national organization and state licensing laws." Although Drown enrolled at the Boston City Hospital School of Nursing three years after its founding, it has been said that she practically created the school. She succeeded Linda Richards (q.v.) as superintendent of the school when Richards left for a new challenge in Japan. Drown founded one of the first nurses' alumnae associations two years after she graduated from training school. This association was one of the first such organizations to band together to create the Associated Alumnae of the United States and Canada, the first national association of its type. She was a charter member of the American Society of Superintendents of Training Schools for Nurses and served as first

treasurer of that society. She also served as first historian of the Massachusetts State Nurses' Association.

REFERENCES: *American Journal of Nursing* (September 1934), pp. 601-602; *Boston City Hospital Nurses' Alumnae Newsletter* (July 1934); Lavinia Dock, *A History of Nursing* (1912); Lavinia Dock and Isabel Stewart, *Short History of Nursing* (1938); Mary Ellen Doona, "Lucy Lincoln Drown," *Massachusetts Nurse* (June 1, 1985), pp. 6-7; papers of the *American Journal of Nursing*, Sophia F. Palmer Historical Collection, Nursing Archives, Mugar Library, Boston University; Mary Riddle, *Boston City Hospital Training School for Nurses: Historical Sketches* (1928); National League of Nursing Education, *Early Leaders of American Nursing* (1922).

ALICE HOWELL FRIEDMAN

E

ELDREDGE, ADDA (November 27, 1864, Fond du Lac, Wisconsin--October 24, 1955, Oconomowoc, Wisconsin). *Educator; organizer.* Daughter of Charles A. Eldredge, attorney, state senator, and congressman, and Ann Maria (Bishop) Eldredge, teacher. Never married. EDUCATION: Attended private school in Fond du Lac; 1899, graduated from St. Luke's Hospital School of Nursing, Chicago; 1915, completed one-year course in public health nursing at Teachers College, Columbia University, New York City. CAREER: 1899-1907, private duty nurse; 1908-1915, nursing arts instructor, St. Luke's Hospital School of Nursing, Chicago; c. 1916, staff nurse, Association for Improving the Conditions of the Poor, New York City; 1917-1920, interstate secretary, American Nurses' Association; 1920, temporary member (seven months) of the New York State Board of Nurse Examiners; 1921, assisted with a study of private duty nursing under a Rockefeller grant; 1921-1934, director of nursing education for the state of Wisconsin; 1934-1938, executive director of Midwest Placement Bureau, Chicago; 1935-1939, taught courses in nursing education and legislation at the University of Chicago; 1939, taught a course in nursing jurisprudence at the University of Minnesota, Minneapolis.

CONTRIBUTIONS: Adda Eldredge's contributions to nursing were many and varied. From the inspiration she gave individual students in her years of teaching to the far-reaching influence she wielded as president of the American Nurses' Association (ANA), Eldredge was a strong presence in her profession. Her tangible contributions were seen in the improvement in the quality of life for nursing students. She encouraged nursing schools to require a high school diploma of their applicants, and she was an advocate of better housing, shorter hours, better health care, and a more-qualified faculty. As director of nursing education for the state of Wisconsin, she inaugurated a program of inspection, evaluation, and accreditation of nursing schools in that state. As an advocate of registration for nurses, she led the effort in Illinois to pass the Nurse Practice Act, and she toured the state speaking in favor of it.

Throughout her career, she was active in various professional organizations. As interstate secretary for the ANA she travelled throughout the United States speaking to groups of nurses in order to inform them of the important work being done by that organization. She was president of the Illinois State Nurses' Association from 1911 to 1912, and she chaired the legislative committee of that organization. She was first vice-president of the ANA from 1913 to 1918, and served as its president from 1922 to 1926. From 1919 to 1922 and 1926 to 1934, she served as a member of the ANA board of directors. She was an expert on legislative matters that had an impact on nursing education and nursing practice. During her tenure as ANA interstate secretary, she worked with the Committee on Nursing of the Council of National Defense to assist with the student-nurse reserve program. In 1935 she received from the ANA the Walter Burns Saunders Memorial Medal for distinguished service in the cause of nursing. In 1940, she was made an honorary member of Sigma Theta Tau, the international honor society of nursing. In addition, the state of Wisconsin established the Adda Eldredge Scholarship Fund in her honor, and in 1986 she was inducted into the ANA's Nursing Hall of Fame.

WRITINGS: "Quality Nursing," *American Journal of Nursing* (November 1932); also numerous articles in various professional journals.

REFERENCES: *American Journal of Nursing* (July 1921), p. 735 and (December 1955), pp. 1456-1458; *American Nurse* (June 1986), p. 10; Francis V. Brink, "Adda Eldredge," information provided by Signe S. Cooper, R.N.; *National League of Nursing Education Biographical Sketches* (1940); Lyndia Flanagan, *One Strong Voice* (1976).

LORETTA P. HIGGINS

ELLIS, ROSEMARY (July 22, 1919, Berkeley, California--October 10, 1986, Cleveland, Ohio). *Researcher; educator.* Never married. EDUCATION: 1937, graduated from Berkeley High School, Berkeley, California; 1941, A.B. in economics, University of California, Berkeley; 1944, B.S. in nursing, University of California, San Francisco; 1953, M.A. in nursing education, University of Chicago; 1964, Ph.D. in human development, University of Chicago. CAREER: 1944-1945 and 1946-1948, head nurse, University of California Hospital, San Francisco; 1945-1946, member, Army Nurse Corps; 1948-1949, supervisor,

University of California Hospital, and lecturer in medical nursing, University of California School of Nursing, San Francisco; 1949-1952, assistant superintendent of nursing, University of California Hospital, San Francisco; 1953-1959, assistant professor of nursing education, University of Chicago; 1963-1964, research assistant, University of Chicago department of psychology; 1964, staff member, Illinois League for Nursing, Chicago; 1964-1968, associate professor of nursing, and 1968-1986, professor of nursing, Frances Payne Bolton School of Nursing, Case Western Reserve University, Cleveland, Ohio; 1964-1986, associate in nursing, University Hospitals of Cleveland; 1976-1980, administrative officer, research, Frances Payne Bolton School of Nursing; July 1-October 10, 1986, professor emerita of nursing, Frances Payne Bolton School of Nursing.

CONTRIBUTIONS: Rosemary Ellis was one of the most distinguished leaders in nursing research and education that this century has yet produced. Her pioneering work in the development of nursing theory and her research on the sensory disturbances of surgical patients relative to light and noise in intensive care units made her an internationally known scholar. Her work played a major role in the National Academy of Sciences' recognition of nursing as a science, a distinction not yet achieved in other nations. Her research reports, begun in the early 1960s, were landmark pieces which set the standard for research in the profession. A prolific writer as well as researcher, some of her articles are classics in the professional literature.

Ellis was also an outstanding teacher, inspiring both students and colleagues to be future oriented in their investigations and serving as a role model for the development of nursing knowledge through her own practice-based research. Although her academic work was initially in economics, Ellis apparently had a change in her career plans either as an undergraduate or shortly after graduation, for she enrolled almost at once in the nursing program at University of California, San Francisco, graduating cum laude in 1944. After a brief time at her "home hospital," she was commissioned as a second lieutenant in the U.S. Army Nurse Corps in March 1945 and served in the Pacific Theater of Operations, on the U.S.S. *Comfort*, a 700-bed hospital ship with the U.S. Navy. She went to the Philippines, Guam, the Caroline Islands, Okinawa, Japan, and Korea. She was promoted to first lieutenant and left the Corps in May 1946. Returning to the University of California Hospital, her teaching abilities must have gained some recognition, for not only did she hold leadership positions as a head nurse, supervisor, and later as assistant superintendent, but she also was a lecturer for her alma mater. Her sound clinical base, as well as her undergraduate training in economics, contributed to the nature of her later research and to her commitment to practice-based research.

Further education led her to Chicago and to her first full-time faculty position. In 1959, she received the Nellie X. Hawkinson (q.v.) Scholarship, enabling her to undertake doctoral studies. During her doctoral program, she was a research assistant for the department of psychiatry, perhaps another impetus for her distinguished research career. Fortunately for nursing and for the Frances Payne Bolton School of Nursing, her career led her to Cleveland where, for over twenty years, she brought distinction to Case Western Reserve University and to the profession.

Besides the magnitude of her contributions as a researcher, author, and teacher, Ellis served on countless school of nursing and university committees, as well as the University Hospitals of Cleveland committee on clinical research (1970-1976). She was a visiting professor at the University of Iowa in December 1968. In 1971, she served as an advisor on nursing research at Tokyo Women's Medical College and was a visiting professor at the University of Edmonton, Alberta, Canada. Even after a stroke in 1972 left her partially paralyzed, she rehabilitated herself, carrying on a full teaching, research, and guest lecturing schedule. She even used her own experiences to write articles for nursing journals about the care of individuals with handicaps. Through the remaining years of her life, she continued to be a prolific author, a researcher, an outstanding teacher, and a much-sought-after guest lecturer. In 1984, she was invited to lecture in Seoul, South Korea, at a conference attended by nurse-researchers from around the world.

Ellis also gave untiringly to the profession. From 1956 to 1966, she served on the Ohio State Nurses' Association committee on continuing education. She was a special consultant to the division of nursing of the U.S. Public Health Service from 1966 to 1968 and a member of the short-term training grants review committee of the Public Health Service from 1967 to 1969. For the council of baccalaureate and higher degree programs of the National League for Nursing (NLN), she was a member of the committee on health and allied profession relations from 1968 to 1970 and on its program commmittee for 1969 to 1971. She was also an NLN accreditation visitor in 1972. Service to the American Nurses' Association (ANA) included membership on the interim certification board for medical surgical nursing from 1968 to 1970 and also in 1972, the convention program committee in 1969, and the commission on nursing research from 1974 to 1978. Beginning in 1979, she was a member of the editorial board of *Advances in Nursing Science* and a review panel member for *Nursing Research* from 1969 and for *Research in Nursing and Health* from 1980. She held membership in and served many professional organizations, including the National Stroke Association's scientific advisory board, the ANA council of nurse researchers, the American Association for the Advancement of Science, the American Public Health Association, the Nursing Theory Think Tank, the Midwest Nursing Research Society, the American Association for Nursing History, the Institute for Society, Ethics, and Life Sciences, the American Association for the Advancement of the Humanities, the Society on Health and Human Values, and the National Task Force on Nursing Diagnosis.

She received numerous honors. She was inducted into Sigma Theta Tau and Alpha Xi Delta. In 1985 she was selected as a fellow of the American Academy of Nursing. That same year, she received the distinguished alumni award of the University of California School of Nursing, San Francisco. On June 16, 1986, the American Nurses' Foundation presented her with its distinguished contribution to nursing science award, and in 1986 she received a congressional citation for her accomplishments, presented at the Greater Cleveland Nurses' Association. In June 1986, the Frances Payne Bolton School of Nursing established the Rosemary Ellis Scholarship for Ph.D. education in nursing.

When a series of small strokes at last provoked her retirement in 1986, Ellis continued her work even during her last five weeks in the hospital, expecting to teach students in the fall while convalescing. She was characterized as an exemplary patient, reminding her nurses that they were not treating a patient but a person who just happened to be a patient. Memorial services were held at the Amasa Stone Chapel of Case Western Reserve University, and she was buried in Arlington National Cemetery.

WRITINGS: Numerous articles in professional journals, including "Symposium on Theory Development in Nursing: Characteristics of Significant Theories," *Nursing Research* (May-June 1968), pp. 217ff.; "The Practitioner as Theorist," *American Journal of Nursing* (July 1969), pp. 1434ff.; "Values and Vicissitudes of the Scientist Nurse," *Nursing Research* (September-October 1970), pp. 440ff.; "Unusual Sensory and Thought Disturbances after Cardiac Surgery," *American Journal of Nursing* (November 1972), pp. 2021-2025; "After Stroke: Sitting Problems," *American Journal of Nursing* (November 1973), pp. 1898-1899; "Research in the Practice Areas," *Nursing Research* (May-June 1977), pp. 177-182.

REFERENCES: *The American Nurse* (November-December 1986); *Campus News* (June 18, November 5, 1986); *Cleveland Plain Dealer* (October 17, 1986); *News from the American Academy of Nursing* (Fall 1986); *Nursing Alumni* (Frances Payne Bolton School of Nursing, Fall 1986); *The Observer*, October 24, 1986; unpublished papers, Nursing Archives, Mugar Memorial Library, Boston University; unpublished papers, archives of the

Frances Payne Boston School of Nursing, Case Western Reserve University.

JOELLEN WATSON HAWKINS

F

FEDDE, ELIZABETH (December 25, 1850, Feda Flekkefjord, Norway--February 25, 1921, Egersund, Norway). *Lutheran Deaconess; pioneer welfare worker.* Daughter of Andreas Villumsen Feda, farmer and sailor, and Anne Marie (Olsdatter) Feda. Married Ola A. P. Slettebo, 1896, in Norway. EDUCATION: 1873, nursing instruction at the Lutheran Deaconess Motherhouse, Christiania, Oslo, Norway. CAREER: 1875-1877, nurse, Government Hospital, Oslo, Norway; 1878, sent to Tromso, northern Norway, and for four years nursed the sick; 1883-1885, Volunteer Relief Society, New York City and Brooklyn; 1885-1889, training program and hospital under Norwegian Relief Society, Brooklyn; 1887-1889, deaconess home, Minneapolis, Minnesota.
CONTRIBUTIONS: In less than a decade in the United States, Sister Elizabeth Fedde made a significant contribution to the development of training programs for nurses and to the care of immigrant Norwegians, the latter during a time when the heavy flow of immigrants into the United States severely strained the health care facilities of the large cities. Her service to the United States began on December 25, 1882, when her brother-in-law, Gabriel Fedde, asked her to serve as a nurse and social worker for Norwegian immigrants in New York City. On April 17, just nine days after she arrived in the United States, she organized the Volunteer Relief Society for the sick and poor Norwegian immigrants living in New York City and Brooklyn, assisted in her work by two pastors and six laypersons. The outdoor relief program was directed from her three-room headquarters in Brooklyn.

Sister Fedde (in the tradition of the time, her family surname was the name of the place where they lived, Feda, and altered to Fedde) was well prepared for her nursing and social work. When her parents died, she spent a brief time in domestic service but also learned to read and then enrolled in the Deaconess Hospital in Oslo, where she received training in nursing and religion. After nursing medical patients in the Government Hospital, she was sent to Tromso, north of the Arctic Circle, to reorganize a small government hospital. Developing septicemia from doing an autopsy, she spent time recuperating until 1882, when she answered the call of the Norwegian seamen's missionary in Brooklyn, conveyed through her brother-in-law. Mrs. Christian Bors, wife of the Norwegian consul to New York City, promised an annual subscription to support part of her work.

When the Christiana motherhouse, where she had trained, refused her request for a deaconess to assist her, she established a deaconess training program in Brooklyn. The Norwegian deaconess authorities apparently insisted that by accepting the invitation to come to America, she had severed her formal ties with the motherhouse and had ceased to be a Norwegian deaconess. Had the call come to the motherhouse rather than directly to Elizabeth Fedde, the sisters might have chosen to support her mission, but that did not occur. But she agreed with the position of the motherhouse, as Reverend Passavant's advice was to train one's own deaconesses, which was precisely what the motherhouse had done and which was what she also decided to do. In 1885, she established a nine-bed hospital and began her training program; in doing so she established the first Norwegian-American deaconess motherhouse, which was dedicated on June 14, 1885.

By 1889, the Norwegian Relief Society, successor to the Volunteer Relief Society she had helped to establish, built a new thirty-bed hospital. In 1892, this institution was renamed the Norwegian Lutheran Medical Center. In that same year, the first Norwegian-American Lutheran deaconesses were consecrated in Sister Elizabeth Fedde's institution. She continued her work, adding an ambulance service and expanding her services to include all residents, regardless of emigrant status. Her agency provided food and clothing, and she and her sisters made house calls. A politically astute individual, in 1894 she successfully petitioned the city to appropriate to her hospital the same amount, $4,000, which was being given to other community hospitals. Learning of her work, in 1885 Pastor W. A. Passavant wanted her to become head of his deaconess hospital in Pittsburgh, but she declined the invitation. She did accept a call to Minneapolis in 1888 to start a deaconess home there (Lutheran Deaconess Home and Hospital), and she remained in Minnesota for two years until her return to Norway in late 1889.

Upon her return to Norway, Sister Elizabeth married Ola A.P. Slettebo, a patient man who had waited thirteen years for her while she accomplished her mission in America. Since she considered the marriage as the highest calling to which women could aspire, it was not

incongruous with the rest of her life that she at last accepted Ola's offer. They settled on a farm near Egersund, where she died in 1921. In 1915 she was presented a silver bowl by the Norwegian Lutheran Deaconesses' Home and Hospital, Brooklyn, New York, and in 1956 she was included on a Johnson and Johnson calendar of famous nurses.
REFERENCES: Beulah Folkedahl, "Elizabeth Fedde's Diary 1883-88," *Norwegian American Studies and Records* (1959), pp. 170-196; *Notable American Women*, pp. 605-606; Meta Rutter Pennock, *Makers of Nursing History* (1940), p. 43.

JOELLEN WATSON HAWKINS

FISHER, ALICE (June 14, 1839, Queen's House, Greenwich, England--June 3, 1888). *Nurse-educator.* Daughter of Rev. George Fisher, instructor of mathematics at the Royal Naval School. EDUCATION: 1875-1876, attended St. Thomas Hospital, London. CAREER: Assistant superintendent, Edinburgh Royal Infirmary; superintendent of the Fever Hospital, Newcastle, England; superintendent (for five years), Addenbroke's Hospital, Cambridge, England; superintendent, Radcliffe Infirmary, Oxford, England; superintendent, General Hospital, Birmingham, England; 1884-1888, founder and superintendent of the training school for nurses, Philadelphia General Hospital, Philadelphia, and chief nurse, Philadelphia General Hospital.
CONTRIBUTIONS: Although she spent only four years in the United States, the work of Alice Fisher lived on in the memories of all who knew her. When she arrived at the Philadelphia General Hospital, previously known as "Old Blockley," she found a scandal of wide proportions. The hospital was really an almshouse and workhouse for the aged and the infirm. Its patients were poor, sick, or insane, and many were orphans, prisoners, or mentally ill. The staff was incompetent, often drawn from the ranks of servants, paupers, or criminals, the only ones willing to work in such surroundings for very small wages. The patients were often abused by the staff, the buildings were filthy and infested with vermin and rodents, and the sanitary facilities were virtually non-existent. There were no laundry facilities, and the heat was inadequate and uneven. Cleanliness and order, comfort and self-respect for patients, and decreased mortality rate all testified to the success of Alice Fisher in transforming a typical almshouse infirmary into something resembling a modern hospital. Although she suffered from a chronic heart problem, she worked hard at the job she loved, even sitting all night with a dying patient and then continuing with her responsibilities the next day.

Fisher was remembered for her high ideals, her sharp intellect, and her striking appearance (being nearly six feet tall with golden hair). Her pupils recalled how she supported them while always maintaining the high standards which were her trademark. She was a stern disciplinarian; there was no recourse once she had decided on an action, but she was remembered as being fair, altruistic, and tolerant. Indeed, she admitted a black student whom she allowed to share her own quarters as an example to the other students who obviously were not nearly as tolerant as their teacher. She was described as being happy with her work, having a charm that endeared her to those with whom she worked.

Rather than return to England for recuperation when she became ill, she continued to work, almost to the end. Even her death was dramatic; because she once had said that the last sound on earth she would like to hear would be the voices of the nurses singing hymns, as they often did on Sunday evenings, an organ was brought into the hall (downstairs from the sickroom), and while she was on her death bed, her students sang hymns. In "The Passing of Old Blockley," Ruth E. Rives described a ceremony by the alumnae of the Philadelphia General Hospital school of nursing in which the nurses placed carnations on the grave of Alice Fisher after a procession and the singing of hymns.

REFERENCES: *American Journal of Nursing* (1964); M. Adelaide Nutting Collection, Columbia University Teachers College (microfiche number 0272); Ruth E. Rives, "The Passing of Old Blockley," *American Journal of Nursing* (June 1927), pp. 747-749; Marion E. Smith, "Alice Fisher," *American Journal of Nursing* (July 1904), pp. 803-808.

LORETTA P. HIGGINS

FITZGERALD, ALICE LOUISE FLORENCE (March 13, 1874, Florence, Italy--November 10, 1962, Bronx, New York). *International relief worker*. Daughter of Charles H. and Alice (Riggs Lawrason) Fitzgerald. Never married. EDUCATION: Educated abroad by governesses and finishing schools in France, Germany, and Switzerland; 1906, received diploma, Johns Hopkins School of Nursing, Baltimore, Maryland; c. 1914, summer course at Teachers College, Columbia University, New York City. CAREER: 1907, head nurse at Johns Hopkins Hospital; 1908, volunteer service with the Italian Red Cross at the Messina earthquake; 1909, charge nurse and then night superintendent, Johns Hopkins Hospital; 1911, reorganized the operating room services, Bellevue Hospital, New York City; 1912, superintendent of nurses, General Hospital, Wilkes-Barre, Pennsylvania; 1914, superintendent of nurses, Robert W. Long Hospital, Indianapolis, Indiana; 1915, head nurse in the student infirmary, Dana

Hall School, Wellesley, Massachusetts; 1916, service with the Nurse Corps, British Army; 1917, staff member, American Red Cross, Paris, France; 1919, chief nurse, commission of the American Red Cross to Europe (later elected the first director of nursing of the League of Red Cross Societies); 1922, advisor on public health nursing to the staff of Governor-General Leonard Wood, the Philippines; 1925, surveyed nursing schools in the Orient for the Rockefeller Foundation; 1927, organized nursing education in Siam; 1929, surveyed nursing conditions in the state for the Maryland Board of Nurse Examiners; c. 1930, head of nurses' residence hall, Sheppard-Pratt Hospital, Baltimore, Maryland; 1948, retired from active nursing.

CONTRIBUTIONS: Alice Fitzgerald was noted for her diplomacy and professional nursing skill in health and welfare work in Europe and Asia following World War I. In the United States, she reorganized the delivery of operating room services, expanded the scope of public health nursing, and organized nursing service for emergency care. She organized and directed relief service following earthquakes in Italy and Japan. She served in World War I with both the British Army and through the American Red Cross with the American Army. As a well-trained nurse and a capable linguist, she was able to secure cooperation between the Allied hospitals when differences in language caused confusion. At the end of the war, through her work with the International Red Cross, she helped expand opportunities for European women to enter nursing schools. She began public health programs using visiting nurses in Germany, Austria, Poland, the Balkans, and Belgium. She created the international public health nursing course at King's College, London. Nurses from eighteen countries attended the first class of that course. She travelled and lectured in America to encourage an international point of view, but she found that the audience was more interested in her war stories.

In 1922, on assignment with the Rockefeller Foundation, she developed public health nursing in the Philippines, and she surveyed nursing care in the Orient for the foundation and then returned to Siam for two years to modernize nursing education in that country.

Through her career, she received numerous awards for her exemplary service. A Massachusetts committee chose her to be the Edith Cavell Memorial Nurse to the British Army Nursing Service. She was awarded the Victory Medal by King George of Great Britain and received a special award from Italy for her disaster work following the Messina earthquake. She also received medals from the governments of Poland, Serbia, Hungary, and Russia. From the French government, she received the French Campaign and Victory medal and the special French Medaille d'honneur with the Rosette. She also received the International Florence

Nightingale Medal. In 1940 she was awarded a medal by the Chinese government for helping to send medical aid to that country. When she retired and moved into the Peabody Home for the remainder of her life, she sent all her medals and decorations to the Johns Hopkins School of Nursing, declaring that they were more properly a credit to her profession than to her personal merit.
WRITINGS: Many articles in the *American Journal of Nursing*, including "Congratulations to Italian Nurses" (1926), p. 30, "Nursing in Siam" (1929, p. 807, "The Nursing Situation in Italy" (1930), p. 292, "Joyful News from Florence" (1930), p. 467, and "New School in Italy" (1932), p. 866.
REFERENCES: *American Journal of Nursing* (1924), p. 1224; Gertrude R. Connolly, "Nurse to Half the World," *Baltimore Sun* (July 28, 1946), sec. A, p. 2; Iris Noble, *Nurse Around the World: Alice Fitzgerald* (1964); Mary M. Roberts, *American Nursing: History and Interpretation* (1964).

ALICE HOWELL FRIEDMAN

FLIKKE, JULIA {OTTESON} (March 16, 1879, Viroqua, Wisconsin--February 23, 1965, Washington, D.C.). *Army Nurse.* Daughter of Solfest Otteson and Kristi (Severson) Otteston. Married Arne T. Flikke, September 11, 1901; two years after he died on October 15, 1912, she attended nursing school. EDUCATION: Graduate of Viroqua High School, Viroqua, Wisconsin; 1912-1915, attended Augustana Hospital Training School, Chicago, graduating in 1915; 1915-1916 and 1925, post-graduate study in administration and nursing education, Teachers College, Columbia University, New York City. CAREER: Taught for two years in Wisconsin; 1916-1918, assistant superintendent of nurses, Augustana Hospital, Chicago; 1918-June 30, 1943, served in the Army Nurse Corps: 1918, Lakewood, Fox Hills, and then 1918-1919, chief nurse, Base Hospital Number 11, France; 1919, head nurse, Nantes Evacuation Unit Number 28 and Hospital Train Number 55, directing care given the Army of Occupation troops being evacuated to the United States; July 1920, stationed at Camp Upton; 1920-1922, tours of duty in the Army and Navy General Hospital, Hot Springs, Arkansas, Fort McKinley, the Philippines, Tientsin, China; 1922-1934, principal chief nurse at Walter Reed General Hospital; 1934-1937, assigned to Fort Sam Houston, Texas; 1927-1937, captain and assistant superintendent of the Army Nurse Corps; 1937-1943, superintendent of the Army Nurse Corps; 1943, retired due to ill health.
CONTRIBUTIONS: Julia O. Flikke's major contribution was in military nursing; she was the sixth superintendent of the Army Nurse Corps. Her service to the corps spanned both world wars, beginning in March 1918

when Augustana Hospital organized an affiliated medical unit in response to the entry of the United States in World War I. Following service during that war, she served in the United States, the Philippines, and China. From 1922 to 1934, she was assigned to Walter Reed General Hospital, where her service earned citations for outstanding service and proficiency. In 1927, she was promoted to captain and appointed assistant superintendent of the Army Nurse Corps. In 1937, she was appointed superintendent of the corps.

Nurses still had only "relative rank," so she was promoted to the relative rank of major. Since the United States was not involved in a major confrontation, her first year as superintendent was spent supervising several hundred nurses at army posts in the United States and abroad. During that time, she worked for increased use of dietitians as well as physical and occupational therapists. World War II necessitated the recruitment, mobilization, and assignment of thousands of additional nurses. A new blue uniform replaced the old olive drab, standards for admission to the corps were revised, and married nurses were accepted into the service. Major Flikke wrote *Nurses in Action* to help educate the public about the responsibilities of army nurses.

In 1942, the superintendent of the corps was finally accorded the rank of colonel, and Colonel Flikke became the first woman to hold that rank in the armed forces. There was considerable controversy, however, about this "temporary" appointment under the provisions of Public Law 252, which was enacted by the Seventy-seventh Congress. It was not until 1947 that Florence Blanchfield (q.v.), Colonel Flikke's successor, received a regular commission in the army.

One of Flikke's last accomplishments, in January 1943, was to ensure that there were changes in the training of Corps nurses so all were prepared to go overseas. When she left her position due to ill health, there were over 29,000 nurses on active duty. Some shadow seems to fall on Flikke in accounts of the corps. She is implied to have been, at times, a weak leader. In 1942, a committee to study the medical department of the army was appointed, and the committee's report seemed to influence Flikke's retirement and Blanchfield's appointment as superintendent. One can only speculate whether some of her weakness can be attributed to the temporary nature of appointments and the unwillingness of military and political authorities to grant military nurses anything other than relative rank.

On June 12, 1945, Flikke received an honorary doctor of science degree from Wittenberg College, Springfield, Ohio. On June 2, 1958 she entered the National Lutheran Home for Aged, Washington, D.C., and after a long illness she died at the home. She was buried in the National Memorial Cemetery, Washington, D.C., with full military honors.

WRITINGS: *Nurses in Action* (1942); numerous articles, including "Invitation to Service," *Journal of the Medical Society of Cape May County, New Jersey* (June 1942), pp. 6-7.
REFERENCES: *American Journal of Nursing* (April 1965), pp. 155-156; Edith A. Aynes, *From Nightingale to Eagle* (1973); *Current Biography* (1942); Meta Rutter Pennock, *Makers of Nursing History* (1940), p. 59; Mary M. Roberts, *American Nursing: History and Interpretation* (1954), and *Army Nurse Corps Today and Tomorrow* (1957); Clark Robinson, "Colonel Julia O. Flikke, Chief of the U.S. Army Nurse Corps," *Journal of the Medical Society of Cape May County, New Jersey* (June 1942), pp. 3-6; Dorothy Schaffter, *What Comes of Training Women for War* (1948); *Who Was Who in America*, vol. 6; letters and unpublished papers, Wittenberg University Library Special Collections.

JOELLEN WATSON HAWKINS

FOLEY, EDNA LOIS (December 17, 1878, Hartford, Connecticut--August 4, 1943, New York City). *Public health nurse.* Daughter of William R. Foley and Matilda (Baker) Foley. Never married.
EDUCATION: Attended grammar and high school, Hartford, Connecticut; 1901, graduated from Smith College, Northampton, Massachusetts; 1904, graduated from Hartford Hospital Training School for Nurses; 1908, post-graduate work in the School for Social Workers, Boston. CAREER: 1904-1905, head nurse, Hartford Hospital, 1904-1905; 1905-1906, chief nurse, Children's Hospital, Albany, New York; 1906-1907, night supervisor, Children's Hospital, Boston; 1907-1909, Municipal Tuberculosis Visiting Nurse, Boston; 1909-1911, nurse for the Chicago Tuberculosis Institute; 1911-1912, superintendent, Municipal Tuberculosis Nurses, Chicago; 1912-1937, superintendent, Visiting Nurse Association, Chicago; 1918-1919, served with the American Red Cross Tuberculosis Commission to Italy; retired to New York City.
CONTRIBUTIONS: Edna Foley's greatest contribution was to the organization and leadership of public health nursing. Early in her career, she became involved in tuberculosis nursing, an important component of the work of public health nursing in the early decades of this century. As a representative of the American Society of Superintendents of Training Schools, she was a member of the committee to study standards for visiting nursing that led to the formation of the National Organization for Public Health Nursing. She served as chairperson of the 1912 meeting in Chicago at which that organization was formally established. Then she served the new organization as its first vice-president, acting president, and president from April 1920 to June 1921. For many years, in two

intervals between 1915 and 1925, she was the editor of the *American Journal of Nursing*'s department of public health nursing. As a member of the National Committee on Red Cross Nursing Service, she helped to direct the activities of Red Cross nurses.

Her reputation and experience in public health nursing led to her call to Italy in October 1918, and in June 1919 she became chief nurse of the American Red Cross Tuberculosis Commission for Italy to undertake the work begun by Mary S. Gardner (q.v.) to organize public health nursing for tuberculosis work through establishment of a course and fieldwork. Public health nurses from the course were assigned to Perugia, Spezia, and Palermo. She served until December 31, 1919, when the American Red Cross withdrew all post-World War I nursing activities from Italy.

Her commitment to the profession and its advancement was exemplified in her ardent support of continuing education and in-service education for nurses and urging nurses to attend conventions of the various nursing organizations. At the 1912 convention of the American Society of Superintendents of Training Schools, she urged leaders in nursing to recognize the need for opportunities for continuing education and in-service education for nurses.

Her reputation as superintendent of the Chicago Visiting Nurse Association (1912-1937) was such that many nurses sought to work in her agency. She was known as a leader who was not only knowledgeable and skilled but also wise and largehearted. As an example of her understanding for the needs of the nurses under her supervision, during the 1920s, she granted the request of one of her nurses to marry. At that time, very few agencies allowed married nurses to serve, for fear that their family responsibilities would detract from their sense of mission to the profession. Her strong commitment to excellence in nursing care for all Americans was demonstrated by the fact that at one meeting she protested when public health officials advocated the use of "nurses" with very brief training. She replied that what she heard them propose was poor nurses for poor people. As director of the Chicago Visiting Nurse Association, she insisted that black nurses were hired and that they had equal opportunities in their profession.

She received recognition for her work in several important ways, including receipt of an honorary doctor of science degree from Smith College (June 18, 1928). She was also awarded the first "citizen fellowship" given by the Chicago Institute of Medicine (1934), and the Forty-seventh Street substation of the Chicago Visiting Nurse Association was named the Edna L. Foley Substation in her honor. After serving as superintendent of the Chicago Visiting Nurse Association for twenty-five years, she retired and eventually moved to New York City to be near her

sister. She died there in her home. Only a few hours before her death, she had attended an air-raid warden's meeting, which indicates that to the end she was serving others.
WRITINGS: *Visiting Nurse Manual* (1914), published by the Visiting Nurse Association of Chicago, under the auspices of the National Organization for Public Health Nursing; also published numerous articles in professional journals.
REFERENCES: *American Journal of Nursing* (April 1923), p. 560, (July 1928), p. 698, and (September 1943), p. 876; American Journal of Nursing Collection, Nursing Archives, Mugar Memorial Library, Boston University; Annie M. Brainard, *The Evolution of Public Health Nursing* (1922); Josephine A. Dolan, M. Louise Fitzpatrick, and Eleanor Krohn Herrmann, *Nursing in Society: A Historical Perspective* (15th ed., 1983); Cordelia W. Kelly, *Dimensions of Professional Nursing* (2d ed., 1968); Portia B. Kernodle, *The Red Cross Nurse in Action, 1882-1948* (1949); *New York Times* (August 5, 1943), p. 15; *Public Health Nursing* (September 1943), p. 522; *Trained Nurse and Hospital Review* (September 1943); *Woman's Who's Who of America* (1914).

JOELLEN WATSON HAWKINS

FOX, ELIZABETH GORDON (December 2, 1884, Madison or Milwaukee, Wisconsin--November 13, 1958, Newington, Connecticut). *Public health nurse.* Daughter of Edwin M. Fox and Frances (Gordon) Fox. Never married. EDUCATION: 1907, B.A., University of Wisconsin at Madison, and inducted into Phi Beta Kappa; 1907-1910, attended Johns Hopkins Hospital Training School for Nurses, Baltimore, Maryland, graduating in 1910. CAREER: 1910-1913, worked as a head nurse of a surgical ward, University Hospital, Minneapolis, Minnesota, and as a staff nurse with the Visiting Nurse Association, Chicago; 1913-1916, superintendent, Public Health Nursing Organization, Dayton, Ohio; 1916-1918, superintendent, Instructive Visiting Nurse Society, Washington, D.C.; April-September 1918, associate director, bureau of public health nursing, American Red Cross; September 1918-August 1919, acting director of the same bureau; 1919-May 1930, national director, bureau of public health nursing, American Red Cross; 1930-49, director, New Haven Visiting Nurse Association, and member of the faculty, Yale School of Nursing, New Haven, Connecticut.
CONTRIBUTIONS: Elizabeth Fox's greatest contribution was in the organization of nursing service under the American Red Cross from an experimental service to one comprised of 636 branches and 795 Red Cross nurses. During the first three months of 1919, she helped to plan and

implement policies for providing public health nursing services in towns and localities where none existed and where there were no plans in place for such. In April of that year, eighteen new public health nursing services were begun in eight districts. In October 1919, she toured the country to interpret the peacetime program of the Red Cross and to learn about local problems and to resolve them. A conference was held in November at national headquarters, which resulted in the production and distribution of guidelines to the chapters, and plans were made for the recruitment and preparation of nurses. In 1921, she appeared at a hearing before the Senate Committee on Education and Labor to testify in support of the Sheppard-Towner maternal health bill. In the aftermath of the April 1927 Mississippi River flood, she took personal charge of the Red Cross nurses in the field, which prepared her for a lecture on disaster nursing that she gave in the post-graduate course at Teachers College, Columbia University, in 1929. In 1930, she gave two of a series of five disaster relief lectures in the same program.

From Washington, Fox moved to New Haven, Connecticut, to serve as the executive director of the Visiting Nurse Association of New Haven and as a member of the faculty of the School of Nursing of Yale University, becoming an associate professor and chairperson of the committee on community nursing. Also, as a senior faculty person, she was a member of the board of administrative officers, responsible for the conduct of the school as a whole. She continued to serve not only on professional committees, including membership on the board of directors of the Connecticut State Nurses' Association (serving as its president in 1941-1942) but also as the only woman on the New Haven Housing Authority. She was a member of the Council of Social Agencies of New Haven from 1938 to 1944 and the nursing advisory committee of the Metropolitan Life Insurance Company.

Fox's contributions were not confined to the American Red Cross or to Yale University; those to the profession were especially significant. She was a member of the Committee on the Grading of Nursing Schools (1920), which was an important part of the work which led to the Goldmark report. She was vice-president of the National Organization for Public Health Nursing (1921), served on its board of directors, and from 1921 to 1926 was its president. In the 1930s, she chaired its education committee. She chaired the provisional public health nursing section of the Public Health Association, was president of the Graduate Nurses' Association (Washington, D.C., 1918-1920), and president of the District of Columbia's Board of Nurse Examiners. She also was active in her support for Johns Hopkins; the "Half-Century Campaign," launched in 1925, included Fox on the committee, as did the special committee of the Alumnae Association in 1926. Finally, she served on the Committee on the Cost of Medical Care, which proposed its five-year program in 1928 and issued its final report in 1932. Even her retirement was an active one; from 1950 to 1958, she was a director of the New Haven Family Service.

During the course of her career, she received many awards, beginning when she was inducted into Phi Beta Kappa while a student at the University of Wisconsin (1907). She also received a senior scholarship while a student at the Johns Hopkins Hospital Training School for Nurses. In 1931, the International Red Cross awarded her its Florence Nightingale Medal, the first time the award was given for extraordinary service in a peace program of a Red Cross society. On November 13, 1958, she received the Charles E.-A. Winslow Award of the Connecticut Public Health Association, and she undoubtedly shocked everyone present when she died at the meeting which was held at the Newington Hospital for Crippled Children for the purpose of presenting her with the award.

WRITINGS: *History of American Red Cross Nursing* (1922); numerous articles on public health nursing; *What the Future Holds for Public Health Nursing under the American Red Cross* (1928).

REFERENCES: *American Journal of Nursing* (January 1923), p. 308; Annie M. Brainard, *The Evolution of Public Health Nursing* (1922); Dorothy Deming, "Elizabeth Gordon Fox," *National League of Nursing Education Biographical Sketches, 1937-1940* (1940); Lavinia L. Dock, Sarah E. Pickett, Clara D. Noyes, Fannie F. Clement, Elizabeth G. Fox, and Anna R. Van Meter, *History of American Red Cross Nursing* (1922); *Hartford Times* (November 13, 1958); Ethel Johns and Blanche Pfefferkorn, *The Johns Hopkins Hospital School of Nursing, 1889-1948* (1949); Johns Hopkins Nurses' Alumni Association, biographical form completed by Fox in 1952; Meta Rutter Pennock, *Makers of Nursing History* (1940), pp. 126-127; James H. and Mary Jane Rodabaugh, *Nursing in Ohio* (1951); *The Trained Nurse and Hospital Review* (July 1931), pp. 55-56; *Who's Who of American Women* (1st ed., 1959), I: 436.

JOELLEN WATSON HAWKINS

FRANCIS, MARGARET E.. See **SIRCH, MARGARET**.

FRANCIS, SUSAN C. (c. 1873, Bridgeport, Pennsylvania--October 18, 1962, Ephrata, Pennsylvania). *Nurse-administrator.* Daughter of a schoolteacher father and a mother who was his cousin. EDUCATION: 1894, graduated from the Reading Hospital School of Nursing, Reading, Pennsylvania. CAREER: 1894-1896, private duty nursing; c. 1896-c. 1905, staff nurse, head nurse, then seven years as superintendent of nurses, City Hospital, Washington, D.C. (later known as Gallinger Hospital); c. 1907, superintendent, Touro Infirmary, New Orleans, Louisiana, resigning after nine months due to ill health; 1909-1917, superintendent of nurses, Jewish Hospital, Philadelphia; 1917-1920, director of nursing of the Pennsylvania-Delaware division of the American Red Cross (during World War I); 1921-1942, superintendent of the Children's Hospital and its school of nursing, Philadelphia.

CONTRIBUTIONS: Susan Francis was best known for her work in nursing organizations and in the American Red Cross during two world wars, and for her skills as superintendent of many hospitals and schools of nursing. She was president of the American Nurses' Association (ANA) from 1934 to 1938, being nominated by Pennsylvania nurses who had observed her talent for leadership when she served as president of the Pennsylvania State Nurses' Association. From 1928 to 1934, she served as secretary of the ANA, and she was secretary and president of the board of directors of the *American Journal of Nursing*. Francis was involved in the historic study of nursing education as the ANA representative on the joint committee on the grading of nursing schools. It is likely that her work as superintendent of Children's Hospital, Philadelphia, brought her to the attention of national political leaders, who appointed her to the subcommittee on nursing of the White House Conference on Child Health and Protection. She also served on the board of directors of the International Council of Nurses. She first joined the National League of Nursing Education when she worked in Washington, D.C., and when she moved to Philadelphia she was the first person to serve as secretary of the newly organized Philadelphia League of Nursing Education.

She served her country during two world wars. In World War I, she was director of nursing of the Pennsylvania-Delaware division of the American Red Cross, working to enroll Red Cross nurses who would serve overseas. During World War II, she was the organizing volunteer director of the American Red Cross nurses' aide program in the southeastern Pennsylvania chapter.

REFERENCES: *American Journal of Nursing* (July 1942), pp. 830-831 and (December 1962), p. 125; Stella Goostray, "Susan C. Francis," *National League of Nursing Education Biographical Sketches, 1937-1940* (1940); *Nursing Outlook* (December 1962), pp. 820-821; M. Adelaide Nutting Collection, Teachers College, Columbia University, (microfiche number 0387).

LORETTA P. HIGGINS

FRANKLIN, MARTHA MINERVA (October 29, 1870--September 26, 1968, New Haven, Connecticut). *Pioneer black nurse.* Daughter of Henry J. Franklin and Marcy (Ganson) Franklin. EDUCATION: attended public schools of Meriden, Connecticut, including high school; 1896-1897, attended Women's Hospital Training School for Nurses, Philadelphia, graduating on December 15, 1897. CAREER: began private duty nursing in 1898, continuing for the remainder of her career as a private duty nurse in Connecticut, where her parents were residents in New Milford.

CONTRIBUTIONS: Martha Franklin was the only black graduate of her class at the Women's Hospital Training School for Nurses, in Philadelphia, and over the next ten years she came to recognize the racial discrimination which existed not only in American society but in the nursing profession as well. She was one of the earliest nurses in Connecticut to pass the state registration examinations (June 17, 1908) and was given registration number 600 (the Connecticut nurse-registration act was not passed until 1905). At the time of registration, she was listed as a resident of New Haven, Connecticut. Her importance, however, was on the national scene rather than in the state of Connecticut.

She was one of the first to campaign actively for racial equality in nursing. She began by gathering together America's black nurses in their own organization, which would provide a network of support for reform and provide black nurses with a forum for sharing information and ideas, therefore enhancing the skills and abilities of America's black nurses. In 1908, Franklin founded the National Association of Colored Graduate Nurses (NACGN), an organization dedicated to promoting the standards and welfare of black nurses and breaking down racial discrimination in the profession. She recognized that opportunities were limited for black nurses, and she realized that the situation would not change unless black nurses joined together to spearhead the movement for reform. From her home in Connecticut, in 1906 and 1907 she sent out letters to nurses, directors of nursing schools, and nursing organizations, and the responses provided her with information on the numbers of black nurses in America and the extent of employment discrimination. The survey also provided evidence that black nurses were interested in establishing an organization of their own, since they were not welcome in the American Nurses' Association (ANA).

In August 1908 Franklin served as chairperson of a meeting of fifty-eight black nurses who gathered at Lincoln Hospital in New York City. At that meeting, the National Association of Colored Graduate Nurses was founded, and, appropriately, Franklin was elected its first president. She continued to remain active in the organization, and in 1921 she attended what was to be her last meeting, which was held at Washington, D.C. Those in attendance were received at the White House by President and Mrs. Warren G. Harding, and after their audience with the president it was resolved to put it on the record that the NACGN was an organization of 2,000 trained nurses who were ready for world service when needed. At the 1976 convention of the ANA, Franklin was one of the first members inducted into the association Hall of Fame, certainly showing that the ANA had come to recognize the important contributions provided by nurses of every race.

REFERENCES: American Nurses' Association, *Nursing Hall of Fame* (1982), p. 14; Vern and Bonnie Bullough, *The Emergence of Modern Nursing* (1969), p. 210; Mary Elizabeth Carnegie, *The Path We Tread* (1986); application for nurse-registration (dated May 1, 1908) provided by the Connecticut Department of Health Services, Hartford; Mariana M. Davis, *Contributions of Black Women to America* (1982), pp. 364-366; Joyce Ann Elmore, "Black Nurses and their Service and Their Struggles," *American Journal of Nursing* (1976); Herbert M. Morais, *History of the Afro-American in Medicine* (1976), p. 73; unpublished manuscripts, records of the National Association of Colored Graduate Nurses, Schonburg Center for Research in Black Culture, New York City; Mary M. Roberts, *American Nursing: History and Interpretation* (1954), pp. 78-79.

ALICE HOWELL FRIEDMAN

FREDERICK, HESTER KING (August 9, 1881, Baltimore, Maryland--June 24, 1950, Baltimore, Maryland). *Nurse-educator.* Daughter of Lawrence N. Frederick and Octavia (Harden) Frederick. Never married. EDUCATION: Attended public school in Baltimore and Girls Latin School for four years; 1906, enrolled at Johns Hopkins Hospital Training School for Nurses, Baltimore, Maryland, graduating in 1912 (1908-1911, recuperated from tuberculosis at Dr. Edward Trudeau's sanatorium at Saranac Lake, New York). CAREER: 1912-1913, head nurse, Trudeau Sanatorium, Saranac Lake, New York; 1913-1916, superintendent of nurses, King's Daughters Hospital, Staunton, Virginia; 1916-1917, private duty nursing; 1917-1919, assistant supervisor of the surgical supply room and nursing school office, Johns Hopkins Hospital; 1919, superintendent of nurses, Fabiola Hospital, Oakland, California; November 1919-1927, instructor in principles and practice of nursing, Johns Hopkins Hospital Training School for Nurses; 1927-1930, superintendent of nurses, Union Memorial Hospital, Baltimore, Maryland; 1930-1941, assistant superintendent, Johns Hopkins Hospital and assistant director of the training school.

CONTRIBUTIONS: Hester Frederick, with her colleague Ethel Northam (q.v.), perhaps made her greatest contribution to nursing after her formal career had ended. Their *Textbook of Nursing Practice* (1928) was an early text and, more important, one that emphasized a theoretical basis for nursing practice. They conceptualized the patient as a care agent, using that term, and they defined nursing as an art, demanding a liberal education and high ideals. Nursing activities, according to their book, must focus on the promotion of the care agent. The textbook is now considered a pioneering early work in the evolution of nursing theory.

During her many years of service at Johns Hopkins, she was characterized as loyal and steadfast, possessing charm and magnetism as an instructor and ability and resourcefulness as an administrator. She always insisted that the well-being of the patient be the foremost consideration. As an instructor, she was demanding of her students, expecting much of them, yet she was generally patient and approachable. She was characterized by those who knew her, including Blanche Pfefferkorn (q.v.), as a beautiful girl and a handsome woman, with a wonderful sense of humor and a joyful and lively spirit. Her photograph in a Johns Hopkins School of Nursing yearbook confirms this description.

She served her alma mater during twenty-one of her twenty-nine years of professional practice. She served on the committee for an endowment fund for the School of Nursing in 1921. From 1921 to 1923, she was president of the alumnae association and chaired its finance committee. In 1930, she was appointed a member of the advisory board of the School of Nursing at Johns Hopkins, representing the staff of the school and serving as its first secretary. With Elsie Lawler, the director, she undertook a series of studies of the school. As a member of the special committee appointed in 1937 to consider a full-time librarian for the school, she was instrumental in preparing the report that recommended not only a full-time position but housing of all reference books in the nurses' home library and enlargement of that library.

Her retirement did not signal the end of her professional activities. From 1941 to 1945, she served with the American Red Cross Home Nursing Program and with the Civilian Defense of Baltimore. She also served on the committee for the history of the Johns Hopkins Hospital School of Nursing from 1946 to 1949.

WRITINGS: *Notes on Practical Nursing Procedures* (1922); *A Textbook of Nursing Techniques* (1928); *A Textbook of Nursing Practice* (with Ethel Northam, 1928, 1938); numerous unpublished reports and studies for the Johns Hopkins Hospital School of Nursing.

REFERENCES: Student records, Alan Mason Chesney Archives, Johns Hopkins Medical Institutions; *American Journal of Nursing* (May 1941), pp. 607-608; *Baltimore Sun* (June 26, 1950); Hester Frederick and Ethel

Northam, *Textbook of Nursing Practice* (2d ed., 1938); Ethel Johns and Blanche Pfefferkorn, *The Johns Hopkins Hospital School of Nursing: 1889-1949* (1954); Laula E. Kennedy, "Hester King Frederick," *Johns Hopkins Nurses Alumnae Magazine* (July 1941), pp. 116-121; Anna D. Wolf, "Hester King Frederick," *Johns Hopkins Nurses Alunmae Magazine* (October 1950), pp. 174-175.

JOELLEN WATSON HAWKINS

FREEMAN, RUTH BENSON (December 5, 1906, Methuen, Massachusetts--December 2, 1982, Cockeysville, Maryland). *Public health nurse; nurse educator.* Daughter of Wilbur Milton Freeman, trucker, and Elsie (Lawson) Freeman. Married Anselm Fisher, September 21, 1927 (but continued using her maiden name throughout her career); one daughter. EDUCATION: 1927, received diploma from Mt. Sinai Hospital School of Nursing, New York City; 1934, B.S., Columbia University, New York City; 1939, M.A., New York University; 1951, Ed.D., New York University. CAREER: 1929-1937, staff nurse, Henry Street Visiting Nurse Service, New York City; 1937-1941, instructor of nursing, New York University; 1941-1946, professor of public health, University of Minnesota, Minneapolis; 1946-1950, director of nursing, American National Red Cross, Washington, D.C.; 1948-1950, consultant to the National Security Resources Board, Washington, D.C.; 1950-1962, associate professor, Johns Hopkins University, Baltimore, Maryland; 1962-1971, professor of public health administration and coordinator of the nursing program, Johns Hopkins University; 1971, professor emeritus. CONTRIBUTIONS: Ruth Freeman was a leader in professionalizing public health nursing, through her many publications, through her teaching at New York University, University of Minnesota, and Johns Hopkins University, and through her extensive work in various professional organizations. Through what one may call on-the-job training as a staff nurse with the Henry Street Visiting Nurse Service, she developed a knowledge of the many public health problems facing twentieth-century American society, as well as an awareness of the ways the public health nurse can help alleviate those problems. She worked to get personnel in public health to accept nurses as full collaborators and helped to prepare nurses to assume that role.

In her teaching and her publications, she tried to use an interdisciplinary outlook, relating academic work to the realities of service in the community. Recognizing the difficulty of coordinating the work of various public health agencies, she worked to improve communication between agencies and between staff members of individual agencies. Her books became widely used texts in public health nursing courses around the country and spread her ideas to professors and public health nurses in virtually every state.

She was active in various professional organizations, serving as vice-president of the National Organization for Public Health Nursing (1946-1950), president of the National League for Nursing (1955-1959), and president of the National Health Council (1959-1960). She also was an active member of the White House Conference on Children and Youth (1958-1960). She was an especially active member of the American Public Health Association, serving as a member of the executive board, governing council, subcommittee on handicapped children, editorial board, technical development board, and awards committee. She received numerous awards for distinguished service, including the Pearl McIver Award for distinguished work in public health nursing (1958), the M. Adelaide Nutting Award (1967), the Bronfman Prize from the American Public Health Association (1971), and the Florence Nightingale Medal given by the International Red Cross (1981). She was made an honorary member of Sigma Theta Tau, the international honor society of nursing.

WRITINGS: *Techniques of Supervision in Public Health Nursing* (1945, 1949); *Health Care for the Family* (with Ramona Todd, 1946); *Public Health Nursing Practice* (1950, 1957, 1963); *Administration in Public Health Services* (with E. M. Holmes, 1960); *Community Health Nursing Practice* (1970); "Developments in Education of Public Health Nurses," *Public Health Nursing* (November 1945), pp. 454-455; "National Security Resources Board and Nursing," *Public Health Nursing* (December 1948), pp. 603-604.

REFERENCES: *American Journal of Nursing* (August 1981), p. 1531; *Contemporary Authors*, vols. 41-44 (1979), pp. 232-233; Ruth Freeman Collection, Nursing Archives, Mugar Memorial Library, Boston University; *Nursing Outlook* (January-February 1983), p. 24; Gwendolyn Safier, *Contemporary American Leaders in Nursing: An Oral History* (1977).

LORETTA P. HIGGINS

FULMER, HARRIET (c. 1877, Fulmerville, Pennsylvania--November 27, 1952, Chicago). *Public health nurse.* Daughter of John Roericke Fulmer and Emma Jane (Beardsley) Fulmer. Never married. EDUCATION: Graduated from high school in Plattsmouth, Nebraska; 1896, graduated from St. Luke's Hospital Training School for Nurses, Chicago. CAREER: 1896-1897, private duty nursing, Chicago; 1898-1900, district nurse, and 1901-1912, superintendent, Visiting Nurse Association of Chicago;

1913-1914, secretary, Illinois State Association for the Prevention of Tuberculosis; 1917-1940, supervisor of rural nursing services, Cook County, Illinois.

CONTRIBUTIONS: Harriet Fulmer was a public health nurse who contributed to nursing history in several important ways. She was superintendent of one of the earliest visiting nurse associations in the United States, that of Chicago. When the association was founded in 1890, it had two nurses on its staff. When Fulmer became superintendent in 1901, the staff consisted of eight nurses; by the time she left the association in 1912, that number had increased to fourteen, with a group of twenty-nine emergency attendants under her direct supervision. She was also the editor for public health nursing reports for the newly established (1900) *American Journal of Nursing*. Although the *Journal* had allocated a certain amount of space for public health nursing, the growth and development of that specialty led to recognition that a magazine devoted exclusively to public health nursing was necessary. Fulmer played a major role in the development of such a journal, *Visiting Nurse Quarterly*, which was forced to suspend publication after two years due to a lack of financial support. Historians of nursing have credited *Visiting Nurse Quarterly* for being the forerunner of a journal of the same name which began publication in 1909 and was sponsored by the Cleveland Visiting Nurse Association. That journal eventually became *Public Health Nurse* in 1918 and, finally, *Public Health Nursing*.

Fulmer also was active in professional organizations and was a pioneer in several important ways. Very early in her career, she became aware of the need for nursing associations. She founded the St. Luke's Alumnae Association and served as its first president. In 1899, she became a member of the committee on periodicals of the Associated Alumnae of the United States and Canada (which became the American Nurses' Association), and her committee planned the *American Journal of Nursing*. Fulmer was also the first president of the Illinois State Nurses' Association, and in 1900 she was one of a group whose work eventually led to passage of the act requiring registration of nurses in the state.

She also played a major role in improving the public health of Illinois. It was due to her efforts that school nurses were provided to the children of Chicago, through the Visiting Nurse Association of Chicago. Later, school nursing shifted to the control and supervision of the city's governing bodies. She also was active in the early public health campaign to control the spread of tuberculosis, and in 1913-1914 she served as secretary of the Illinois State Association for the Prevention of Tuberculosis. She was an ardent supporter of the organization of statewide public health nursing, and she is credited with being the person who brought public health nursing to Illinois. For many years, she was the supervisor of rural nursing for Cook County, until she retired in 1940.

Fulmer was an active member of a great many organizations; she was a member of the American Red Cross Society, the Consumer's League, and the American Public Health Association. In 1901 she served as a delegate to the International Congress of Women, which was held in Berlin, Germany, and in 1906 she was a delegate to the International Congress of Nurses, which met in Paris, France. The following year, 1907, she attended the fortieth anniversary of district nursing, a celebration held in Liverpool, England.

WRITINGS: "History of Visiting Nurse Work in America," *American Journal of Nursing* (1901), pp. 411-418.

REFERENCES: Harriet Fulmer, "History of Visiting Nurse Work in America," *American Journal of Nursing* (1901), pp. 411-418; "Report of the A.N.A. Delegates and Societies: Visiting Nurses' Association of Chicago," *American Journal of Nursing* (1901), pp. 882-884; *Who's Who in Chicago and Illinois* (1950).

ALICE HOWELL FRIEDMAN

G

GABRIEL, SISTER JOHN (born Ryan, Cumberland Hill, Rhode Island--?). *Educator*. Never married. EDUCATION: Studied pharmacy, Columbus Hospital, Great Falls, Montana; 1906, graduated from Columbus Hospital School of Nursing; graduated from St. Vincent Hospital School of Nursing, Portland, Oregon; post-graduate work at University of California, Catholic University of America, Marquette University, University of Oregon; 1927, B.A., University of Washington, Seattle; 1937, M.A., Seattle College. CAREER: 1899, entered the Sisters of Charity of Providence, Rhode Island; 1904, passed the Montana State pharmacy examination and began work as a pharmacist, Columbus Hospital, Great Falls, Montana; public health nursing in a variety of settings; 1912, pharmacist and teacher in the school of nursing, St. Vincent Hospital, Portland, Oregon; established school of nursing, Cranbrook, British Columbia, Canada; ?-1938, general supervisor of all schools of nursing in the Pacific Northwest conducted by the Sisters of Charity of Providence (including British Columbia, California, Montana, Oregon, and Washington); 1932, taught summer school, Loyola University, Chicago; 1935, taught summer school, Holy Name College, Oakland, California; 1936 and 1937, taught summer school, Creighton University, Omaha, Nebraska; 1936 and 1937, taught in the fall session, Seattle College.

CONTRIBUTIONS: Sister John Gabriel was one of the leading Catholic nurse-educators, and she was known for valuing education and for her willingness to share knowledge with her colleagues and with nursing students. She encouraged the superiors of her order to elevate the standards of nursing education for the members of that order, which ran hospitals and nursing schools throughout the country. In addition to her teaching and her many speeches, Sister John wrote a number of books on nursing education, books which consistently received praise in the *American Journal of Nursing*. In addition, she was active in professional organizations. From 1931 to 1935, she served as a member of the board of directors of the *American Journal of Nursing*, chaired the ethical standards committee of the American Nurses' Association, and was a member of the council of the Western Hospital Association and of the board of directors of the Washington State Nurses' Association. She was on the advisory editorial staff of *Hospital Management* and *Modern Hospital*, a member of the council of community relations and administration of the American Hospital Association, and a member of the Washington State Public Health Association.

After she studied pharmacy but before she attended nursing school, she and other sisters of her order were called upon to provide health care for people in the isolated communities of the Pacific Northwest. She nursed patients in their homes, in lumber camps and mining towns, and railroad crews where they lived in box cars. The sisters cared for people in outlying areas who were suffering from communicable diseases--nursing the sick and trying to prevent the disease from spreading. While caring for members of Indian tribes in the region, she perfected the skills needed to teach health and hygiene.

She was recognized for her contributions by the American College of Hospital Administrators, which in 1935 conferred on her the degree of honorary fellowship. In 1938 she was made honorary president of the Washington State Hospital Association.

WRITINGS: *Practical Methods of Study* (1930); *Teacher's Work Organization Book* (1931); *Professional Problems* (1932; 2d ed. 1937); *Through the Patient's Eyes* (1935); "Undergraduate Nurses at the University of Oregon," *American Journal of Nursing* (March 1932), pp. 265-268.

REFERENCES: *American Journal of Nursing* (March 1931), pp. 388-389, (October 1931), p. 1227, (January 1933), pp. 90-91, (August 1935), p. 810, and (August 1938), p. 945; Margaret Felton, National League of Nursing Education sketch (n.d.); M. Adelaide Nutting Collection, Teachers College, Columbia University, microfiche number 2440.

LORETTA P. HIGGINS

GAGE, NINA DIADAMIA (June 9, 1883, New York City--October 18, 1946, Syracuse, New York). *Nurse; educator; superintendent.* Daughter of Charles Gage and Sarah Ann (Perrin) Gage. Never married. EDUCATION: c. 1900, attended training department, Normal College, New York City; 1905, A.B., Wellesley College, Wellesley, Massachusetts; 1908, diploma, Roosevelt Hospital School of Nursing, New York City; 1925, M.A., Teachers College, Columbia University, New York City. CAREER: 1909-1917 and 1925-1927, principal and then superintendent of nurses, Hunan-Yale Hospital, Changsha, China; 1918, professor of nursing, Training Camp for Nurses, Vassar College, Poughkeepsie, New York; 1920, in charge, Infirmary Annex, Yale University, New Haven, Connecticut; 1928-1931, executive secretary, National League of Nursing Education; 1931-1935, instructor, Jersey City Medical Center, then director of nursing services at Willard Parker Hospital, New York City, and Hampton Institute, Virginia; 1935-1936, superintendent of nurses, Newport Hospital, Rhode Island; 1943-1945, director of nurses, Protestant Hospital, Nashville, Tennessee.
CONTRIBUTIONS: Nina Gage helped to develop nursing education in China. After her brother's survey of the possibilities for Yale schools in China, she prepared for her lifetime work by training to be a graduate nurse. She went to China in 1909, studied Chinese, and began to translate nursing texts into Chinese for use in Chinese nursing education. She set curricular standards for training Chinese nurses, and the Hunan-Yale Hospital became one of the leading nursing schools in China, a country which only twenty years earlier had no Chinese word for nurse. When she left in 1927, there were sixty-five graduates of the Hunan-Yale school serving as nurses in China. From 1910 to 1914, she served as president of the Nurses' Association of China, and in that capacity she was influential in the development of the American-style nursing curriculum and method of licensing nurses.

Her competencies in the basic nursing arts and sciences led to a faculty position at Vassar during World War I, when a shortened program for college graduates was offered to increase the number of trained nurses for military service. Her continued interest in the quality of nursing education was demonstrated in the report (with Alma Haupt {q.v.}) "Observation of Negro Nurses in the South." That report, published in 1932, documented the poor quality of nursing education provided to black nurses during the segregation era and how that limited their professional mobility. From 1925 to 1929, she served as president of the International Council of Nurses (ICN), and in 1929 she presided over the ICN Congress in Montreal. That meeting was originally scheduled to be held in Shanghai, but it had to be moved due to riots against foreigners in China. On December 1, 1946, the trustees of the Yale-in-China Association

(New Haven) adopted a resolution expressing "profound gratitude for a fruitful life of their comrade, Nina Diadamia Gage, who died October 18, 1946, after a courageous and uncomplaining fight against malignant disease."
WRITINGS: Many of her articles about nursing in China were published in the *American Journal of Nursing*, the *Medical Missionary Magazine of China*, the *Quarterly Review of the Nurses' Association of China*, and the *International Nursing Review*. She was co-author of two textbooks, including *Communicable Diseases* (with John L. Laudow, 1939). She also revised L. Seymour's *A Guide to the History of Nursing* for an American edition (1932); "Observation of Negro Nurses in the South," *Public Health Nursing* (1932), p. 674. The Nursing Archives at the Mugar Memorial Library, Boston University, has a collection of articles by and about Nina Gage.
REFERENCES: *American Journal of Nursing* (November 1943), pp. 1045-1046, and (December 1946), p. 892; Alumnae Office, Wellesley College, Wellesley, Massachusetts; *American Women, 1935-1940*, p. 316; G. Champpison, *Vassar's Rainbow Division* (1964); *Index to Women of the World* (19XX); E. Hume, *Doctors East, Doctors West* (19XX); Meta Rutter Pennock, *Makers of Nursing History* (1928); Mary M. Roberts, *American Nursing: History and Interpretation* (1954).

ALICE HOWELL FRIEDMAN

GARDNER, MARY SEWALL (February 5, 1871, Newton, Massachusetts--February 21, 1861, Providence, Rhode Island). *Public health nursing leader*. Daughter of William Sewall Gardner and Mary (Thornton) Gardner, a descendant of Matthew Thornton of New Hampshire, a signer of the Declaration of Independence. Never married.
EDUCATION: 1890, graduated from Miss Porter's School, Farmington, Connecticut; 1905, graduated from Newport Hospital Training School for Nurses, Newport, Rhode Island. CAREER: 1905-1931, director, Providence District Nurse Association, Providence, Rhode Island; while on leave from that position, 1917, American Red Cross town and country nursing service; 1917-1919, director of the nursing department, American Red Cross commission for tuberculosis, serving in Italy; 1920, special advisor on child health programs, American Red Cross.
CONTRIBUTIONS: Mary Sewall Gardner made three major contributions to the field of public health nursing: she was the director of an outstanding visiting nurse association, the author of the first public health nursing textbook, and the founder of the National Organization for Public Health Nursing (NOPHN). She began her career with a tiny district

nursing agency in Providence, Rhode Island, and as the agency grew, it became noted for its contributions to the development of district (public health) nursing. As that occurred, others began to seek Gardner's advice about administrative practices and about future advances in the field. She was always willing to assist others who sought her advice in developing their agencies, and even in her retirement she was an informal consultant to public health nurses around the world.

Gardner's textbook, *Public Health Nursing* (1916), was for many years the only publication on the subject, and it remained useful to several generations of visiting nurses. A second edition of the book came out in 1924, followed by a third edition in 1936; in addition, it has been translated into a number of foreign languages, including Chinese, French, Japanese, and Spanish, and undoubtedly has had a profound influence on public health nursing in a number of foreign countries. After she retired, she wrote and published a book on the administration of public health nursing (1942).

Gardner might be best remembered, however, as the force behind the creation of the National Organization for Public Health Nursing (1912). Previously, she had been the secretary of the joint committee of the American Nurses' Association and the National League of Nursing Education which was directed to look into the need to establish an organization on public health nursing. Although some were opposed to the creation of a third nursing organization, she persuasively addressed the national nursing meeting of 1912 regarding the need to establish the NOPHN, and she was successful in getting the endorsement of M. Adelaide Nutting (q.v.), professor at Columbia University's Teachers College and the most influential nursing leader of her time. Gardner became a member of the board of directors of the new organization, and she was its second president (1913-1916). She also represented the NOPHN on the public health education subcommittee of the National League of Nursing Education. In addition, she served as chairperson of the public health nursing section of the International Council of Nurses, she was a fellow of the American Public Health Association, and she was a member of the board and executive committee of the Social Hygiene Association.

She was a prolific writer, publishing more than fifty articles during her career, mostly in *Public Health Nursing* but also in the *Visiting Nurse Quarterly*, a publication of the Chicago Visiting Nurse Association which preceded *Public Health Nursing* as the forum for writings on the newly developing field of public health nursing.

During World War I, she responded to the request from the American Red Cross for her contribution to public health crises which continued in the postwar period. Wishing to maintain her services after the war, the Providence District Nurse Association granted her a leave of absence to fulfill the assignment with the Red Cross. From 1917 to 1919, she served in Italy as director of the nursing department of the Red Cross commission for tuberculosis, and in 1920 she served as a special advisor to the American Red Cross on child health programs.

Over the course of her career, she received a number of honors and awards in recognition of her contributions to the field of public health nursing. In 1918, she was awarded an honorary M.A. degree from Brown University, Providence, Rhode Island. In 1931, the year of her retirement, she was named honorary president of the NOPHN and received the Walter Burns Saunders Medal for distinguished service to the cause of nursing. She was also made honorary director of the Providence District Nurse Association. In 1986, she was elected to the Nursing Hall of Fame of the American Nurses' Association.

WRITINGS: *Public Health Nursing* (1916, 1924, 1936); *So Build We* (1942); *Katharine Kent* (1946); numerous articles in journals of public health nursing.

REFERENCES: *American Journal of Nursing* (1926), p. 390; M. Louise Fitzpatrick, *The National Organization for Public Health Nursing* (1975); Sophie Nelson, "Mary Sewall Gardner," *Nursing Outlook* (1953), p. 54; *Notable American Women*, IV: 262-264; Meta Rutter Pennock, *Makers of Nursing History* (1940), p. 70; Mary M. Roberts, *American Nursing: History and Interpretation* (1954); *Who Was Who in America*, vol. 5 (1969-1973).

ALICE HOWELL FRIEDMAN

GEISTER, JANET M. (June 17, 1886, Illinois--December 8, 1964, Evanston, Illinois). *Nurse-author.* Daughter of Henry Geister and Sophie (Witte) Geister. Never married. EDUCATION: 1910, graduated from Sherman Hospital School of Nursing, Elgin, Illinois; post-graduate studies at the Chicago School of Civics and Philanthropy, now the University of Chicago. CAREER: 1910, private duty nursing; 1911-1917, infant welfare nurse, medical social worker, and supervisor of visiting nurses, Cook County Hospital, Chicago; 1917, member of the nursing staff, U.S. Children's Bureau, Washington, D.C.; 1919-1922, field secretary and educational secretary, National Organization for Public Health Nursing, New York City; 1923-1926, staff researcher, Committee on Dispensary Development; 1927-1933, executive secretary, American Nurses' Association; 1933, writer, consultant to *RN* magazine, and editor, *Trained Nurse and Hospital Review.*

CONTRIBUTIONS: A prolific writer, Janet Geister was author of some 300 articles. She worked hard to produce articles which were not only well written but interspersed with wit and humor that managed to make an important point soundly and subtly. Her articles were based on study, as well as on experiences, curiosity, and her power of creativity. For instance, she presented a report which described the findings of an independent study of employment conditions of 14,000 nurses. She made the point in the report that the poor working conditions of private duty nurses would have been in much better condition if the leaders had devoted as much time to that problem as they did to reducing the working hours of the nursing student. She believed that the practice of nursing suffered because of the undue attention paid to nursing education and service provided by student nurses and that the profession should focus attention on improving the conditions of the private duty nurses around the country.

Her views were presented in the *Trained Nurse and Hospital Review* when she became associate editor and then editor after her years as executive secretary of the American Nurses' Association. Her columns "Plain Talk" in the *Trained Nurse and Hospital Review* and "Candid Comment" in *RN* magazine were well received by young practicing nurses, an indication that her ideas reflected the conditions in the profession at large. Her special interest was in public health nursing, and in pediatric nursing. For several years she worked for a specialized agency in infant welfare, and when Julia Lathrop, the head of the U.S. Children's Bureau, asked her to look into the problems of children in rural areas and to establish health clinics, she jumped at the opportunity to do so. For this project, she was assigned to the New Orleans Child Welfare Association, where she helped reorganize public health nursing in that city. In 1918, along with an engineer, she designed and outfitted a mobile van equipped to travel through rural areas bringing clinic services to the rural children of Louisiana. She practiced with the belief that the public health nurse existed to provide education about personal hygiene and home sanitation. She believed that this personalized approach was essential for improving health in a way that providing clean water and sewage systems, for instance, could not do without the focus on personal hygiene and household sanitation.

At the suggestion of Ella Phillips Crandall (q.v.), the first executive director of the National Organization for Public Health Nursing (NOPHN), Geister resigned from the Children's Bureau to join the NOPHN. Her task was to implement the high standards of public health nursing practice which had been adopted by the organization. She did so by providing a series of short courses in public health nursing, but she was especially concerned that the courses be of the highest quality possible.

She was loaned to the committee which studied nursing and nursing education in the United States (and which resulted in the Goldmark report) and to the city of Cleveland where she helped evaluate the work of public health nurses in clinics and homes (1918). Although she found that the diploma school education had prepared the nurse to function with multifaceted problems, in fact the nurse was poorly prepared in school health, industrial hygiene, and home maternity service. She insisted that supervisors of public health nursing actually observe their nurses function in the clinic as well as the home, yet she recognized that supervision could easily become "snoopervision" and impair the effectiveness as well as the morale of the nurse in the field. She was quite satisfied with her work in Cleveland; for a five-month period, she made home visits with visiting nurses and went into the homes of people of a variety of races and cultures. She believed that the assistance being provided to families by the visiting nurse was of crucial importance, especially for the health of children.

In another study, she worked with the staff of an organization studying the services of the dispensary. This turned into a six-year evaluation of out-patient systems and the philosophy behind them. She enjoyed working with researchers, declaring that she had the greatest respect for the recognition that diverse opinions served to help find the correct answers and to improve public health services in the process.

At one point in her career, she volunteered to serve as secretary of a medical society committee which was trying to legislate a reduced program of nursing education. After a great deal of testimony and study, it was apparent that the sponsors had no real understanding of the problems of nursing education or the needs of the public for trained nurses, and the bill was withdrawn. From her study of 14,000 nurses in the New York State Nurses' Association, she was able to demonstrate the appalling economic and employment conditions facing nurses, and in the process she helped to educate the medical profession about the needs and problems of America's nurses. Her report was reprinted in full by the American College of Surgeons.

As the executive director of the American Nurses' Association, Geister was a strong supporter of the private duty nurse. Although it was at a time when leaders of professional nursing believed that private duty nursing was dying and that the energies of the association had to be focussed on hospital nursing, she insisted that the needs of the private duty nurse be addressed by the association. The result was a conflict over philosophy, and the dispute ended with another nurse completing the remaining years of her term as executive secretary. She resigned rather

than devote the rest of her term in any way which would abandon the private duty nurse. Her remaining year (1933-1934) as executive director was temporarily filled by Alma Ham Scott (q.v.), when Geister resigned her position.
WRITINGS: More than 300 articles in various nursing journals; in the latter half of her career, virtually every issue of the *Trained Nurse and Hospital Review* contained one of her articles or a column she wrote.
REFERENCES: Personal papers of Janet Geister, Nursing Archives, Mugar Memorial Library, Boston University.

ALICE HOWELL FRIEDMAN

GLADWIN, MARY ELIZABETH (December 24, 1862, Stoke-on-Trent, Staffordshire, England--November 22, 1939, Akron, Ohio). *Red Cross nurse; military nurse.* Never married. EDUCATION: 1887, Ph.B., Buchtel College (now University of Akron), Akron, Ohio; July 1895-c. 1897, attended Boston City Hospital Training School for Nurses, returning October 9, 1900 after service as a Red Cross nurse in the Spanish-American War; January 9, 1902, graduated from Boston City Hospital Training School for Nurses. CAREER: c. 1888-c. 1895, science teacher, Norwalk High School, Norwalk, Ohio; 1898, teacher in a private school, New York City; 1898, volunteer, Spanish-American War; 1898-1900, Red Cross nurse, serving during and immediately after the war; 1902-1904, supervisor, Boston City Hospital; 1905, volunteer nurse in the Russo-Japanese War; c. 1906-c. 1911, superintendent of Nurses, Beverly Hospital, Beverly, Massachusetts; c. 1911-1912, superintendent, Woman's Hospital, New York City, and Cleveland City Hospital, Ohio, and welfare worker, B. F. Goodrich Rubber Company, Akron, Ohio; 1912-1914, director, George R. Perkins Visiting Nurse Association, Akron, Ohio; 1914-1922, Red Cross nurse, serving in Europe during World War I; 1922-1923, director of nursing education, state of Indiana; 1923-1927, director of nursing education, Minnesota State Board of Nurse Examiners; 1927-1930, superintendent, St. Mary's Hospital, Minneapolis, Minnesota, and St. Mary's Hospital School, Rochester, Minnesota.
CONTRIBUTIONS: Mary Gladwin's contributions were twofold: she was a leader in Red Cross nursing and military nursing, and she was a leader in organizing nursing services and in educating the public about nursing as a profession. Her war service began with the Spanish-American War. She had already had some training at Boston City Hospital Training School for Nurses where she enrolled on July 6, 1895, but she interrupted her education to provide nursing care to an ill friend and to support herself by teaching in a private school in New York City. She

volunteered when war was declared, and she was accepted and enrolled as Red Cross Sister No. 2. She sailed from Tampa on the U.S. transport S.S. *Lampasas*, arriving in Cuba just after the destruction of the Spanish fleet at the mouth of Santiago Bay. When the ship arrived, the staff were not allowed to disembark; Santiago was under quarantine with a yellow fever epidemic underway. She and the other nurses were invited by General Miles to become part of his expeditionary force to Puerto Rico.

When they landed, the transport was converted into a hospital ship, and Gladwin provided nursing care to the ill soldiers and sailors who were brought to the ship. Toward the end of the war, she was sent to the U.S. field hospital Sternberg, Chickamauga Park, Georgia, as a representative of Red Cross Auxiliary Number 3; she became a chief nurse and was responsible for closing the hospital. From there, in December 1898 she became chief nurse of a small nursing unit in a division hospital at Macon, Georgia. Auxiliary Number 3 then requested that she go in February 1899 to Manila with three nurses and supplies. They traveled on the U.S. transport *Sheridan* along with army forces and the wives and children of non-commissioned officers. In 1900, upon her return to the United States, she attended a meeting of Spanish-American War nurses. There, Lavinia Dock (q.v.) persuaded her to reapply to Boston City Hospital Training School and wrote a letter on her behalf. Gladwin returned to school on October 9, 1900, graduating cum laude in January 1902. Following graduation, she worked for two years as a staff nurse at Boston City Hospital and then accepted a position as superintendent of nurses at Beverly Hospital, Beverly, Massachusetts. Her five years there were interrupted in 1905 when she travelled to Hiroshima, Japan, to serve as one of twelve nurses in the Japanese Military Hospital during the Russo-Japanese War.

After a year as superintendent of nurses at Woman's Hospital, New York City, she returned to Akron, Ohio, to care for her ailing mother. During her time there, she worked as a welfare worker for women in the B. F. Goodrich Rubber Company and served briefly as superintendent of nurses at City Hospital, Cleveland. She left to organize and supervise the George R. Perkins Visiting Nurse Association of Akron, whose services included school nursing and a milk station and which conducted the Christmas Seal campaign that raised funds needed to support the work of the tuberculosis nurse.

Gladwin did not abandon Red Cross service during the years between 1900 and 1914, however. In 1908, she gave a lecture on home nursing in a series sponsored by the Brooklyn branch of the Red Cross, and in 1913 she volunteered to assist in the aftermath of a flood which devastated Dayton, Ohio. At Dayton, she was placed in charge of the 110 nurses who for five weeks provided relief work. She also worked closely with Jane Delano (q.v.), helping to organize state and local Red Cross committees, and from 1913 to 1938, Gladwin served on the National Committee on Red Cross Nursing Service, representing the American Nurses' Association toward the end of that period. She was for many years a member of one or another state or local Red Cross committees as well.

When war broke out in Europe in 1914, Gladwin was one of the first Red Cross nurses to volunteer. Early in September 1914, she sailed for Europe with the first Red Cross unit which participated in the war effort. They were stationed on the Danube River in Belgrade, where they worked in the American Military Hospital. During that time, the hospital was under constant danger of being shelled, and eventually it was captured by Austrian and German forces late in 1915. The unit went home, and in 1916 and 1917, Gladwin spoke on behalf of the Red Cross before high school and college audiences, urging graduates to enter nursing during the wartime emergency. She returned to Europe in 1917, when she was stationed in Salonika and where she provided nursing care to the Serbs. It was not until 1919, after the armistice, that Mary Gladwin finally returned to the United States. She continued her work with the Red Cross in Ohio until 1922.

In that year, perhaps because of her active work as president of the Ohio State Nurses' Association from 1911 to 1913 and her effort for passage of a nurse-registration law to regulate the profession, she was called to Indiana to assume the directorship of nursing education for the state board. Her responsibilities included the inspection of the schools of nursing in Indiana. In 1923, she accepted a similar position with the State Board of Nurse Examiners in Minnesota. She also conducted an inspection of schools of nursing in Arkansas between 1922 and 1927. Her last two positions were superintendent of nurses for St. Mary's Hospital in Minneapolis and then St. Mary's Hospital, Rochester, Minnesota, where she was educational director for the hospital's nursing school.

In 1930, Gladwin retired to her home in Akron, Ohio, where she and her family had settled after emigrating from England. Her retirement years were filled with another kind of service to the profession; in 1930, she was nominated as a candidate for the presidency of the American Nurses' Association, but she graciously withdrew when the acting president was nominated from the floor and consented to serve. In her retirement, Gladwin continued to respond to invitations to speak and also held many workshops in which she shared with other nurses her wealth of knowledge and experience. Her writing during this time included two important books on ethics and a tribute to her friend and colleague Jane Delano.

Over the course of her career, Gladwin received a number of awards in recognition of her service to humankind and to the nursing profession. Following the Spanish-American War, she was given the Spanish-American War Medal, and following the Russo-Japanese War of 1905, she was given life membership in the Japanese Imperial Red Cross and was awarded several medals by Japan in recognition of her service during that war. In 1921, the International Red Cross awarded her its Florence Nightingale Medal. Following her service during World War I, King Alexander of Serbia named her to the Serbian Order of St. Sava, and she received the Serbian Royal Red Cross Medal as well as the Serbian Cross of Charity. She also received the Russian medal and ribbon of St. Anne. Finally, the University of Akron awarded her an honorary doctor of laws degree and in the process honored one of its most distinguished graduates (Buchtel College had become the University of Akron).

WRITINGS: *Ethics, Talks to Nurses* (1930); *The Red Cross and Jane Arminda Delano* (1931); *Ethics, A Textbook for Nurses* (1938); numerous articles in professional journals, including an account of her experiences during the Dayton, Ohio, flood of 1913: "The Red Cross in Dayton," *American Journal of Nursing* (August 1913), pp. 829-831.

REFERENCES: *American Journal of Nursing* (January 1940), pp. 105-106; Boston City Hospital Training School Records, Nursing Archives, Mugar Memorial Library, Boston University; Celia Cranz, *National League of Nursing Education Biographical Sketches 1937-1940* (1940); Mary Gladwin, *The Red Cross and Jane Arminda Delano* (1931) and typed resume (1933), *American Journal of Nursing* Collection, Nursing Archives, Mugar Memorial Library, Boston University; Portia B. Kernodle, *The Red Cross Nurse in Action, 1882-1948* (1949); Meta Rutter Pennock, *Makers of Nursing History* (1940), pp. 68-69; *Trained Nurse and Hospital Review* (December 1939), pp. 526-527; Mary M. Riddle, *Boston City Hospital Training School for Nurses--Historical Sketch* (1928).

JOELLEN WATSON HAWKINS

GOLDMAN, EMMA (June 27, 1869, Kovno, Lithuania--May 14, 1940, Toronto, Ontario, Canada). *Private duty nurse; midwife; leader in birth control movement; anarchist.* Daughter of Abraham Goldman, innkeeper, theater manager, grocer, and factory worker, and Taube (Bienowitch) Goldman, garment worker. Married Jacob Kerschner, February 1887 (divorced in 1888 or 1889, remarried, and then separated); married James Colton (Welsh miner), June 1925; no children. EDUCATION: Three and a half years in Realschule, Konigsberg, Prussia; 1881, attended school for six months in St. Petersburg, Russia; October 1, 1895-1896, studied nursing at Allgemeines Krankenhaus, Vienna, Austria, receiving certificates in nursing and midwifery. CAREER: 1882, knitted shawls at home, worked in a glove factory, and then a corset factory, St. Petersburg, Russia; December 1885, migrated to the United States, and worked in a clothing factory, Rochester, New York; 1887, worked in a corset factory, New Haven, Connecticut; 1889, worked in sweatshops in New York City; from 1889 to the end of her life, devoted herself to the anarchist movement, lecturing in North America and Europe on the anarchist movement, labor, social problems, theater, and birth control and supported herself by garment work, nursing, and various commercial schemes, including an ice cream parlor in Worcester, Massachusetts (1892); 1893-1894, imprisoned at Blackwell's Island, New York City, where she worked as a nurse in the prison hospital; 1906-1917, editor of *Mother Earth*, an anarchist publication; 1920, deported during the Red Scare with her U.S. citizenship revoked for her political activities and beliefs; spent the rest of her life writing, lecturing, and residing in various foreign countries.

CONTRIBUTIONS: Emma Goldman has been called the mother of anarchy in America, the archetypal new woman of the second decade of the twentieth century, and one of the most significant women in America in the years before World War I. The Haymarket Square riot and bombing of November 11, 1887 (in Chicago) fired her interest in political radicalism. When she moved to New York City in August 1889, she attended anarchist rallies, where she heard a speech by Johann Most, America's leading anarchist, and where she met Alexander Berkman. She became a lifelong friend and comrade of Berkman and a protege of Most. In 1890, she was elected to the Anarchist Executive Board and began her lecture career, spending the next few years travelling with fellow anarchists, holding rallies, and supporting herself with garment work and other schemes to make money, including a brief attempt at prostitution. In October 1893, she was arrested for inciting a riot as the result of a speech to striking workers, and she was sentenced to one year in Blackwell's Island prison. After her release, she resumed her political activities, did some nursing work for Dr. White, the prison doctor, and worked at Beth Israel Hospital, New York City.

Recognizing that she needed formal training, she spent a year studying nursing in Vienna, where she also attended lectures on sexuality by Sigmund Freud. In the fall of 1896, she returned to New York City, where she worked as a private duty nurse and as a midwife. Through a friend, she became acquainted with the Henry Street Settlement, and she met Lillian Wald (q.v.), Lavinia Dock (q.v.), and other nursing leaders. Her nursing work helped support her continued political activities.

Unlike many of her contemporaries, Goldman used nursing to support herself and as a point from which to attack the ills of society as a whole. Her nursing activities, as well as her previous work in American factories, exposed her to the profound poverty of the have-nots and inflamed her sense of commitment to the larger cause. Upon her return to America, she supported herself and her anarchist activities with income from private duty nursing and midwifery. In 1899, during a second European lecture tour, she was introduced to the ideas of the neo-Malthusians, and she received information on birth control.

In 1901, she served as manager for Peter Kropotkin's lecture tour of the United States and in 1905-1906 for the Orleneff Troupe. From March 1906 to 1917, she served as editor of *Mother Earth*, a radical journal. During this time she continued to lecture and began to write the first of several books. On March 28, 1915, she gave her first public lecture on birth control methods, although she had been giving information privately for several years. In the first issue of *Woman Rebel*, Margaret Sanger's publication, in March 1914, an excerpt from Goldman's essay on love and marriage was included. On February 11, 1916, Goldman was arrested for a birth control lecture, spending fifteen days in jail. On July 9, 1917, she was convicted for her activities in an anti-conscription campaign (during World War I), and sentenced to two years in Jefferson City Prison, Missouri.

During her imprisonment and after her release in September 1919, the government continued its relentless pursuit of a means to deport her and Berkman (who earlier had tried to assassinate industrialist Henry Clay Frick during the Homestead Steel strike). On December 21, 1919, she and Berkman were deported, arriving at the Finnish-Russian border in January 1920, and at Riga, Latvia, on December 1, 1921. From there, she went to Estonia, Sweden, Germany, and England, a woman without a country, continuing her lecturing and writing. In 1928, she went to France, where she worked on her autobiography. In 1934, she was granted a ninety-day visa to visit the United States, her only visit after her deportation. In 1936 she went to Spain to aid the cause of revolution, working there until 1939. On February 17, 1940, while in Toronto, she suffered a stroke, and she died on May 14. She was buried near the graves of the Haymarket martyrs, in Waldheim Cemetery, Chicago.

WRITINGS: Voluminous papers, articles, and pamphlets, notable among them *Why and How the Poor Should Not Have Many Children* (c. 1910); *Marriage and Love* (1914); *Anarchism and Other Essays* (1911); *The Social Significance of the Modern Drama* (1914); *My Further Disillusionment in Russia* (1924); *My Disillusionment in Russia* (1925); *Living My Life* (1931); *Voltairine De Cleyre* (1933).

REFERENCES: *Dictionary of American Biography* (supplement 2); Richard Drinnon, *Rebel in Paradise* (1961); Candace Falk, *Love, Anarchy, and Emma Goldman* (1984); Emma Goldman, *Living My Life* (1931); Linda Gordon, *Woman's Body, Woman's Right* (1977).

JOELLEN WATSON HAWKINS

GOODNOW, MINNIE (1871, Albion, New York--February 9, 1952, Boston, Massachusetts). *Nurse-author; administrator.* Never married. EDUCATION: Attended high school, Denver, Colorado; attended University of Denver; 1899, graduate of Las Vegas Hot Springs (New Mexico) Sanitarium School of Nursing; post-graduate courses at General Memorial Hospital and the New York Infant Asylum, both in New York City. CAREER: Draftsperson, Denver, Colorado; 1889-1901, private duty nursing, Denver; 1902-1906, superintendent of nurses, Denver Woman's Hospital; 1907, superintendent of nurses, Milwaukee County Hospital, Wauwatosa, Wisconsin; 1908, superintendent of nurses, Park Avenue Hospital, Denver; 1909-1911, superintendent, Bronson Hospital, Kalamazoo, Michigan; c. 1912-1914, hospital architectural work, Boston; 1915-1917, nursing with the Harvard Unit, at Camiers, France, then St. Valery-en-Caux, Normandy, and Paris; 1917-1920, army nursing, then civilian work in Wheeling, West Virginia; c. 1920, factory survey work, Institute for Crippled Men, New York City; 1920-1925, superintendent of nurses, Children's Hospital, Washington, D.C.; 1925-1928, director of nurses, School of Nursing, Hospital of the University of Pennsylvania Graduate School of Medicine, Philadelphia; 1929-1935, superintendent, Newport Hospital, Newport, Rhode Island; 1935-1938, travelled around the world and revised *Outlines of Nursing History*; 1938-1941, superintendent of nurses, Somerville Hospital, Somerville, Massachusetts; 1941-1943, Massachusetts state supervisor of schools of nursing; 1943-retirement, superintendent of nurses, Pratt Diagnostic Hospital, Boston.
CONTRIBUTIONS: Minnie Goodnow is known as a prolific writer, who turned out book after book aimed at the nursing student. Because she worked in a number of small hospitals and recognized the problems of teaching in those institutions, she tailored her textbooks so they were easy to study and easy to teach from. As early in 1911, she published the first textbook on chemistry for nurses, *Ten Lessons in Chemistry* (1911). As a result of her military nursing during the early years of World War I, she wrote *War Nursing: A Text-Book for the Auxiliary Nurse* (1917). The previous year, she had published a textbook on nursing history, *Outlines of Nursing History*, which went through at least nine editions from 1916

to 1953. She also wrote a shorter version, *Nursing History in Brief*, which went through three editions from 1938 to 1950.

In many ways, Goodnow was far better educated than many others who entered nursing during that time. Her father was an architect, and as a student, she studied classics and Greek, winning prizes for her essays. Her artistic abilities launched her into a career in illustrating, but that was short-lived due to economic necessities. She then began to do drafting work with her father, intending to become an architect. But the financial panic from 1893 to 1896 intervened, severely reducing building construction and forcing her to seek another career. At this point, she decided to be a nurse and thereafter would devote her artistic and writing ability, her knowledge of form and architecture, and her talents as an administrator to the nursing profession. Throughout her long career, she held positions as superintendent of nurses in many prestigious institutions and guided others in their professional development.

From 1912 to 1914, she returned to her love of architecture, working for a Boston architect who specialized in hospital design. She helped to plan many hospitals, including the selection and placement of equipment. The war intervened, however, and Goodnow served for several years, first in France and then in the United States. In late 1917, she returned to the United States to take up occupational therapy, anticipating the needs of veterans returning home. Her last position connected with the war effort was finding jobs for disabled veterans in New York, working for the Institute for Crippled Men. In connection with that position, she undertook a survey of factory work which would be suitable for the handicapped.

After the war, she served as superintendent of nurses at the Children's Hospital of Washington, D.C., of the University of Pennsylvania Graduate School of Medicine Hospital, the Newport, Rhode Island, Hospital, the Somerville Hospital, and the Pratt Diagnostic Hospital, in Massachusetts. She often took ocean cruises, using the time aboard ship to write, revise, or plan new books. For instance, in February and March 1925 she cruised the Mediterranean Sea, planning *The Technic of Nursing*, published later that year. For three years, from 1935 to 1938, she travelled once again, this time around the world, for first-hand information to revise her book *Outlines of Nursing History*. On that trip, she visited New Zealand, Japan, China, Siam, India, Palestine, Turkey, and Greece, and she attended the International Council of Nurses meetings in London and Scotland.

Goodnow gave time to the profession in other ways, serving in 1922-1923 as president of the League of Nursing Education in the District of Columbia. For two years, she was chairperson of the committee that established and carried on the central school in

Washington. Retiring from Pratt, she remained in Boston and died at the hospital in 1952.
WRITINGS: *Ten Lessons in Chemistry* (1911); *First Year Nursing* (2nd ed., 1916); *Outlines of Nursing History* (1916, 1919, 1923, 1928, 1933, 1938, 1942, 1953); *War Nursing: A Text-Book for the Auxiliary Nurse* (1917); *Practice Physics for Nurses* (1919); *The Technic of Nursing* (1925); *Outline for Teaching* (1933); *Nursing History in Brief* (1938, 1943, 1950); numerous articles in professional journals, including "In the Heart of China," *Trained Nurse and Hospital Review* (January 1937), pp. 21-30, and "In the Land of Egypt," *American Journal of Nursing* (1925), pp. 755-758.
REFERENCES: *American Journal of Nursing* (April 1952), p. 511; Meta Rutter Pennock, *Makers of Nursing History* (1928), pp. 84-85.
JOELLEN WATSON HAWKINS

GOODRICH, ANNIE WARBURTON (February 6, 1866, New Brunswick, New Jersey--December 31, 1954, Cobalt, Connecticut). *Nurse-educator; leader.* Daughter of Samuel Griswold Goodrich, representative for the Equitable Life Assurance Society, and Annie (Butler) Goodrich. Never married. EDUCATION: Tutored by a governess until age eleven, then enrolled in Miss Churchill's Private School, Berlin, Connecticut; 1880, attended Miss Budd's School, London, England; also attended Miss Goldie's Day School, Tunbridge Wells, England, and Pere Hycinthe Loyson's School, Paris, France; November 5, 1890-September 30, 1892, attended New York Hospital School of Nursing, where Lillian Wald (q.v.) was the senior student who gave her an initiation on Ward G. CAREER: 1880s, companion of Miss A.S.C. Blake of Boston, when Annie's father's health caused a setback in family finances; returned to Hartford, Connecticut, to care for her ailing maternal grandparents; September 1892-May 1893, head nurse, New York Hospital, New York City; May 1893-May 1, 1900, superintendent of nursing, Post-Graduate Hospital, New York City; 1895, became director of the training school at Post-Graduate Hospital; May 1, 1900-1902, superintendent, St. Luke's Hospital School of Nursing, New York City; 1902-1907, superintendent, New York Hospital; 1904-1913, part-time lecturer at Teachers College, Columbia University, New York City; 1907-1910, general superintendent for nurses, Bellevue and Allied Hospitals, New York City; September 1, 1910-September 1, 1914, inspector of training schools, New York State Education Department; 1914-1923, assistant professor, Department of Nursing and Health, Teachers College, Columbia University; January 1917, director, Visiting Nurse Service of Henry Street Settlement, New

York City; February 18, 1918, became chief inspecting nurse of army hospitals at home and abroad, and May 27, 1918-July 19, 1919, dean of the Army School of Nursing; 1919, returned to Henry Street and Teacher's College; 1923-1934, dean, Yale University School of Nursing, New Haven, Connecticut; 1930, for the Rockefeller Foundation, conducted a study of nursing in the Orient; 1934-1937, served as consultant to the Institute of Living, Hartford, Connecticut; 1940, lectured at Western Reserve University School of Nursing, Cleveland, Ohio; 1942, at the request of the surgeon-general, served as special nursing education consultant to the U.S. Public Health Service.

CONTRIBUTIONS: Annie Goodrich's most important contribution to nursing was her leadership in education, exemplified through her service as first dean of the Yale University School of Nursing. When the Rockefeller Foundation gave Yale a grant of $150,000 for an experiment in nursing education, she seemed the natural choice as dean. While at Yale, she not only brought the school into being from the ground up but dealt with those in the hospital administration who were less than pleased that the Connecticut Training School was being subsumed by the new school. She also dealt with the university administration; she fought for granting a degree to the graduates and won, not an insignificant accomplishment, for Yale had never before granted degrees to women. By 1932, she achieved her dream of the baccalaureate as minimum requirement for admission, and the granting of a master's degree in nursing.

Goodrich was one of the "great trio" or "great triumvirate" in American nursing in the first quarter of the twentieth century, along with M. Adelaide Nutting (q.v.) and Lillian Wald (q.v.). Beginning with her first superintendent position at the Post-Graduate Hospital in New York City, she gave classes for students, instituted graduation from high school as a requirement for admission, and arranged an affiliation for students with Sloane Maternity Hospital, beginning in 1899. At St. Luke's, she introduced the idea of a graduation ceremony, and the first was held on June 8, 1901. Throughout her career, she instituted changes that were far ahead of her time but eventually became standard practice. These included educational requirements for admission, a probationary period, time off for students, and more varied clinical experiences, such as in obstetrics and public health. She expanded and systematized nursing curriculum, advocated state regulation and licensure, campaigned in the medical community for recognition of nursing, and always fought for high standards.

Her deanship of the Army School of Nursing led her to fight for rank for army nurses. She also served on the advisory committee on curriculum for the Vassar Camp. She was very active in professional organizations, serving as president of the American Federation of Nursing (1909), first vice president of the American Society of Superintendents of Training Schools for Nurses (1910), and chair of the committee to finance a course in hospital economics at Teachers College, Columbia University. From 1912 to 1915 she was president of the International Council of Nurses and continued as honorary president from 1915 to 1954. In 1914, she was chairperson of the National League of Nursing Education committee on education. From 1915 to 1918, she was president of the American Nurses' Association. She served on the Committee for the Study of Nursing Education (the Goldmark report, 1923), and was first president of the Association of Collegiate Schools of Nursing (1933). In 1934, she told a nursing audience that within a decade, every school of nursing should have a college or university affiliation or be discontinued.

In 1934, upon her retirement from Yale, she became consultant to the Institute of Living (originally the Hartford Retreat), in Hartford, Connecticut, devoting three years to develop a better training program for nurses. Her maternal grandfather was Dr. John Butler, a pioneer in the treatment of the mentally ill and head of the Hartford Retreat for thirty years. During World War II, she was invited by the surgeon-general to serve as special nursing education consultant to the U.S. Public Health Service. She believed that the Army School of Nursing should be revived, but that was not to be, and the U.S. Cadet Nurse Corps was organized.

Goodrich received numerous honors during her lifetime. In 1920, she was awarded a medal by the National Institute of Social Science, and in 1923 she received the Distinguished Service Medal of the United States. She received the Silver Medal of the Ministry of Social Welfare of France and the Bronze Medal of Belgium. She received honorary degrees from Mt. Holyoke College (Sc.D.), Yale University (M.A.), and Russell Sage College (L.L.D.). In 1949, she received the M. Adelaide Nutting Award of the National League of Nursing Education. The Annie W. Goodrich Professorship at Yale was named in her honor. On the occasion of her eightieth birthday, the Yale School of Nursing had an engagement calendar for 1946 printed showing her at various stages in her career and gave her a birthday dinner. The Yale School of Nursing *Alumnae News* was dedicated to her for that year, and she received tributes from all over the United States, including from President Harry S. Truman. On February 26, 1946, more than 500 nursing leaders held a testimonial luncheon at the Waldorf-Astoria Hotel, New York City, sponsored by the *American Journal of Nursing*. Actress Helen Hayes joined in the occasion to represent the average American at that luncheon. In 1976, Goodrich was elected to the American Nurses' Association Hall of Fame.

After the war, she studied, wrote letters, and entertained, feeling that she had earned her retirement. She lived in the house in Westchester Center, Colchester, Connecticut, that she had dubbed "Far Hills," across the street from her sister, Grace. During her last year of life, she lived at a nursing home in Cobalt, Connecticut.
WRITINGS: *Social and Ethical Significance of Nursing* (1932); collections of essays and extensive contributions to journals, especially the *American Journal of Nursing* and *Modern Hospital*, on whose boards she served.
REFERENCES: *American Journal of Nursing* (July 1910), pp. 710-711, (March 1918), p. 447, (December 1922), p. 210, (July 1934), pp. 669-680, (April 1946), pp. 215-218, and (February 1955), pp. 158-159; Daisy Caroline Bridges, *A History of the International Council of Nurses, 1899-1964: The First 65 Years* (1967); *Dictionary of American Biography*, supp. 5: 251-252; Lyndia Flanagan, *One Strong Voice: The History of the American Nurses' Association* (1976); Virginia Henderson, "Annie Warburton Goodrich," *American Journal of Nursing* (December 1955), pp. 1488-1492; Harriet Berger Koch, *Militant Angel* (1951); *Notable American Women: the Modern Era*, pp. 286-288; *National Cyclopedia of American Biography*, XLII: 326-327; *Nursing Outlook* (January 1955), pp. 107-108; Meta Rutter Pennock, ed., *Makers of Nursing History* (1928); Mary M. Roberts, *American Nursing: History and Interpretation* (1954), and "Annie Warburton Goodrich," *American Journal of Nursing* (February 1955), p. 163; Esther A. Werminghaus, *Annie W. Goodrich: Her Journey to Yale* (1950); Edna Yost, *American Women of Nursing* (rev. ed., 1965).

JOELLEN WATSON HAWKINS

GOOSTRAY, STELLA (July 8, 1886, Boston--May 8, 1969) *Nurse-educator; historian.* Daughter of Job Goostray and Jane (Wyllie) Goostray. Never married. EDUCATION: 1919, graduated from the Children's Hospital School of Nursing, Boston; 1926, B.S., Teachers College, Columbia University, New York City; 1933, M.Ed., Boston University. CAREER: c. 1905-1916, assistant to the editor of diocese publications, Episcopal Diocese of Massachusetts, Boston; 1919-1921, private duty nursing; 1921-1922, instructor in science, Philadelphia General Hospital School of Nursing; 1922-1927, educational director, Philadelphia General Hospital School of Nursing; 1927-1946, director of the school of nursing and the nursing service, Children's Hospital, Boston; 1946, director emeritus, Children's Hospital School of Nursing; 1939, 1941-1942, 1946-1947, 1951, part-time instructor, Boston University.
CONTRIBUTIONS: Stella Goostray was influential in strengthening the nursing service at Boston's Children's Hospital to such an extent that it

became world renowned. For nineteen years, which included the financial difficulties resulting from the Great Depression and the shortage of nurses produced by U.S. involvement in World War II, she provided the leadership that resulted in recognition of the Children's Hospital School of Nursing as one of the best schools in the country. Her success can be measured by the fact that when the National League of Nursing Education (NLNE) directed its committee on the grading of nursing schools to evaluate all of America's schools from 1926 to 1934, the Children's Hospital School of Nursing received one of the highest ratings nationwide.

Like many other renowned nurse-educators, she believed that "a school of nursing exists primarily for the education of students rather than for providing a nursing service" for the hospital, and she insisted that the needs of students take precedence over the staffing needs of the hospital, even during the difficult years of the Depression and the war. Prior to assuming the position as director of the program at the Children's Hospital, she had several years of experience at the Philadelphia General Hospital, where she was recognized as a gifted teacher and where she began to publish textbooks. When she accepted the position at the Children's Hospital in 1927, she was still relatively new to the profession, having only eight years of experience after graduation. She did not have a lack of experience, however; having entered nursing school at the age of twenty-nine, she was far more mature than others at the same stage of their careers, and her early editorial experience with the Episcopal Diocese of Massachusetts provided her with the skills necessary for a successful writing career.

Goostray was a leader in reviving interest in the history of nursing. While a student at Columbia University Teachers College, she began to collect historical materials. Some of her early collections have since become part of the extensive M. Adelaide Nutting Collection at Teachers College. She was one of three members of the committee on early source materials, which Isabel Stewart (q.v.) organized at Teachers College in 1948. That committee later developed into the National League for Nursing's committee on historical source material in nursing. From 1952 to 1964, she served as regional consultant for the North Atlantic history group, and she was a member of the committee on nursing archives of Boston University's Mugar Memorial Library (1966-1969). In 1965, she wrote an inspirational article for *Nursing Outlook* in which she encouraged the systematic preservation of important nursing documents and in which she described a "Nationwide Hunt for Nursing Historical Treasures."

In addition to her interest in historical preservation, she was an active researcher and writer of numerous articles on the history of nursing. Her book, *Memoirs*, which was not originally intended for the general public, provides an inside look at a number of significant events in the history of American nursing during the twentieth century. Due to her knowledge of the history of nursing, she was invited to join the advisory committee for the vitally important biographical dictionary, *Notable American Women.* She also served on the advisory committee of the Elizabeth and Arthur Schlesinger Library on the History of Women in America, Radcliffe College, Cambridge, Massachusetts, which was to become the largest repository of its kind in the United States.

Goostray was also a national leader of the nursing profession, serving on countless committees of the American Nurses' Association, the National League for Nursing, and the National Organization for Public Health Nursing. Indeed, she served on a number of the most important joint committees of those organizations which made decisions profoundly influencing the direction of American nursing. She was on the board of directors of the *American Journal of Nursing* for more than twelve years, including seven years as its president (1931-1938). She was secretary and then a director of the NLNE, and from 1940 to 1944 she served as its president. She was a consultant to the committee on the grading of nursing schools, for which she took a seven-month leave of absence from Children's Hospital. Her experience with the committee made her an ardent advocate of accreditation, and her master's thesis at Boston University focused on this subject. Then she became a member of the NLNE accrediting committee.

She is well remembered as the president of the National Nursing Council for War Service, from the date of its incorporation in 1942 until 1946. The Council was involved in making decisions regarding the profession's attitude and actions concerning the draft of nurses into the military service, the position of black nurses in the armed forces, and the question of increasing enrollment in America's nursing schools to fill the hospital positions which were vacated by trained nurses who rushed to the service of their country. In 1930, Goostray was chairperson of the committee on nursing of the White House Conference on Child Health. She also served the commonwealth of Massachusetts as chairperson of the Massachusetts Nurses' Association's central registry for nurses (District 1, Boston) and as chairperson of the state Board of Registration for Nurses (1940-1948).

Even after her retirement, she continued to be active in a number of important organizations. She was the first nurse to serve on the board of directors of the United Community Services (of Boston, 1949-1951), and she continued to serve on the board of directors of the nursing council of that same organization (1950-1953). She was chairperson of the advisory committee to the regionalization project in nursing education, which was developed by the nursing council of the United Community Services of Metropolitan Boston (1956-1959). The project resulted in the establishment of the first junior college nursing program in New England, at Newton Junior College.

Over the course of her career, Goostray received numerous awards in recognition of her service to the profession and to society. In 1955, the National League for Nursing bestowed upon her its M. Adelaide Nutting Award for leadership in American nursing. That same year, the Massachusetts League for Nursing granted her a citation and honorary membership in recognition of her contributions to the health and welfare of the public and to the advancement of nursing and nursing education. In 1962, the United Community Services of Metropolitan Boston gave her a citation for meritorious service to the community. In 1965, the Massachusetts Nurses' Association gave her a citation in recognition of her outstanding leadership in improving the image of professional nurses in the state. In 1967, Columbia University's Teachers College gave her the Louise McManus Medal for distinguished service to nursing, and Boston University granted her an honorary degree of doctor of science.

WRITINGS: *Drugs and Solutions* (1924), revised as *Introduction to Materia Medica* (1939) and as *Mathematics and Measurement in Nursing Practice* (1963); *Fifty Years of the School of Nursing, the Children's Hospital, Boston* (1941); *Applied Chemistry for Nurses* (co-author with Walter G. Karr, 1924. The 9th edition of this book became Goostray and Schwenck, *A Textbook of Chemistry* (1966); *Memoirs: Half a Century in Nursing* (1969); numerous articles in professional journals.

REFERENCES: Mary E. G. Bliss, "Stella Goostray," published by the National League of Nursing Education (n.d.); Stella Goostray, *Memoirs: Half a Century in Nursing* (1969), and her personal papers, Nursing Archives, Mugar Memorial Library, Boston University; Mary M. Roberts, "Stella Goostray," *American Journal of Nursing* (1958), pp. 352-355; *Who's Who in American Women* (1958-1959), p. 491.

ALICE HOWELL FRIEDMAN

GORMAN, ALICE AMELIA (1864--?) *Nurse-administrator.* Never married. EDUCATION: August 9, 1887-August 9, 1889, attended Boston Training School, Massachusetts General Hospital, Boston, graduating in 1889; 1899-1900, attended post-graduate course in hospital economics, Teachers College, Columbia University, New York City, graduating in 1900. CAREER: 1889-1890, superintendent, Touro Infirmary, New Orleans, Louisiana; January 1890-January 1891, head nurse, men's surgical ward, St. Luke's Hospital, New York City; 1891-1896, private duty nursing; 1896-1899, superintendent, Mercer Hospital, Trenton, New Jersey; 1900-1902, assistant superintendent, Training School for Nurses, Massachusetts General Hospital; 1902-1905, superintendent, Training School for Nursing, Bridgeport Hospital, Bridgeport, Connecticut; 1905, matron, Susrun Club, New York City; served for four months as superintendent, Auburn City Hospital, Auburn, New York; September 24, 1908-December 1909, superintendent, Lawrence General Hospital, Lawrence, Massachusetts; 1913-1914, superintendent, Baptist Memorial Hospital, Memphis, Tennessee.

CONTRIBUTIONS: Alice Gorman had the distinction of being one of the first two students (Anna Alline {q.v.} was the other) in the course in hospital economics at Teachers College, Columbia University, that was formally undertaken in 1899 under the direction of Isabel Hampton Robb (q.v.). The post-graduate course was developed to provide special preparation for nurses who wanted to prepare to be heads of schools and teachers of nurses. When the program was begun at Teachers College, it was with the understanding that the American Society of Superintendents of Training Schools for Nurses would supply and maintain the special courses dealing with training school and hospital practice.

Little is known of Alice Gorman before she entered the Boston Training School of the Massachusetts General Hospital (1887). We do know that she was twenty-three years old when she enrolled in what was then a two-year course and also that she was not a high school graduate. On August 6, 1899, when she had been superintendent of nurses at Mercer Hospital (Trenton, New Jersey) for sixteen months, responsible for nine pupil nurses and thirty-three beds, the thirty-five-year-old nurse-educator applied for admission to the newly developed program in hospital economics at Teachers College. The handwritten application was sent to Isabel Hunter Robb along with a letter describing her previous experience.

After successfully completing the course at Teachers College, Gorman returned to her alma mater in Boston where she was assistant superintendent for two years, moving then to a number of similar positions in Connecticut, Massachusetts, New York, and Tennessee. In 1908, she was forced to retire due to ill health, and then she resumed her career as a superintendent.

REFERENCES: Lavinia L. Dock and Isabel M. Stewart, *A Short History of Nursing* (4th ed., 1938); unpublished records, Massachusetts General Hospital Training School for Nurses, 1896-1940, Countway Library of Medicine, Harvard University Medical School, Boston; unpublished documents, the M. Adelaide Nutting Historical Nursing Collection, Teachers College, Columbia University; Thomas W. Leavitt, *A History of Lawrence General Hospital* (1975).

JOELLEN WATSON HAWKINS

GOWAN, SISTER MARY OLIVIA, O.S.B. (May 15, 1890, Stillwater, Minnesota--April 2, 1977, probably in Duluth, Minnesota). *Educator.* Daughter of William Gowan and Margaret (Lawler) Gowan. Never married. EDUCATION: Graduated from Roosevelt High School, Virginia, Minnesota; 1912, graduated from St. Mary's Hospital Training School for Nurses, Duluth, Minnesota; 1925, B.S., College of St. Scholastica; post-graduate studies, Catholic University of America, Washington, D.C.; 1933, M.A., Columbia University. CAREER: 1912-1914, entered the order of the Sisters of St. Benedict; 1914-1916, general duty nurse, St. Mary's Hospital, Duluth, Minnesota; supervisor of the operating room, St. Joseph's Hospital, Brainerd, Minnesota, returning to St. Mary's to teach nursing students in a variety of foundation courses; 1916-1926, superintendent, St. Mary's Hospital (while studying part time at the College of St. Scholastica); 1926-1932, while continuing her education at Catholic University of America, worked with Dr. Thomas Verner Moore to found St. Gertrude's School for the retarded and became head of the school; 1933-1935, director of the newly organized department of nursing education, Catholic University of America; 1935-retirement, dean of the school of nursing education, Catholic University of America.

CONTRIBUTIONS: Although Sister Mary Gowan had strong administrative skills, she has been remembered primarily for her work as an educator. As the head of the new department of nursing education and then the school of nursing at Catholic University of America, she brought the school through the trying years of early development, especially since it occurred at the height of the Great Depression, when institutions of higher education everywhere had great difficulty providing needed financial support for their programs. She enlisted the support of local hospitals and heads of other nursing schools to ensure the success of the new program at Catholic University. During the first five years of its existence, the school grew from 36 to 162 students, and it developed a program of graduate studies as well as the baccalaureate program.

Her talents were recognized early by religious leaders, who appointed her superintendent of St. Mary's Hospital, Duluth, Minnesota, when she was twenty-nine years old, just four years after she graduated from nursing school. As head of that institution, she instituted many reforms, including developing a department of medical records and pathology, increasing the x-ray and laboratory services, and overseeing an addition to the hospital as well as acquiring a new nurses' residence. In

1947, when the Jesuits were in the process of founding the Boston College School of Nursing, Sister Mary Gowan was called upon as a consultant. Her contributions were obviously significant, for in June 1949 she was granted an honorary doctor of laws degree by Boston College, in the same year in which the first class of registered nurse students graduated.

Sister Mary Gowan was active in professional organizations on both the state and national levels. She was a director of the District of Columbia League of Nursing Education and served as chairperson of its curriculum committee. She was a member of the curriculum committee of the National League of Nursing Education (NLNE) and served as a member of the sisters' committee of the NLNE, in the process working to bring about a closer relationship between lay and religious nurses. She also served as president and treasurer of the Association of Collegiate Schools of Nursing, as well as on its membership and executive committees, and she was a strong advocate of that association as the best mechanism to advance the cause of nursing education in the college or university setting.

She regularly spoke before professional organizations, her talks often provoking a great deal of discussion and thought which had an impact nationwide. For instance, in June 1935 she spoke on "What Changes in Standards of Nursing Practice?" before the convention of the NLNE, and in her paper she urged that nurses be prepared in the areas of health promotion and disease prevention and that nurse-educators include out-patient and social service departments as clinical sites for nursing students. Her position, a forward-looking one, eventually was accepted by many schools across the country.

In 1940, she served as a member of the subcommittee on nursing under the health and medical committee of the Council of National Defense, and she also was a member of the National Nursing Council for War Service. Her expertise continued to be recognized on the national level, when in 1948 along with three other nurses she was appointed to the training committee's subcommittee on psychiatric nursing, an advisory committee to the National Advisory Mental Health Council.

WRITINGS: "Nursing Education at the Catholic University of America," *American Journal of Nursing* (April 1934), p. 343; with Sister M. Maurice Sheehy, "Contributions of Religious Communities to the Development of Nursing Education," *Trained Nurse and Hospital Review* (April 1938), pp. 404-409, 469; "Influence of Graduate Nurses on the Formative Years of a University School of Nursing: A Memoir," *Nursing Research* (Summer 1967), pp. 261-266.

REFERENCES: *American Journal of Nursing* (July 1935), p. 683, (March 1939), pp. 327-328, (December 1940), p. 1374, (March 1941), pp. 366-367, (March 1943), p. 315, and (May 1948), p. 38 adv.; Boston

College honorary degree citation, 1949; information provided by the dean's office, Catholic University of America School of Nursing; Mary A. Somers, *National League of Nursing Education Calendar* (n.d.).

LORETTA P. HIGGINS

GRACE, SISTER MARY GONZAGA (born Anne Grace, February 22, 1812, Baltimore, Maryland--October 8, 1897, Philadelphia). *Civil War nurse; orphanage administrator.* Daughter of a sailor who died in 1814; her mother died of yellow fever in 1816. Although both parents were Protestants, she was adopted by a seventeen-year-old Catholic woman, Elizabeth Michel, who had cared for Anne's mother during her terminal illness. Never married. EDUCATION: 1823-1827, St. Joseph's Academy, Emmitsburg, Maryland. CAREER: March 11, 1827, received into the Community of the Sisters of Charity; 1828, helped to open a school in Harrisburg, Pennsylvania; March 28, 1830, took final vows; May 1830, assigned to St. Joseph's Asylum (orphanage), Philadelphia; 1843-1844, director of the orphanage during a time of anti-Catholic sentiment in Philadelphia; 1844, sent to Donaldsonville, Louisiana, as assistant at the Sisters of Charity Novitiate; 1845, transferred to New Orleans, where she helped work toward the affiliation of the Mother Seton Community of the Sisters of Charity and the French sisters known as the Daughters of Charity of St. Vincent DePaul, an affiliation which occurred in 1850; 1851-1855, again placed in charge of St. Joseph's Asylum; 1855-1856, sent in an administrative capacity to the mother house in Paris, France; 1856, returned to Emmitsburg; 1857, went back to St. Joseph's Asylum; 1862, when the Sisters of Charity were asked by Surgeon-General William Hammond to take charge of Satterlee Hospital, West Philadelphia, she and others Sisters of Charity began caring for the Civil War wounded while continuing as director of St. Joseph's Asylum; 1887, recalled to Emmitsburg, but after rousing protests from her friends in Philadelphia, culminating in a petition drive signed even by Archbishop Ryan, she was returned to Philadelphia; July 26, 1896, at the age of eighty-four, fell in her room and fractured her hip, never walking again; afflicted with cataracts causing blindness in the months before her death; died at St. Joseph's Asylum.

CONTRIBUTIONS: Sister Mary was an indefatigable nurse during the Civil War years. She and other sisters cared for from 50,000 to 80,000 wounded and ill soldiers in their three years of service. They ministered to the physical and spiritual needs of their patients, and their selfless devotion did much to help dispel the prejudice directed against Catholics in the mid-nineteenth century. Their devotion was made obvious from the fact that some of the hospitalized soldiers suffered from smallpox and other infectious diseases, and traditionally the isolation of infectious disease cases was in "pesthouses" without anything resembling adequate nursing or medical care. That clearly was not the case with the sisters who provided nursing care to Civil War soldiers. In August 1862, over 1,500 wounded soldiers from the Battle of Bull Run were taken to Satterlee Hospital. Occasionally during the war, the space required exceeded the capacity of the hospital, and tents were set up on the hospital grounds to accommodate the overflow. After her death, an orphanage was constructed in Germantown, Pennsylvania, and was named the Gonzaga Memorial Asylum. Five thousand people came to honor her by their attendance at the laying of the cornerstone on September 25, 1898, and the building was formally dedicated on June 21, 1899.

REFERENCES: George Barton, *Angels of the Battlefield* (1898); Ellen Ryan Jolly, *Nuns of the Battlefield* (1927); Eleanor C. Donnelly, *Life of Sister Mary Gonzaga Grace* (1900).

LORETTA P. HIGGINS

GRANT, AMELIA HOWE (September 23, 1887, Utica, New York--August 8, 1967, Amsterdam, New York). *Nurse-executive; public health nurse.* Daughter of George A. Grant and Allie (Stowell) Grant. Never married. EDUCATION: 1910, graduated from Faxton Hospital School of Nursing, Utica, New York; 1917, completed one-year public health nursing course at Simmons College, Boston; 1922, B.S., and 1923, A.M., Teachers College, Columbia University, New York City. CAREER: 1910-1916, private duty nursing; c. 1917, supervisor, Henry Street Nursing Service, New York City; 1920, assistant instructor, department of nursing education, Teachers College, Columbia University; 1923-1926, assistant professor of nursing education, Yale School of Nursing, and director of the nursing service, New Haven Dispensary, New Haven, Connecticut; 1926-1928, assistant director in charge of public health nursing program of the Bellevue-Yorkville Health Demonstration, New York City (supported by the Milbank Memorial Fund), and lecturer at Teachers College; 1928-1943, director, bureau of public health nursing, New York City Department of Health.

CONTRIBUTIONS: Amelia Howe Grant's greatest contribution to nursing was as director of the New York City bureau of public health nursing during the years of the Great Depression. This was a major administrative responsibility and perhaps the most complex position in the country for a nurse-administrator. She had approximately 700 nurses under her supervision, and she was an integral part of the largest official health agency in the country at the time. For almost fifty years, public health nursing had been considered to be that of the visiting nurse working for a non-official or private agency. Grant demonstrated that the public health nurse had an important role to play in the municipal board of health. She defined the place of the nurse in the health department and provided professional leadership to the staff, inspiring them to take pride in their work and to see the value of it. Instead of specialization, she assigned supervisors to the generalized programs so that all shared the experts' knowledge. She worked out plans for staff education programs and secured scholarships for post-graduate training of the nurses under her supervision. She worked to improve the relationship between the various private agency services and the city's department of health.

Grant was elected president of the National Organization for Public Health Nursing (NOPHN) for two terms (1934-1938). Fiscal problems were of great concern to all public health nursing agencies because of the depression, and her speeches and writings addressed the budgetary issues of public as well as private nursing agencies. She was credited with helping to find solutions to the problems of one agency through her knowledge and understanding of how other agencies responded to similar problems. During her terms of office, the passage of the Social Security Act and its health amendments increased the number of nurses employed in public health nursing agencies and also the number returning for one-year collegiate programs in public health nursing. Funds had been made available through the federal legislation, and Amelia Grant's work with the NOPHN developed more public health nursing student experiences in a variety of agencies. She continued her interest in the NOPHN and served as chairperson of the national membership committee.

Another outstanding contribution of Grant, although earlier in her professional career, was in the educational field. When the school of nursing at Yale University opened in 1925, she was put in charge of the public health component of the undergraduate program. Her contribution to both the Yale school and to nursing education was unique. It was she who saw the possibilities for enriching the student's learning through experiences in the out-patient department of hospitals and clinics, believing it to be the proper place for the student to see the connecting link between the hospital and the family. That was an innovative idea in nursing education at the time, which primarily took place at the patient's bedside in the hospital. Annie Goodrich (q.v.), the first dean of the Yale nursing school, claimed that Amelia Grant was one of the pioneers in nursing and that her keen, analytical mind enabled her to enrich the experiences of students.

As a result of her experience at Yale and her work with the New York City bureau of public health nursing, she had a major impact on the development of public health nursing education, publishing many articles, particularly in *Public Health Nursing*, the journal of the NOPHN. She also served as chairperson of a joint committee of the American Social Hygiene Association and the National League of Nursing Education. She was responsible for curriculum study regarding the inclusion of social hygiene issues in nursing education, which was not part of the typical nursing school curriculum of the time. Consistent with her interest in this subject, she contributed a chapter to the text *Social Hygiene*, edited by Long and Goldberg.
WRITINGS: *Nursing: A Community Health Service* (1942); many articles in nursing journals.
REFERENCES: *American Women: 1935-1940*, p. 347: *New York Times* (August 15, 1967), p. 39; *Nursing Outlook* (October 1967), p. 13; *Trained Nurse and Hospital Review* (1938), p. 423; Marguerite Wales, "Amelia Grant," *National League of Nursing Education Biographical Sketch* (n.d.).

ALICE HOWELL FRIEDMAN

GRAY, CAROLYN ELIZABETH (1873, New York City--December 29, 1938, Florida). *Nurse-educator; author.* Never married. EDUCATION: Attended St. Mary's Academy, Newburgh, New York; 1893, diploma from City Hospital School of Nursing, Blackwell's Island, New York City; 1917, B.S., Teachers College, Columbia University, New York City; 1920, M.S., Teachers College. CAREER: 1889, taught in a country school, Croton Falls, New York; 1893-1895, superintendent, Gouverneur Hospital, New York City; 1895-1907, superintendent, Fordham Hospital, New York City; 1907-1911, instructor, City Hospital School of Nursing, New York City; 1911-1913, superintendent of nurses, Pittsburgh Homeopathic Hospital; 1914-1919, superintendent, City Hospital School of Nursing, New York City; 1919-1920, secretary, State Board of Nurse Examiners, Albany, New York; 1920-1921, assistant secretary, Committee on Nursing and Nursing Education (funded by the Rockefeller Foundation); 1921-1923, associate professor of nursing education, College for Women, Western Reserve University, Cleveland, Ohio; 1923-1924, professor and dean of School of Nursing, Western Reserve University; 1925-1926, lecturer, department of nursing education, Teachers College, Columbia University; 1926-1931, consultant in problems of nursing service and education; 1931-1932, principal, School of Nursing, City Hospital, New York City; 1932, retired. CONTRIBUTIONS: Carolyn Gray was a knowledgeable nurse-educator who was successful in bringing about changes in nursing education.

While superintendent of the only school of nursing in western Pennsylvania, she upgraded education by raising admission requirements, establishing set times for entering classes, and organizing students into four distinct graded classes (senior, intermediate, junior, and preparatory). The last was a revolutionary idea at the time (1911-1913). She also added dietetics to the curriculum and increased instruction in general.

By the time Gray became superintendent of the City Hospital School of Nursing (1914-1919), she was becoming well known within the circle of pioneering nurse-educators, evidenced by the fact that she was appointed by M. Adelaide Nutting (q.v.) to serve on the committee to arrange the curriculum for the Vassar Training Camp during World War I. Gray became the first dean of the School of Nursing of Western Reserve University (1923), one of the earliest collegiate programs in nursing. That she was chosen reflects her high reputation as a nurse-educator. She developed a sound basis for this school, and in 1928 when the school had been well established within the university community, it was renamed the Frances Payne Bolton School, after the benefactress. The school continues to be one of the leading academic institutions in nursing education. She increased the length of the nursing course in the schools where she was superintendent. She also revised the curriculum, improved the course content, and increased and diversified clinical experience by arranging affiliations with other hospitals. She was among the first to inaugurate the eight-hour day for nursing students, and she encouraged self-government and supported the development of student councils. She wrote about the evils of overwork for students in hospitals, and she showed the detrimental effects this had on the health of student nurses.

She was a pioneer in publicizing nursing schools. She travelled to talk with many groups of young women and to explain student nurse training. After World War I, the National League of Nursing Education saw a need to attract more students to nursing, and she was active in this campaign, particularly in New York City. As part of the campaign, she showed a series of lantern slides of the life of a student nurse. As a consultant in nursing education between 1925 and 1935, she gave courses relative to nursing education in at least seven different colleges and universities throughout the country. In 1928, the National League of Nursing Education appointed her chairperson of a committee to study nursing education in colleges and universities. As an advocate of collegiate-level nursing education, she created a scholarship for the graduates of New York's City Hospital School of Nursing who went on to Teachers College for advanced training in public health nursing. The scholarship was named the Darche-Kimber scholarship, after two of her instructors.

Beginning in 1909, she was co-author of *Anatomy and Physiology for Nurses.* When this text was first written by Diane Kimber (q.v.), it was probably the second of the earliest permanent textbooks prepared by a nurse and for a nurse. This text was used by generations of students; Caroline Stackpole later became an author, and a total of seven editions were published. She was also associate editor (with Annie Goodrich, {q.v.}) of *The Modern Hospital* and served as editor from 1918 to 1925.
WRITINGS: *Textbook of Anatomy and Physiology* (with D. E. Kimber and C. E. Stackpole, many editions, beginning in 1909); "Health, Hours, and Assignments," *American Journal of Nursing* (June 1935), p. 529; "Tentative Standards for Schools of Nursing Seeking Connections with Colleges or Universities," *American Journal of Nursing*, (July 1931), p. 856.
REFERENCES: Vern and Bonnie Bullough, *The Emergence of Modern Nursing* (1960); Harriet Gillett, "Carolyn E. Gray," *National League of Nursing Education Biographical Sketch* (n.d.); Nursing Archives, Mugar Library, Boston University; Mary M. Roberts, *American Nursing: History and Interpretation* (1954); G. Sellew and M. Ebel, *A History of Nursing* (1955); S. Wallace, *Dictionary of North American Authors* (1951).
ALICE HOWELL FRIEDMAN

GREGG, ELINOR DELIGHT (1889--March 24, 1970, Santa Fe, New Mexico). *Indian health nurse.* Never married. EDUCATION: 1895-1901, attended grammar schools in Colorado Springs, Colorado; 1901-1905, attended Cutter Academy, Colorado Springs; 1905-1906, attended Colorado College; 1907-1911, studied at the Waltham Training School for Nurses, Waltham, Massachusetts; 1914, completed Massachusetts General Hospital's four-month course on institutional management; 1919-1920, attended public health nursing course at Simmons College, Boston. CAREER: 1911-1913, factory nurse, Boston Manufacturing Company, Waltham; 1913-1914, six months of private duty nursing; 1914-1915, assistant superintendent of nurses, Cleveland (Ohio) City Hospital; 1915-1917, superintendent of Infants Hospital, Boston; 1917-1919, Red Cross Army nurse overseas during World War I; summer 1919, American Red Cross Chautauqua lecturer; 1921, public health nursing in New Hampshire; 1922-1924, American Red Cross nurse, working with the Indian Bureau in Rosebud and Pine Ridge agencies; 1924-1939, supervisor of public health nursing, Medical Division of the Bureau of Indian Affairs.

CONTRIBUTIONS: An intrepid traveller who enjoyed primitive living conditions, Elinor Gregg used the knowledge and experience she had gained early in her career to become a leader in Indian health care. She spent two years working with the Sioux Indians in South Dakota (1922-1924), and working without policies or guidelines, she carved out a role for public health nurses on Indian reservations. She faced many challenges in her work with the Indians. As a Red Cross nurse "on loan" to the Indian Service, she was resented by some of the Indian Service employees, and as a result they failed to give her their wholehearted cooperation. In addition, she had to make decisions about ways to assist the Indians at a time when she had little knowledge of the Indian culture and beliefs, all of which required not only scientific knowledge but also common sense and a strong belief in nursing and what it encompassed.

In 1924, Gregg became supervisor of public health nursing in the medical division of the Indian Bureau, working in Washington, D.C., and administering a far-reaching nursing service aimed at improving the health of American Indians. Her colleagues in Washington were many of the nursing leaders of the time, including Josephine Beatrice Bowman (q.v.), Elizabeth Fox (q.v.), Mary Hickey (q.v.), Lucy Minnigerode (q.v.), and Clara D. Noyes (q.v.), who helped her become accustomed to and find her way through the governmental bureaucracy. During her many years as an administrator with the Bureau of Indian Affairs, she learned how to deal with the Washington bureaucracy while she established qualifications for public health nurses and recruited them to work for the Indian Health Service. Because of poor living and working conditions on Indian reservations, recruitment of qualified nurses was perhaps her greatest challenge. On behalf of her recruitment effort, she spoke at meetings of state nurses' associations and published articles in nursing journals, always emphasizing the moral and ethical obligation to work where one was most needed, and that certainly was on America's Indian reservations.

Instead of remaining in her office in Washington, D.C., with all the amenities of civilization, she insisted on making extensive field trips to visit Indian reservations and meet medical directors, field matrons, and nurses working in her agency. In this way she was able to observe the problems encountered in attempting to provide health care for the American Indian and to make changes which may have been required to improve the level of care. While she was at Rosebud, the Indians gave her the name "Helper Woman," which indicates the respect they had for Elinor Gregg. By the late 1920s, governmental leaders apparently came to recognize the good work being done by public health nurses under her control, and as a result she was assigned her own secretary, as well as an assistant, Sallie Jeffries, who also was a trained nurse.

Under the New Deal, President Franklin Delano Roosevelt's response to the Great Depression, more funds were made available for Indian health care. As a result, progress was made in the control of tuberculosis, and at the same time, she became involved in making decisions about how construction funds should be spent. After seventeen years of working to improve Indian health, her sister persuaded her to retire, which she did in 1939, not regretting her decision to devote her professional life to the needs of the American Indian.
WRITINGS: *The Indians and the Nurse* (1965); articles in *American Journal of Nursing* and *Public Health Nursing Journal*; numerous newspaper articles describing her work with the American Indians.
REFERENCES: *American Journal of Nursing* (June 1970), p. 1327; Elinor Gregg Collection, Nursing Archives, Mugar Library, Boston University; Elinor D. Gregg, *The Indians and the Nurse* (1965); Meta Rutter Pennock, *Makers of Nursing History* (1928).

LORETTA P. HIGGINS

GRETTER, LYSTRA E. (1858, Ontario, Canada--February 27, 1951, Detroit, Michigan). *Nurse-educator.* While she was young, her parents moved to North Carolina where they became American citizens. Married, c. 1877, had one daughter, and was widowed a few years later. After her husband's death, she took up nursing. EDUCATION: 1888, received diploma, Buffalo General Hospital Training School for Nurses, Buffalo, New York. CAREER: 1889-1907, principal, Farrand Training School for Nurses, Detroit, Michigan; 1908-1923, director, Detroit Visiting Nurse Association, Detroit.
CONTRIBUTIONS: As director of the Farrand School, which was associated with Harper Hospital, Lystra Gretter made many significant changes. She was noted for her efforts to secure better educational opportunities for students and better nursing care for patients. Many of her ideas about nursing education were followed by other directors of nursing schools. Before she left the school, an assistant principal had been appointed, there were a sufficient number of supervisors, and there was at least one graduate nurse employed on every floor. She originated the eight-hour day for student nurses, discontinued student private duty nursing in patients' homes, proposed that the hospital no longer pay students, lengthened the program from eighteen months to three years, required medical examinations of incoming students, included in the curriculum experience in the diet kitchen, began the school's reference and fiction library, and provided for a three-month probationary period

for beginning students. The last change was financed as the result of her successful drive for an endowment for the school.

Isabel Stewart (q.v.), the well-respected nurse-educator and writer, was impressed with Gretter's ability to put into practice her innovative ideas about nursing education. For Gretter, a nurse's education had come to mean more than the preparation of the nurse to be either a private duty nurse or an assistant to the physician in the care of hospitalized patients. She was among the first to recognize that nursing included public health nursing, helping achieve social reforms and philanthropy, as well as scientific research. She believed that as the field of nursing was expanding, the training schools had to update their curriculum and their teaching methods, and she was a leader in initiating these changes.

Gretter was the chairman of the committee which composed the Florence Nightingale Pledge, which she first administered to the graduating class of the Farrand School in 1893. Historians have considered this modified Hippocratic Oath to be nursing's first code of ethics which provided early nurses with a guide to assist in practice. In 1893, she founded the Farrand Training School Alumnae Association, and she helped establish a nurses' registry on a sound business basis so graduates could be assisted in finding positions as private duty nurses. Gretter was one of the few training school superintendents to be called upon by the War Department to assist in recruiting nurses for the army during the Spanish-American War. During the war she kept in contact with all of the graduates of the Farrand School who had enlisted.

Gretter left the Farrand School to become the director of the Detroit Visiting Nurse Association, which had been founded in 1894. She had been a trustee of the association, and when she began as director in 1908, the staff consisted of eight nurses. When she resigned in 1923, that had increased to sixty-seven. Many innovative ideas in district nursing resulted from her leadership, most notably agency involvement in the community, with the Babies' Milk Fund, and with visiting housekeepers for the sick and poor. In addition, visiting nurses were assigned to the hospital's Social Service Department, and there was staff follow-up of crippled children of Ford Motor Company employees.

She was a charter member of the Michigan branch of the Red Cross, and in 1910 when Jane Delano (q.v.) was organizing the Red Cross Nursing Service, Gretter was appointed chairperson of the Michigan state committee. She was a delegate at the International Conference of Red Cross Societies at which the Florence Nightingale Medal was instituted. Gretter was a charter member of the National Organization for Public Health Nursing, the first president of the Michigan State Nurses' Association, and president of the National League of Nursing Education

(1902). After her retirement in 1923, she continued as a member of the Detroit Visiting Nurse Association board, living with her daughter until her death in 1951.
REFERENCES: *American Journal of Nursing* (1951), p. 352; National League of Nursing Education, *Early Leaders of American Nursing* (1923); Nursing Archives, Mugar Memorial Library, Boston University; Meta Rutter Pennock, *Makers of Nursing History* (1940), p. 71; Victor Robinson, *White Caps: The Story of Nursing* (1946), p. 282; Isabel Maitland Stewart, *The Education of Nurses* (1943), p. 123.

ALICE HOWELL FRIEDMAN

H

HALL, CARRIE M. (July 5, 1873, Nashua, New Hampshire--November 17, 1963, Norwell, Massachusetts). *Nurse-educator.* Daughter of John K. Hall and Caroline (Rogers) Hall. Never married. EDUCATION: 1901-1904, attended Massachusetts General Hospital Training School for Nurses, Boston, graduating in 1904; 1911-1912, post-graduate studies at Teachers College, Columbia University, New York City. CAREER: 1904-1905, head nurse, Massachusetts General Hospital; 1905-1906, assistant matron, Quincy Hospital, Quincy, Massachusetts; 1906-1911, superintendent, Margaret Pillsbury Hospital, Concord, New Hampshire; 1912-1937, director of the hospital and school of nursing, Peter Bent Brigham Hospital, Boston; 1917-1918, chief nurse, Base Hospital Number 5, Harvard Medical School and Peter Bent Brigham unit; May-November 1918, chief nurse, American Red Cross, England; November 1918-1919, chief nurse, American Red Cross, France; 1931, five-month leave from Peter Bent Brigham to be field representative of the Harmon Association for the Advancement of Nursing.

CONTRIBUTIONS: As the founding director of the school of nursing at the Peter Bent Brigham Hospital, Carrie Hall made the most of her opportunity to advance the cause of nursing education. She succeeded in developing a school which was to become highly respected across the nation and acknowledged as a leader in the education of nurses. She was able to put into effect the most modern ideas about nursing education, including the requirement of a high-school education or its equivalent for admission, increasing the length of study to three years, arranging for affiliations in maternal-child nursing, specialties not available at that time at the hospital, and district (public health) nursing as an elective, and she had her students work an eight-hour day, after a six month probationary period during which they attended classes in subjects which were basic to the practice of nursing.

Hall did not confine her leadership skills to her position with the Peter Bent Brigham Hospital. She was active in state and local nursing organizations, serving as president of the Massachusetts General Hospital Alumnae Association from 1915 to 1918 and again from 1921 to 1922, as president of the Massachusetts Nurses' Association from 1921 to 1925, as a member of the board of the National League of Nursing Education (NLNE) from 1922 to 1932, and as president of the NLNE from 1926 to 1927. She was most interested in the problem of security for nurses in their retirement years, and she was an active member of various committees which dealt with that subject. For five months in 1931, she even served as a field representative of the Harmon Association for the Advancement of Nursing, an annuity plan, and she travelled across the country meeting with groups of nurses to encourage them to plan for their retirement years. Since most nurses never married, they would not have family to care for their needs as they grew older, and low salaries of hospital as well as private duty nurses restricted their opportunity to save for the future. During the years following her work with the Harmon Association, many of Hall's publications dealt with retirement planning. She served for many years as a member of the board of directors of the Harmon Association.

During World War I, Hall's administrative skills were used in the service of her country. She was the chief nurse of the Harvard Medical School and Peter Bent Hospital Unit Number 5, which took over General Hospital Number 11 of the British Expeditionary Forces in Dannes Camiers, France. The unit then moved to General Hospital Number 13, at Boulogne. In May 1918, Hall was appointed to the new position of chief nurse for the American Red Cross in England. Her job included the enrollment, assignment, and supervision of Red Cross nurses. While there, she organized a local committee on Red Cross nursing, and she enrolled more than one hundred American nurses. She also established two convalescent homes, one catering to army, navy, and Red Cross nurses, as well as other female workers who needed rest and recuperation. Another of her contributions was the establishment of a budget system and a procedure which ensured a better-equipped headquarters.

In September 1918 she left England to return to France as chief nurse. While in France, her correspondence to Clara Noyes (q.v.) reflected her concern about Jane Delano (q.v.), who fell ill and died on April 15, 1919, a few days after the Cannes conference which she was unable to attend. Hall participated at that meeting, which laid the groundwork for a League of Red Cross Societies. When the war ended, Hall oversaw the demobilization of American Red Cross nurses in France, urging their speedy deployment, since (as she wrote to Clara Noyes), the French people no longer needed or wanted such a large American presence in their country. In March 1919 Hall asked to be relieved of her European duties, as she had been overseas for two full years. Her recommendations for the future operation of the Red Cross Nursing Bureau abroad were accepted and promulgated throughout Europe. They addressed various issues, including lines of command, support with advisory services, adequate personnel, and the maintenance of nursing records.

Hall's ideas were carried to others through numerous speeches and articles in professional journals. As chairperson of the committee that published the *Quarterly Record*, the alumnae journal of the Massachusetts General Hospital Training School for Nurses, she made some improvements such as establishing better business procedures and adding a reporter to the committee.

Hall has been honored for her contributions to the profession and to humanity. In 1929 the International Red Cross awarded her the Florence Nightingale Medal, and from France she received La Medaille de la reconnaisance. She also received awards for distinguished service from the Royal Red Cross of England. In June 1937, the Peter Bent Brigham *Alumnae Journal* was dedicated to her. At the 1956 convention of the Massachusetts Nurses' Association, a special citation honoring Hall was read by Stella Goostray (q.v.), the well-known nursing historian. Hall died at the age of ninety, after a long illness.

WRITINGS: "Taking Courage: The Presidential Address--1926," *American Journal of Nursing* (July 1926), pp. 547-550; "The Effect of the Grading Committee Report on Schools of Nursing," *American Journal of Nursing* (February 1929), pp. 129-134; "Security and Contentment," *American Journal of Nursing* (February 1931), pp. 175-176; "Protected Retirement Income," *American Journal of Nursing* (February 1932), pp. 177-179; "Success of the Harmon Plan," *American Journal of Nursing* (April 1933), pp. 313-315.

REFERENCES: *American Journal of Nursing* (July 1925), p. 582, (July 1926), pp. 578-580, (June 1937), pp. 686-687, and (February 1964), p. 55; Emily Bax, "The Harmon Association's Field Representative Reports Progress," *American Journal of Nursing* (January 1931), pp. 70-71; Sally Johnson, *National League of Nursing Education Biographical Sketch* (n.d.); Portia B. Kernodle, *The Red Cross Nurse in Action: 1882-1948* (1949); Marilyn King, "Nursing Education at Peter Bent Brigham Hospital: The Carrie M. Hall Years, 1912-1937," abstract of a talk about Hall, generously provided by King; Massachusetts General Hospital Training School for Nurses Collection, 1896-1940, Rare Book Room, Francis A. Countway Library of Medicine, Boston; M. Adelaide Nutting Collection, Teachers College, Columbia University, (microfiche number AN 0387); *Nursing Outlook* (January 1964), p. 8; Meta Rutter Pennock, *Makers of*

Nursing History (1928); Sylvia Perkins, *A Centennial Review: The Massachusetts General Hospital School of Nursing, 1873-1973* (1975).

LORETTA P. HIGGINS

HAMPTON, ISABEL ADAMS. See **ROBB, ISABEL ADAMS {HAMPTON}.**

HARMER, BERTHA (?, Port Hope, Ontario, Canada--December 14, 1934, Toronto, Ontario, Canada). *Nurse-educator; author.* Daughter of Mr. and Mrs. John Harmer. Never married. EDUCATION: Attended Jarvis Collegiate Institute, Toronto, Ontario, Canada; 1913, graduated from Toronto General Hospital School of Nursing; post-graduate study in social case work at the School of Philanthropy, New York City; c. 1916-1918, attended Teachers College, Columbia University, New York City, receiving a B.S. in 1918; c. 1920-1928, M.A., Teachers College, Columbia University. CAREER: 1913-1915, head nurse, instructor, and supervisor, Toronto General Hospital School of Nursing; 1918, taught at Vassar Training Camp, Poughkeepsie, New York; 1918-1923, head nurse and instructor, St. Luke's Hospital School of Nursing, New York City; 1923-1927, assistant professor of nursing, Yale University, New Haven, Connecticut, and assistant superintendent of nurses, New Haven Hospital; 1928-1934, director of the McGill University School of Graduate Nurses, Montreal, Canada; resigned because of ill health and died shortly after.

CONTRIBUTIONS: Bertha Harmer was a woman of many talents, which she had successfully demonstrated before she entered the nursing profession. Trained as a teacher, she became involved in business before she had an opportunity to practice that profession. Although she enjoyed her work and received rapid promotion, she eventually sought a more personally satisfying career. After a trip abroad, she entered the School of Nursing at the Toronto General Hospital. Her intellectual gifts were obvious when she was a student at Toronto General Hospital; by the last year, she was often placed in charge of wards, and she graduated first out of a class of forty. She is best known as the author of the highly successful and influential book, *Textbook of the Principles and Practice of Nursing* (1922). Her books became known all over the world, as they were translated into a number of foreign languages and served as the basis for nursing education in many countries. She expressed herself eloquently in her books, where she defined nursing and included roles still seen as important today. Her focus was on the importance of disease prevention, health promotion, and teaching, as well as caring for the sick. Her second book, *The Principles and Methods of Teaching the Principles and Practice of Nursing* (1926), has been considered the first book written for teachers of nursing rather than for their students.

As one of the first professors of nursing at Yale University, Harmer was involved in the early development of that prestigious school, where she was able to influence the shape and content of the curriculum. After her time in New Haven, she returned to Canada, and as director of the McGill School for Graduate Nurses, she nurtured it through the financially trying years of the Great Depression, never wavering in her optimism that the school would outlast the financial troubles of the time. She was a private person, shy and uncomfortable in groups, which probably explains the fact that in spite of her important positions and exceptional research and writing ability, she did not participate in nursing organizations, although she often was asked to become involved in leadership positions.

WRITINGS: Listed above.

REFERENCES: *American Journal of Nursing* (May 1928), p. 465 and (January 1935), pp. 90-91; American Journal of Nursing Collection, Nursing Archives, Mugar Memorial Library, Boston University; *Canadian Nurse* (September 1928), p. 463, (September 1934), p. 415, and (January 1935), p. 18; Meta Rutter Pennock, *Makers of Nursing History* (1928).

LORETTA P. HIGGINS

HASSON, ESTHER VOORHEES (?, Baltimore, Maryland--March 8, 1942, Washington, D.C.) *Military nurse.* Daughter of Colonel Alexander Hasson, member of the U.S. Army Medical Corps, and Mrs. Hasson. Never married. EDUCATION: 1897, graduated from Connecticut Training School, New Haven. CAREER: 1897, private duty nursing; June 1, 1898, contract nurse, U.S. Army; 1900, chief nurse, U.S. Army Nurse Corps; 1901, nurse, Letterman General Hospital, San Francisco; 1901, discharged from the army upon her request; c. 1904-1908, nurse, Isthmian Canal Service, Panama Canal Zone; 1908-1911, superintendent of the Navy Nurse Corps; 1917, active duty with the Army Nurse Corps reserve force; 1917-1918, active duty as a member of the Army Nurse Corps, serving in France.

CONTRIBUTIONS: Esther Hasson was one of the few nurses who served with both the army and navy nurse corps. In 1898, she was asked by Dr.

Anita Newcomb McGee, acting assistant surgeon-general in charge of the army nurse division, if she would accept an assignment within the division. The assignment was with the hospital ship *Relief*, which was dispatched to evacuate the sick and wounded from Cuba during and immediately after the Spanish-American War. The military personnel who were being evacuated by the *Relief* were not only those suffering from battlefield wounds but also those who contracted yellow fever, malaria, typhoid fever, and dysentery. After a year on the hospital ship, Hasson was assigned to provide nursing service for the military in the Philippines. Upon her return to the United States after her tour of duty in the Pacific, she was assigned to hospitals in the San Francisco area. Since the war was over and she did not see any need for her to continue as a military nurse, she requested a discharge from the service. Shortly afterwards, Esther Hasson became a staff nurse and then chief nurse on the public health team of Dr. William C. Gorgas in the first years of the building of the Panama Canal. Nurses who had cared for patients with tropical diseases such as those who had served in the Philippines and Cuba during the Spanish-American War were eagerly recruited for these positions.

In 1908, she was again asked to assume a position with the armed forces, this time as superintendent of the newly created Navy Nurse Corps. She was active in that position for the next three years, during which she developed practice manuals and protocols for naval nursing service, including standardized uniforms, benefits, and personnel practices. She is well remembered as the one who designed the insignia of the naval nurses. Before being authorized to wear the insignia, naval nurses had to complete successfully a six-month trial assignment in the military.

In 1909, she wrote two articles on the Navy Nurse Corps which were published in the *American Journal of Nursing*, and she was explicit about the stringent requirements for admission to the corps but encouraging to the well-qualified recent graduates of America's nursing schools. She oversaw the development of the Navy Nurse Corps from its beginnings with the first twenty nurses who were inducted, and before she left her position, naval nurses were receiving assignments around the world. By 1911 some who were stationed in Guam had started a nursing school for the natives of that region.

Once again, during World War I, she was recalled into active duty, this time with the Army Nurse Corps. She served overseas with Base Hospital Number 12 and with the Army Red Cross Military Hospital, in France. She left active service on June 21, 1918. Hasson was secretary of the Spanish-American War Nurses' Association, and she

was active in fighting for the interests of those who had served with her in Cuba and the Philippines.
WRITINGS: "The Navy Nurse Corps," *American Journal of Nursing* (1909), pp. 262-264, 410-415.
REFERENCES: *American Journal of Nursing* (1908), pp. 91-92 and (1942), pp. 602-603; Josephine Dolan et al., *Nursing in Society: A Historical Perspective* (1983), p. 288; Meta Rutter Pennock, *Makers of Nursing History* (1928), p. 72.

ALICE HOWELL FRIEDMAN

HAUPT, ALMA CECELIA (March 19, 1893, St. Paul, Minnesota--March 14, 1956, San Francisco). *Public health nurse.* Daughter of Rev. Charles Edgar Haupt, Episcopal minister, and Alexandra (Dougan) Haupt. Never married. EDUCATION: Attended local schools in St. Paul, Minnesota; 1915, B.A., University of Minnesota, Minneapolis; 1916-1918, attended University Hospital School for Nurses, University of Minnesota; 1919, post-graduate work, Johns Hopkins Hospital School of Nursing, Baltimore, Maryland. CAREER: 1919-1924, public health nurse and 1922-1924, superintendent, Visiting Nurse Association of Minneapolis; 1922-1924, part-time faculty in public health, University of Minnesota; 1924-c. 1927, associate director of child health program, Vienna, Austria, under the Commonwealth Fund; 1927-1929, associate director of the Commonwealth Fund's division of rural hospitals; 1929-1935, associate director of the National Organization for Public Health Nursing; 1935-1953, director, nursing bureau, Metropolitan Life Insurance Company; 1941-1943, on leave to serve as nursing consultant and executive secretary of the nursing subcommittee, Office of Defense Health and Welfare Services; 1950-1951, faculty member, New York University, New York City.
CONTRIBUTIONS: Alma Haupt was a pioneer and expert in public health nursing. As a graduate of the first class at the University of Minnesota, she helped develop courses for the School of Public Health and taught "Field Practices in Infant Welfare," "Practice in County Nursing," "Mental Hygiene," and "Field Service in Visiting Nursing." Her major contributions came as director of the Nursing Bureau of the Metropolitan Life Insurance Company, where she helped to establish a model home nursing program, providing nursing service to insured individuals in communities where there were no nursing services available or where standards were low. Policy holders and group certificate holders were eligible for the nursing services, including visiting nursing, bedside

care, and home health teaching. By 1939, Metropolitan affiliated with 850 local public health nursing services and employed 700 nurses of its own, in over 400 centers covering 7,500 cities and towns in the United States and Canada. Through her leadership, Metropolitan provided many benefits to its staff, including illness, disability, and retirement protection and assistance in purchasing an automobile.

During World War II, Haupt served the nation's war effort by coordinating nursing activities of twelve government agencies, also serving on the advisory staffs of the War Manpower Commission and the American Red Cross. She served for four years as treasurer of the Joint Committee on the Structure on National Nursing Organizations (c. 1948-1952), which examined the existing nursing organizations and formulated the plan for the National League for Nursing as it evolved from the National League of Nursing Education.

In June 1949, she visited Great Britain in the company of Alice Girard of the Canadian office of the Metropolitan Life Insurance Company, to study the National Health Service. Her entire life was devoted to nursing care for the underserved and to the advancement of the profession and its organizations. She believed in continuing education for nurses as an important aspect of professional growth. She lived to witness the conferring of professional status on nurses under the classifications of the U.S. Census Bureau in 1940.

WRITINGS: Numerous articles on public health and public health nursing, the most important of which was "Forty Years of Teamwork in Public Health Nursing," *American Journal of Nursing* (January 1953), pp. 81-84.

REFERENCES: *American Journal of Nursing* (May 1956), p. 564; *Dictionary of American Biography*, supp. 6: 283-284; James Gray, *Education for Nursing: A History of the University of Minnesota School* (1960); Alma C. Haupt, "Forty Years of Teamwork in Public Health Nursing," *American Journal of Nursing* (January 1953), pp. 81-84; *New York Times* (March 17, 1956); *Nursing Outlook* (June 1953), p. 365 and (April 1956), p. 235.

JOELLEN WATSON HAWKINS

HAWKINSON, NELLIE XENIA (May 20, 1886, Webster, Massachusetts--October 7, 1971, Evanston, Illinois). *Nurse-educator.* Daughter of Sven Hawkinson and Agnes (Olson) Hawkinson. Never married. EDUCATION: 1909, diploma, Framingham Hospital School of Nursing, Framingham, Massachusetts; 1919, B.S., Teachers College, Columbia University, New York City; 1923, M.A., Teachers College; 1932-1933,

Rockefeller Foundation Traveling Fellowship, studying nursing activities in Europe and public health nursing programs in the United States; 1933-1934, advanced study in general education, Teachers College.
CAREER: 1909-1913, private duty nursing and assistant superintendent of nurses, Milford Hospital, Milford, Massachusetts; 1913-1916, superintendent of nurses, Union Avenue Hospital, Framingham, Massachusetts; summer 1918, instructor, Vassar Training Camp for Nurses, Vassar College, Poughkeepsie, New York; 1918-1919, assistant, department of nursing education, Teachers College, Columbia University; 1919-1923, instructor, Massachusetts General Hospital, Boston; 1923-1927, assistant professor of nursing education and assistant to the dean, Western Reserve University School of Nursing (now the Frances Payne Bolton School of Nursing), Cleveland, Ohio; summer 1934, instructor of advanced nursing education, University of Chicago; fall 1934, professor of nursing education, Illinois Training School for Nurses' Foundation, Chicago; 1934-1951, professor and chairperson of nursing education, University of Chicago.
CONTRIBUTIONS: Nellie Hawkinson was a teacher and administrator of several outstanding programs in nursing education, including the schools of nursing at Western Reserve University, the University of Chicago, and the Massachusetts General Hospital. She was successful in establishing programs in nursing education for graduate nurses, which were seen as offering a golden opportunity to the nurses of the Midwest. She applied her wide experience to the organization and development of nursing education within a university setting. Her own philosophy of nursing education influenced the curriculum, the selection of faculty, and the definition of faculty programs and policies. She established cooperative student-faculty associations, which she saw as an effective means of providing opportunity for the personal development of the students and for normal and stimulating student-faculty relationships.

Hawkinson was one of the most active and influential members of the National League of Nursing Education, serving as president from 1936 to 1939. She also served as vice-president and was on the league's curriculum committee and its board of directors. She was chairperson of the league's committee on standards at the time it was responsible for the preparation of the influential document, *Essentials of a Good School of Nursing* (1936). She helped to organize the committee on accrediting of schools of nursing, for which she first studied the accrediting practices in other general and professional agencies. In 1942 she became chairperson of the league's newly created committee on educational problems in wartime, which was concerned with the double challenge that schools of nursing faced: how to maintain patient service and uphold educational standards while trying to train a larger number of students than ever before and while many of the more experienced nurses had left the hospitals for military service. The committee also was responsible for ensuring that auxiliary personnel were wisely used and for informing the public about nursing and nursing education. She was chairperson of a special committee which produced a bulletin, "Nursing Education in War Times," which was considered to be the National League of Nursing Education's "tour de force." She was a member of the early Association of Collegiate Schools of Nursing, and she attended congresses of the International Council of Nurses.

In recognition of her contribution in the 1920s to the educational program of the Massachusetts General Hospital School of Nursing's educational program, she was chosen as the main speaker at that school's seventy-fifth anniversary of its founding, which was held in June 1947. Her own extensive involvement in nursing and nursing education was reflected in her speech, urging that schools of nursing change according to society's needs and challenging nurses to continue to update their skills and knowledge through post-graduate courses. Rather interestingly, less than a decade before that time, she had served as chairperson of the alumnae committee of Columbia University Teachers College, which organized a program commemorating the fortieth anniversary of nursing education in Teachers College. As president of the National League of Nursing Education, she gave the opening address on October 13, 1939.

Over the course of her career, she received numerous awards in recognition of her fine work. In June 1931, the Western Reserve University School of Nursing alumnae association made her an honorary member and presented her with the school insignia. At the Jesuit Centennial in 1957, she received a citation as one of Chicago's outstanding citizens. She was an honorary member of the National and of the Illinois League of Nursing Education. She was an honorary member of Sigma Theta Tau, the national scholarship association for nurses. In 1950, upon her retirement, she was named professor emeritus of nursing education of the University of Chicago.

WRITINGS: "Western Reserve School of Nursing," in *Methods and Problems of Medical Education* (1932).

REFERENCES: *American Journal of Nursing* (November 1971), p. 2220, and (October 1934), pp. 980-981, Margaret Carrington, "Nellie X. Hawkinson," *National League of Nursing Education Biographical Sketch* (n.d.); Meta Rutter Pennock, *Makers of Nursing History* (1940), p. 84; Sylvia Perkins, *A Centennial Review of the Massachusetts General Hospital School of Nursing: 1873-1973* (1975); Mary M. Roberts, *American Nursing: History and Interpretation* (1954).

ALICE HOWELL FRIEDMAN

HAY, HELEN SCOTT (1869, Lanark, Illinois--November 25, 1932, Savannah, Illinois). *Nurse-educator; Red Cross nurse.* Daughter of Scottish father and Pennsylvania mother. Never married. EDUCATION: 1889, graduated from Northwestern Academy, Illinois; 1893, received B.Lit. degree, Northwestern University, Evanston, Illinois, and initiated into Phi Beta Kappa; 1893-1895, attended Illinois Training School for Nurses, Chicago; 1900, graduate studies at the University of Chicago. CAREER: Taught in rural ungraded schools, and in high schools, and was principal of Savannah High School, Illinois; superintendent, Southwestern Iowa Hospital for the Insane, Clarinda, Iowa, then at a private sanatorium in Los Angeles; superintendent of nurses, County Institute for Insane and Indigent, Chicago; superintendent of the hospital and training school, Pasadena Hospital, Pasadena, California; private duty nursing; 1906-1912, superintendent of nurses, Illinois Training School; 1912-1913, travelled for eighteen months; 1913-1914, organized West Suburban Hospital and School for Nurses, Oak Park, Illinois; 1913-1925, Red Cross Nursing Service, including 1913-1917, chief nurse serving in Eastern Europe; 1917-1918, director of the bureau of elementary hygiene and home care of the sick, Washington, D.C.; 1918, special assignment with the Army School of Nursing; 1918-1919, director of nursing under the Balkan Commission; 1919-1922, director of American Red Cross nursing in Europe; 1922-1925, director of the bureau of instruction, department of nursing, American Red Cross.

CONTRIBUTIONS: Helen Scott Hay's greatest contribution came as a result of her role as chief nurse of the Red Cross in establishing educational standards for nursing in Europe. When she joined the Red Cross in 1913, she brought with her more than ten years of experience in nursing practice and education and as a hospital administrator. She organized the first Red Cross nursing school in Eastern Europe (1915), and she served as an advisor to new schools of nursing in Europe following World War I. Her work in Europe began on September 12, 1914, when she became general superintendent of the 126 nurses on the "mercy ship" S.S. *Red Cross* bound for Kiev, Russia. Once there, she assumed responsibility as senior supervisor of Red Cross nursing units in Kiev. She and her nurses set up a hospital in a wing of the Polytechnic Institute, and in December, the American hospital was formally opened, first with fifty patients and increasing to 800 in the spring of 1915. When the order came to withdraw all units, she journeyed to Sofia, Bulgaria, in June 1915, to explore the possibility of establishing a school there. In 1913, Queen Eleanora had made such a request to the Red Cross, but action was deferred due to the outbreak of World War I. Although the European war was continuing, a decision was made to begin at once and, with the queen furnishing the nurses' home, uniforms, and allowances, eight pupils were admitted on September 15, 1915. Bulgaria's entrance into the war as an ally of Germany brought an end to the experiment a year and a half later. Although the school was abandoned by the Red Cross, Hay remained, demonstrating the value of professional nursing through her activities as a district nurse among the Bulgarians, Spaniards, Jews, Greeks, and Turks in Philippopolis; she finally returned to the United States when it became obvious that there was no end in sight to the European war.

Returning to Europe on October 4, 1918, she served as director of nursing under the Balkan Commission, organizing a nursing unit for the Balkans and sending nurses to Albania, Greece, Rumania, and Serbia. Her work included directing relief work for orphans and destitute persons, who were so numerous in postwar Europe. In November 1919, she was appointed director of American Red Cross nursing in Europe, a post she held until her return to the United States on June 4, 1922. During her tenure in that position, she travelled numerous times from headquarters in Paris to the Balkans, Czechoslovakia, Poland, and the Baltic states in order to support her staff and oversee the work of her nurses. She became known as "Sister Helen" to the women in Sofia, Bulgaria, and to peasants in Tirana, Albania. She also provided an advisory service to new schools of nursing in Bulgaria, Czechoslovakia, Greece, and Poland and to the Florence Nightingale School at Bordeaux, France. After her return to the United States, she continued Red Cross work until 1925. Thereafter, ill health permitted her only intermittent periods when she could resume her local Red Cross work and other community activities.

She received many honors for her work in international nursing. She was given the honor of representing the American Red Cross Nursing Service at the laying of the cornerstone for the American Nurses' War Memorial in Bordeaux. In addition she received numerous decorations from the countries in which she served, including the first order of decoration conferred on a foreign woman by the Bulgarian Red Cross, the jeweled Cross of the Good Samaritan from Queen Eleanora of Bulgaria, the third order of the Cross of St. Sava of Serbia, and the Gold Cross of St. Anne by the Russian government, and she was one of six Americans to receive the Florence Nightgale Medal for distinguished service in peace and war conferred by the International Committee of the Red Cross (1920). In 1922, Northwestern University conferred on her an honorary doctor of humane letters degree.

In addition to her international work, she demonstrated her concern for the educational standards of nursing education, through reforms she instituted while serving as superintendent of the Illinois Training School for Nurses at Chicago. During her tenure, a number of wards came under the aegis of the training school, the Nurses' home was enlarged and provided with new baths and lavatories, and the nursing staff was expanded to meet the demand for the nursing service. Hours on duty were reduced, and nurses who were ill were attended by a graduate resident nurse in the nurses' home. The curriculum was enlarged by the addition of dietary instruction, massage, and physical education, and a preliminary instructor was added for the probationers. Awards and scholarships were established to recognize achievement by the hardworking nurses. Recognizing the need for social events, Hay began to schedule musicals, receptions, and social teas. In effect, she considered herself as a mother, with the training school her household.

In addition to her work in Illinois and in Europe, she served her profession as an active member of the National League of Nursing Education. When she died, she was buried in the family cemetery near Savannah, Illinois, with full military honors arranged by the American Legion.

WRITINGS: Numerous letters and reports, some of which are published in the history of the Illinois Training School and in histories of the American Red Cross; also countless unpublished reports and letters.

REFERENCES: *American Journal of Nursing* (April 1920), pp. 561-562 (October 1920), p. 39, and (January 1933), pp. 67-68; American Journal of Nursing Collection, Nursing Archives, Mugar Memorial Library, Boston University; *British Journal of Nursing* (February 10, 1912), pp. 105-106; *Daughters of the American Revolution Magazine* (November 1929), pp. 642-644; Lavinia L. Dock, Sarah E. Pickett, Clara D. Noyes, Fannie F. Clement, Elizabeth G. Fox, and Anna R. Van Meter, *History of American Red Cross Nursing* (1922); Portia B. Kernodle, *The Red Cross Nurse in Action, 1882-1948* (1949); National League of Nursing Education, *Leaders of American Nursing* (1924); *Pacific Coast Journal of Nursing*, (July 1914), p. 219; *Pacific Coast Nursing Journal* (January 1933), pp. 25-26; Meta Rutter Pennock, ed., *Makers of Nursing History* (1928), pp. 68-69; Grace Fay Schryver, *A History of the Illinois Training School for Nurses, 1880-1929* (1930); *Trained Nurse and Hospital Review* (January 1933), p. 44.

JOELLEN WATSON HAWKINS

HEIDE, WILMA SCOTT (February 26, 1921, Ferndale, Pennsylvania--May 8, 1985, Norristown, Pennsylvania). *Feminist leader.* Daughter of William Robert Scott, brakeman for the Baltimore and Ohio Railroad, and Ada (Long) Scott. Married Eugene Heide, May 27, 1951 (divorced in 1972); two daughters. EDUCATION: 1942-1945, attended Brooklyn State

Hospital nursing school, Brooklyn, New York, graduating in 1945; c. 1950, A.B. in sociology and psychology and Litt.M. in sociology and nursing, University of Pittsburgh; 1978, Ph.D., Union for Experimental Colleges and Universities, Cincinnati, Ohio. CAREER: 1938-1942, clerk in department store, attendant in mental hospital, worker in electrical instrument factory; 1945-c. 1947, nurse, state mental hospital, Torrance, Pennsylvania; c. 1947-1948, nurse, Mayview State Hospital, Pennsylvania; 1948-1950, nurse, Pennsylvania College for Women (now Chatham College, Pittsburgh); 1951, taught health education and was school nurse at campus elementary school, Oswego, New York; 1950s, a variety of positions, including night supervisor at Lankenau Hospital, sociology instructor at Pennsylvania State University, administrator of a training program for Head Start staff members, teaching a community-based course on mental health; 1960s, associate research scientist, American Institutes for Research, Pittsburgh; 1975, feminist in residence, Wellesley College, Wellesley, Massachusetts; 1978, taught in adult degree program at Goddard College, Plainfield, Vermont; c. 1979-1982, teaching and administration, Sangamon State University, Springfield, Illinois, leaving because of health problems; 1982-1985, lived in Norristown, Pennsylvania and served as a consultant to many organizations, and as an invited speaker across the nation.

CONTRIBUTIONS: From her earliest days in the working world, Wilma Heide tried to make changes when she saw injustices. Returning to the same mental hospital in which she had earlier worked as an aide, she believed that because she was a registered nurse, she would be able to implement needed changes, but she felt frustrated at many times. She was always unwilling to remain silent in the face of wrongdoing, and her life is to some extent a history of risk taking for her beliefs. While living in the South from 1953 to 1955, for instance, she and her husband became deeply involved in the struggle for civil rights of the black. She actively participated in the National Association for the Advancement of Colored People, and helped in the League of Women Voters' drive to register blacks. She even was willing to put her life on the line for her beliefs. While walking through town alongside a black man, he was felled by a bullet. Heide believed that she was the object of that attack; Southern whites were angrier at whites who supported the blacks, than at the blacks, whom they viewed as pawns being used by Northerners to drastically change the Southern way of life.

Heide was a leader during the second stage of the feminist movement of the 1970s. Her participation in the National Organization for Women (NOW) began when she lived in Pittsburgh in 1967, where she organized and became president of the NOW chapter in that city. With that valuable experience, she was sought by the national organization to become national membership coordinator, a position that included chapter development. She was elected chairperson of the NOW board in 1970, and the following year she was elected president of the organization, serving until 1974. Under her leadership, NOW grew from 3,000 to over 50,000 members and became the world's largest feminist organization. While she was president, NOW took on giants such as American Telephone & Telegraph and the broadcast media in order to eliminate what were considered to be sexist policies. NOW members went to court, picketed, wrote letters, and used numerous other tactics in order to change the status quo and to advance the cause of the American woman. In some instances, they were successful in court but found that they had to be vigilant to ensure that the court decrees were followed. Heide helped to persuade the American Nurses' Association (ANA) to support the equal rights amendment to the U.S. Constitution, and she helped to convince the ANA and the International Council of Nurses not to hold their conventions in Georgia and Missouri, states which failed to ratify the amendment.

Heide became known throughout the world. In 1973 she was invited by the Swedish government to take part in its Opinion Builders national program; she accepted and toured the country, speaking with enthusiastic audiences. In her desire to help others and to generate feminist organizations, she never forgot nursing or her roots in the profession. Because of her support and her work with the ANA, for instance, N-CAP was born. Standing for the Nurses' Coalition for Action and Politics, it became the political action arm of the ANA, an important development in a governmental system which required intensive lobbying to ensure that no state or federal legislation is adopted which may prove harmful to an organization or a profession.

During her leadership years in the NOW, Heide worked hard for the economic betterment of the poor, for the inclusion of all women, not just whites, in the fight for equality, and for the rights of lesbians. In 1975, after her tenure as president of NOW had ended, she became feminist in residence at Wellesley College, where she did a great deal of teaching and lecturing in the greater Boston area. Among her countless activities, she served as a human rights commissioner for Pennsylvania, on the American Civil Liberties Union, the National Women's Political Caucus, the Corporation for Public Broadcasting, and the national board of the Coalition for Human Needs and Budget Priorities. She was also a member of the editorial board of *Social Policy* magazine.

WRITINGS: *Feminism for the Health of It* (1985); among many articles are "Women's Liberation Means Putting Nurses and Nursing in Its Place," *Imprint* (May-June 1971), pp. 4-5, 16; "Feminism and the 'Fallen Woman,'" *Criminal Justice and Behavior* (December 1974), pp. 369-373;

"The Struggle for Peaceful Conflict Resolution," *Feminist Forum* (June 1982), pp. 16-17.
REFERENCES: *American Nurse* (July-August 1985), p. 26; Eleanor Humes Haney, *A Feminist Legacy: The Ethics of Wilma Scott Heide and Company* (1985); *The Network* (Spring 1985); *Nursing Outlook* (November-December 1985), p. 309.

LORETTA P. HIGGINS

HIBBARD, M(ARY) EUGENIE (1856, Montreal, Quebec, Canada--June 7, 1946, Malvern, Jamaica, British West Indies). Parents were of New England stock. EDUCATION: 1886, graduate of St. Catharine's General Hospital Training School, St. Catharine's, Ontario, Canada. CAREER: principal, Grace Hospital School of Nursing, Detroit, Michigan; 1898, Spanish-American War nurse; 1899-1900, hospital ship nurse, Boer War, South Africa; 1900-1904, superintendent of training schools for nurses, Cuba; 1904-1907, superintendent, Ancon Hospital, Panama Canal Zone; 1908-1909, inspectress-general and superintendent of nurses, Republic of Cuba; 1909-1917, head of department of nursing, tuberculosis section of health, Havana, Cuba; 1919-1927, chief of Bureau of Nurses of the Republic of Cuba; 1927, retired.
CONTRIBUTIONS: Eugenie Hibbard is best known for her long service in the tropics and for her role in the completion of the Panama Canal. Born in Canada, she was nonetheless an American; her parents had come from New Hampshire where their families had settled in the seventeenth century. She was introduced to tropical nursing in 1898 when the United States entered into war with Spain. Her first assignment was in Jacksonville, Florida, where she was chief nurse for the Second Division of the Seventh Army Corps. Except for a brief period in the office of the surgeon-general in Washington, D.C., the remainder of her career was in the tropics.

When the Spanish-American War ended, she was appointed superintendent of nurses on the hospital ship *Maine*, sailing under the flags of the United States, Great Britain, and the Red Cross. She was on the ship when it sailed to aid the South Africans in the Boer War in 1900, and she wrote her accounts of that experience in a series of articles for the *American Journal of Nursing*. She was also in a party received by the queen on December 4, 1899, and she had luncheon at Windsor Castle for her work on the *Maine*.

With the U.S. military government established in Cuba, the Spanish nursing sisters returned home, and U.S. nurses were invited to help develop a national health program for Cuba, which was now under the influence of the United States. Hibbard became a leader in the development of nursing in Cuba. Her earlier experience as the first principal of Grace Hospital School of Nursing served her well as she undertook the establishment of training schools for nurses which were so necessary in order to replace the nursing sisters. Altogether, seven schools were established under the Cuba Department of Charities, and Hibbard served as superintendent of the entire program. The provision for licensure of Cuban nurses was secured in 1902, thus predating licensure in the United States. While in Cuba, she also served as superintendent of the Santa Isabel Hospital, Mantanzas, and of Hospital Number 1, Havana. As superintendent, Hibbard became a member of the American Society of Superintendents of Training Schools for Nurses (which later became the National League for Nursing).

In June 1904, Hibbard was one of four persons who sailed to Panama aboard the *Allianco.* Upon arrival, they set out for Ancon (later Gorgas) Hospital, which had been established by the French and which was still operating under the Sisters of Charity, who were not trained nurses. Hibbard's courageous spirit was severely tested by many problems, including the fact that the seventy-five buildings had suffered from fifteen years of neglect, as well as the lack of supplies needed to treat a large number of patients who suffered from a variety of diseases ranging from leprosy to beriberi. Within six months, however, she and the two nurses who accompanied her had created a well-equipped hospital which was capable of handling 600 patients, and two years later in 1906 it could hold 1,000 patients. In addition, she put together a staff prepared to provide care for the crews engaged in the mammoth engineering project which resulted in the construction of the Panama Canal.

As superintendent of the hospital, she demonstrated her tremendous abilities as both an organizer and an administrator. The greatest challenge lay in convincing the U.S. government of the need for mosquito netting and similar supplies. But at last she and Dr. William C. Gorgas, the physician in charge, succeeded in creating a hospital that could serve the needs of canal workers but which no longer was needed to deal with the epidemics of yellow fever which had struck the region for centuries. By 1913 the death rate was less than five percent of what it had been under French control. Hibbard and her nurses had helped the medical authorities to prove that yellow fever was indeed spread by the mosquito.

Hibbard demonstrated her progressiveness in the organization of nurses at the hospital. She established eight-hour day shifts and ten-hour night shifts, and she was concerned with the need for recreation for the members of the nursing staff. The important role being played by the U.S. nurses was so obvious that they received a great deal of credit for their contributions. Indeed, even the U.S. minister on the isthmus considered her role to be so important that she was invited to social events which had traditionally been restricted to diplomats and other governmental leaders. Now, as a result of the excellent work being done by the U.S. nurses, a nurse was accorded that high a social role. Her stay in Panama, therefore, included social gatherings which had previously not included any nurses.

After two and a half years in Panama, Hibbard returned to Cuba where she was appointed inspectress-general of nurses and where in 1909 she helped to established Cuba's first tuberculosis dispensary. As inspectress-general, she was responsible for all matters pertaining to the seven schools for nurses, including inspecting hospitals, and keeping a register of nurses. She remained in Cuba for a number of years, doing public health nursing. She retired in 1927 and went to Canada, where she had been born and raised.

Over the course of her life, she received recognition in various ways. She received a medal for her service in the Spanish-American War, and the British Parliament authorized her to receive a medal for her work during the Boer War. At her retirement in 1927, she was awarded a gold medal by the National Association of Nurses of Cuba. In addition, there is a bronze plaque in Gorgas Hospital, Ancon, to honor Hibbard for her important contributions to the Panama Canal Zone.

WRITINGS: Numerous articles for professional journals, including "With the Maine to South Africa," *American Journal of Nursing* (October 1900), p. 1, (February 1901), pp. 319-324, (March 1901), pp. 395-400, and (June 1901), pp. 615-620; "The Queen's Reception of American Nurses and Doctors," *American Journal of Nursing* (March 1901), pp. 401-402; "The Establishment of Schools for Nurses in Cuba," *American Journal of Nursing* (September 1902), pp. 987-999.

REFERENCES: *American Journal of Nursing* (May 1907), p. 665, (October 1908), p. 92, (April 1909), p. 510, (August 1927), p. 660, and (September 1946), p. 640; Document Files, 1894-1917, Office of the Surgeon General, Record Group 112, National Archives, Washington, D.C.; Janet M. Geister, "Mary Eugenie Hibbard, Whose Nurses Helped to Build the Panama Canal," *Trained Nurse and Hospital Review* (June 1941), pp. 417-421, 473; Minnie Goodnow, *Nursing History* (7th ed., 1942); M. Eugenie Hibbard, "The Establishment of Schools for Nurses in Cuba," *American Journal of Nursing* (September 1902), pp. 985-999; Mary M. Roberts, *American Nursing: History and Interpretation* (1954); St. Catharine's General Hospital Archives, Ontario, Canada.

JOELLEN WATSON HAWKINS

HICKEY, MARY A. (c. 1874, Springfield, Massachusetts--February 15, 1954, Fort Howard, Maryland). *Public health nurse; military nurse.* Daughter of Daniel McCarthy and Ellen McCarthy. After completing post-graduate studies at Lying-in Hospital, New York City, married Dr. James Eli Hickey, physician who was her high-school classmate (he died at a young age). No children. EDUCATION: Graduated from Cathedral High School, Springfield, Massachusetts; 1900, graduated from St. Mary's Hospital Training School for Nurses, Brooklyn, New York; post-graduate work at Lying-in Hospital, New York City, and public health nursing courses at Teachers College, Columbia University, New York City. CAREER: c. 1911-1917, nurse, Springfield Public Schools, Springfield, Massachusetts (at the same time served as tuberculosis and child welfare nurse); 1917, nurse with the American Red Cross children's bureau, Paris, France, then served with the U.S. Army Nurse Corps, also in France; November 7, 1918, staff nurse, U.S. Public Health Service, then a number of other positions with the Public Health Service until 1921 (chief nurse of Fort McHenry, Maryland, chief nurse in District 4 {comprising the District of Columbia, and the states of Maryland, West Virginia, and Virginia}, and assistant superintendent of nurses); 1922-1942, superintendent of nurses, U.S. Veterans Administration; January 1, 1943, retired.

CONTRIBUTIONS: From the earliest days of her career as the first school nurse in Springfield, Massachusetts, to her last position as superintendent of nurses for the Veterans Administration, Mary Hickey devoted her talents and energies to government service. During World War I, she went to Europe with the American Red Cross, but she enlisted in the Army Nurse Corps because of the acute need for nurses when the United States entered the conflict. She served with the Fourth French Army in a surgical unit close to the front lines, where she often had to work under fire. When she returned to the United States, she began what was to become an illustrious career in nursing with the federal government.

Beginning as a staff nurse in the U.S. Public Health Service, Hickey worked her way up the ranks. As chief nurse in District 4, she supervised public health nurses in their work of case finding; they were authorized to locate ex-servicemen and women who were in need of health care. Then, as assistant superintendent of nurses in the public health service, she was in an excellent position when the Veterans Administration took responsibility for the hospitals which were caring for veterans of the world war, and she was appointed superintendent of nurses in the Veterans Administration. Her responsibilities then included the supervision of almost 2,000 nurses, mostly working in the forty-seven hospitals under her jurisdiction while about 400 were public health nurses in the field. With the assistance of an advisory committee, which she requested, she established courses for nurses in specialty areas such as tuberculosis management, and she also developed courses for attendants.

The demanding nature of her work did not deter Hickey from active participation in numerous nursing organizations. She served as president of the District of Columbia League of Nursing Education and as a member of its board. She also was a board member of the District of Columbia Graduate Nurses' Association. Her work for the American Nurses' Association (ANA) included national secretary (1938-1942), chairperson of the federal government section, member of the committee on federal legislation, and ex-officio member of the Nursing Council on National Defense (during World War II). She was the ANA representative on the American Committee on Maternal Welfare. She was also active in the American Legion and was a trustee of the Washington Community Chest. She served as a member of the national committee of the American Red Cross Nursing Service.

WRITINGS: *Bulletin on Tuberculosis Nursing* (c. 1927); articles in nursing journals.

REFERENCES: *American Journal of Nursing* (December 1924), p. 1209, (April 1938), p. 676, (March 1940), p. 344, (April 1942), p. 437, (February 1943), pp. 129, 222; *National League of Nursing Education Biographical Sketches, 1937-1940* (1940); Meta Rutter Pennock, *Makers of Nursing History* (1928, 1940); *New York Times* (February 16, 1954), p. 25; *Springfield Daily News* (February 15, 1954); *Springfield Union* (October 29, 1922 and February 15, 1954); *Springfield Republican* (February 16, 1954); archives of the nursing service, Veterans Administration, Washington, D.C.

LORETTA P. HIGGINS

HITCHCOCK, JANE ELIZABETH (August 1, 1863, Amherst, Massachusetts--April 8, 1939, Northampton, Massachusetts). Daughter of Dr. Edward Hitchcock, physician and professor who taught hygiene and physical education at Amherst College for fifty years, and Mary Lewis (Judson) Hitchcock. She was a direct descendant of Peregrine White, the baby born on the *Mayflower*, through her grandmother Orra (White) Hitchcock. Never married. EDUCATION: Graduated from Amherst High School; 1882-1884, attended Mt. Holyoke Seminary (now Mt. Holyoke College), South Hadley, Massachusetts; 1885-1888, special student at Cornell University, Ithaca, New York; 1889-1891, attended New York Hospital Training School for Nurses, New York City, graduating in 1891. CAREER: 1891-1896, rest at home and two years

(1891-1893) as head nurse, Newton Hospital, Newton, Massachusetts; 1896-1922, public health staff nurse, head nurse, and then supervisor, Henry Street Settlement, New York City; 1917, instructor in public health, Lincoln Hospital School for Nurses, New York City; 1922-1928, special lecturer in public health nursing for several schools in New York State; 1928, retired to Amherst, Massachusetts, where she devoted her time to correspondence and converting a New England barn into a home.
CONTRIBUTIONS: At the National Conference of Charities and Corrections held in 1904, Jane Hitchcock, a staff member of Lillian Wald's (q.v.) Henry Street Settlement, gave an address about public health nurses and their work with other health care professionals who were engaged in charitable work. Indeed, her whole career was devoted to the development of public health nursing and to improvement of the basic preparation of nurses for public health work. After graduation, she devoted a short time to hospital nursing but soon took up residence at Henry Street Settlement, as one of the first four nurses. During her tenure there, which lasted until the autumn of 1922, she was a staff nurse and then assumed a supervisory role as the visiting nursing program grew more extensive in work and in numbers of nurses. While there, she inaugurated the nursing service given to policyholders of the Metropolitan Life Insurance Company. Only once during the twenty-six years did she leave for a brief time, to respond to a call to serve in Ithaca, New York, during a severe epidemic of typhoid fever which struck over 1,500 people. At that time, Hitchcock went to Ithaca, where she established and directed visiting nursing during the emergency.

Hitchcock produced many important articles on public health nursing, which furthered the development of that field as an important specialization for the profession. In 1902, she wrote of the nursing care of 500 cases of pneumonia, detailing the role of the visiting nurse and providing statistics about the cases.

In addition to her role in the development of public health nursing, Hitchcock had a second major contribution to the profession and its development. From the establishment of the New York State Board of Nurse Examiners in 1903, she served as its secretary (until 1919). She was responsible for questions on public health nursing which appeared in the state's licensing examinations. In 1913, she was responsible for the state's civil service examinations which were given to nurses applying for city and state positions. She was also an active member of the National Organization for Public Health Nursing and of the New York Hospital Alumnae Association, serving for two years each as president and secretary.

For two years after World War I, she conducted the public health nursing division of the bureau of placement under the American Red

Cross and the joint nursing committee. Between February 10 and September 15, 1919, she reported that 366 different public health organizations had applied for assistance in securing public health nurses.

In 1922, Hitchcock embarked on a new venture, one she had begun part time in 1915. She moved from the Henry Street Settlement, where she had resided for more than twenty-five years, to Brooklyn, and she devoted full time to lecturing on public health nursing to students in training schools in the greater New York area and then throughout the state.

WRITINGS: Numerous articles in professional journals, including "Five Hundred Cases of Pneumonia," *American Journal of Nursing* (December 1902), pp. 169-174, and "How Much Does the Graduating Nurse Know about Public Health Nursing?" *American Journal of Nursing* (December 1921), pp. 894-895.

REFERENCES: Alumni Association of Mt. Holyoke College, *One Hundred Year Biographical Directory of Mount Holyoke College, 1837-1937* (c. 1937), p. 169; *American Journal of Nursing* (December 1904), p. 171, (January 1922), p. 289, (May 1939), pp. 587-588; American Journal of Nursing Collection, Nursing Archives, Mugar Library, Boston University; Annie M. Brainard, *The Evolution of Public Health Nursing* (1922); M. Louise Fitzpatrick, *The National Organization for Public Health Nursing, 1912-1952: Development of a Practice Field* (1975); Martin Kaufman et al., *Dictionary of American Medical Biography* (1984), vol. 1 (under Edward Hitchcock); archives, Mt. Holyoke College, South Hadley, Massachusetts; National League of Nursing Education, *Biographical Sketches of Leaders in Nursing* (1923); Meta Rutter Pennock, *Makers of Nursing History* (1940); *Springfield {Massachusetts} Republican* (April 10, 1939).

JOELLEN WATSON HAWKINS

HODGINS, AGATHA COBOURG (?, Canada--March 24, 1945, Chatham, Massachusetts). *Nurse-anesthetist; educator.* Daughter of affluent parents. Never married. EDUCATION: Graduated from a junior college; 1900, graduated from Boston City Hospital training school for nurses; post-graduate study at Boston Lying-in Hospital, and studied anesthesia with Dr. George W. Crile, surgeon-in-chief of Lakeside Hospital, Cleveland, Ohio. CAREER: 1909-1914, director of anesthesia services, Lakeside Hospital; 1914-1915, service as chief anesthetist in France, with the Western Reserve University surgical unit; 1915, with Dr. George Crile, founded school of anesthesia at Lakeside Hospital;

1915-1934, director of school of anesthesia, Lakeside Hospital; 1934, retired due to a heart condition.

CONTRIBUTIONS: Agatha Hodgins was an innovator and an inventor in the field of anesthesiology, and she was also an educator, serving as a pioneer in the training of nurse-anesthetists. Not only did she observe and participate in ground breaking techniques in the field, but she tirelessly trained other nurses, physicians, and dentists, both at the battlefront during World War I and at the Lakeside Hospital school of anesthesia. In the science and art of anesthesia administration, she and Dr. Crile conquered the problem of cyanosis with nitrous oxide anesthesia by administering oxygen along with nitrous oxide. She also worked with Dr. C. W. Clarke, who had invented an anesthesia machine, and she made important contributions to the improvement of that machine.

Before the United States entered World War I and after having studied anesthesia at the Lakeside Hospital, she, as chief anesthetist, and Dr. Crile, as chief surgeon, left for France with a special American hospital unit, known as the Lakeside Unit or the Western Reserve Unit. They served in Neuilly, at the American Ambulance Hospital. It was there that Hodgins and Crile introduced the use of nitrous oxide for surgery during wartime. It was an important application because men who had experienced the horrors of gas warfare found the inhalation of ether intolerable. When the Lakeside Unit was replaced by the Harvard Unit, Agatha Hodgins was asked by Dr. Harvey Cushing to remain in order to instruct members of that unit in the new technique for administering anesthesia.

When she returned to Cleveland in 1915, she and Dr. Crile organized what was probably the first school of anesthesiology in the United States, and perhaps in the world. The first class was organized in 1916 and included physicians, dentists, and nurses. Rather than return to Europe when the United States entered the war, she remained in Cleveland and contributed to the war effort by training a great many nurse-anesthetists for military service. Her earlier experiences in France were invaluable in explaining the conditions that her students would find in Europe and in describing how to administer anesthesia in field hospitals. Over the years, the curriculum changed and expanded as new methods of administering anesthesia were developed; by 1930 over 500 people had graduated from the school.

Hodgins was the founder of the American Association of Nurse Anesthetists. She believed that such an organization would help to strengthen the professional position of nurse-anesthetist, and in a 1945 editorial she stated that such organizations were "designed to dispense and perpetuate good to humanity." She called a meeting of nurse-anesthetists in 1931, which led to the organization of the association, originally called the National Association of Nurse Anesthetists. In 1933, she was made honorary president, which was appropriate since she had provided the education for so many nurse-anesthetists and had pioneered in the new specialty for American nurses. She served on the association's board of trustees from its founding in 1931 until her death in 1945.

After her retirement, she continued to serve as consultant to the school and association she had founded, and she was active in the community, supporting the work of the Red Cross, the Boy Scouts and Girl Scouts, her church, and other civic groups.

WRITINGS: "An Evaluation of Anesthetic Drugs and Methods," *Bulletin of the National Association of Nurse Anesthetists* (August 1935), pp. 6-18; "Introducing the Department of Education," *Bulletin of the American Association of Nurse Anesthetists* (May 1940), pp. 102-105; "Permanent Values in Organization," *Bulletin of the American Association of Nurse Anesthetists* (May 1941), pp. 106-108; several editorials, chapter on nitrous oxide/oxygen anesthesia in Frederick F. Burghard, ed., *Oxford Surgery* (1926).

REFERENCES: *American Journal of Nursing* (September 1930), pp. 1163-1165 and (June 1945), p. 502; American Journal of Nursing Collection, Nursing Archives, Mugar Memorial Library, Boston University; Agatha C. Hodgins, letter to the editor, *Bulletin of the National Association of Nurse Anesthetists* (August 1939), p. 211; Clara R. Moore et al., "Agatha Cobourg Hodgins," *Journal of the American Association of Nurse Anesthetists* (May 1946), pp. 32-35; *Trained Nurse and Hospital Review* (June 1945), p. 435.

LORETTA P. HIGGINS

HOGAN, AILEEN I. (November 10, 1899, Ottawa, Ontario, Canada--January 7, 1981, Whiting, New Jersey). *Nurse-midwife.* Daughter of James Hogan and Christina (MacMasters) Hogan. EDUCATION: 1940, graduated from Columbia-Presbyterian Hospital School of Nursing, New York City; 1946, B.S., and 1948, M.A., Teachers College, Columbia University, New York City; 1947, nurse-midwifery certificate, Maternity Center Association, New York City. CAREER: 1915, secretary, Federal War Department, Ottawa, Canada; c. 1920, medical secretary, New York City; 1940-1942, staff nurse and then head nurse, Sloane Hospital for Women, Columbia-Presbyterian Hospital, New York City; 1942-1945, member, Army Nurse Corps, serving in England, France, and Ireland; 1948-1951, assistant professor and chairperson of the department of obstetrical nursing, Frances Payne Bolton School of Nursing, Case Western Reserve University, Cleveland, Ohio; 1951-1965, consultant and director of workshops, Maternity Center Association, New York City; 1966-c. 1970, member of the faculty, Catholic Maternity Institute, Santa Fe, New Mexico; 1970-1972, lecturer, Atlantic Community College, Mays Landing, New Jersey.

CONTRIBUTIONS: Aileen Hogan was a founding member of the American College of Nurse-Midwives (ACNM), served as its first executive secretary, and helped organize its first convention, which was held in November 1955 at Kansas City, Missouri. She was a board member of the ACNM and served on many committees, most important being the publications committee. She helped prepare the early issues of the *ACNM Bulletin.* In 1972, she helped organize the fiftieth anniversary congress of the International Confederation of Midwives (ICM), which was held in Washington, D.C., the first time the ICM met in the United States.

In addition to her work for the American College of Nurse-Midwives, Hogan was a pioneering childbirth educator. When she left her faculty position at the Frances Payne Bolton School of Nursing (1951), more than one hundred parents who had participated in her natural childbirth preparation classes met to pay tribute to her guidance. Hogan was successful in teaching students a positive approach to family-centered maternity care and to preparation for childbirth. This was at the time, in the 1950s, when an intrusive approach to obstetrics and obstetrical training was dominant. She fostered the advance of the concept of family-centered maternity care during her fifteen years with the Maternity Center Association (New York City, 1951-1965). She conducted workshops on this subject throughout the United States and Canada and thereby spread her ideas to other nurses and nurse-midwives, as well as to other health-care providers. Her audiences, most frequently public health nurses, were especially attentive to her message that they could make a significant contribution toward improving the health care of the pregnant woman and her entire family. Hogan's message was that the family must remain the focus of care during the entire maternity cycle.

Hogan was a leader in the development of nurse-midwifery in the United States, and she inspired many students not only to consider nurse-midwifery as a proper role for the nurse-clinician but to continue their studies in the field, a difficult endeavor at a time when nurse-midwifery was a very limited practice in the United States. Not only was the concept of the nurse-midwife revolutionary in a nation which had removed obstetrics from women during the nineteenth century, but the role of the nurse as family health-care advocate was equally revolutionary at a time when the vast majority of nurses were either private duty nurses or members of hospital staffs. In the 1950s, Hogan was one of the very few nurses who supported the natural childbirth movement, although her main emphasis was that it was part of a broad educational program and not simply childbirth without medication.

She received her certificate as a midwife seven years after she became a registered nurse. Prior to her advanced studies at the Maternity Center Association, she had rotated through all the obstetrical services at the Sloane Hospital, then the only way one could prepare to be a nurse-specialist. Following World War II, she took advantage of the GI Bill, which provided educational support for veterans, and as a result of this support she was able to study for her bachelor's and master's degrees in nursing education. Later, she credited three nursing professors for having influenced her choice of a specialty: Virginia Henderson, the respected teacher-researcher, Frances Reiter (q.v.), and Hattie Hemschemeyer, another pioneer midwife.

In 1966, Hogan joined the faculty of the Catholic Maternity Institute, a twenty-year-old program which was one of the few places in the United States which awarded the certificate in midwifery as well as a master's degree. In addition to her work on behalf of various organizations and her educational services provided to nurse-midwifery, she published a number of articles which had a great influence on future developments of her field. Perhaps her most famous publication was "Bomb Born Babies" (1951), in *Public Health Nursing*, which addressed the issue of emergency birth and which was based on her experience during World War II. She also helped to compile a national register of nurse-midwives, but her labor of love was her volunteer work in 1970 which led to the establishment of the archives of the American College of Nurse-Midwives, now housed at the National Library of Medicine, Bethesda, Maryland.

WRITINGS: "Bomb Born Babies," *Public Health Nursing* (1951), pp. 383-385; "A Tribute to the Pioneers," *Journal of Nurse Midwifery* (1975).

REFERENCES: *Briefs* (March 1981); *Cleveland Plain Dealer* (July 19, 1951); Elizabeth Hosford and Teresa Marsico, "Aileen Hogan: In Memoriam," *Journal of Nurse Midwifery* (1981), pp. 12-13; Sally Austen Tom, "Spokeswoman for Midwifery: Aileen Hogan," *Journal of Nurse-Midwifery* (May-June 1981), pp. 7-11.

ALICE HOWELL FRIEDMAN

HOLMAN, LYDIA (January 5, 1868, Philadelphia--February 25, 1960, Oteen, North Carolina). *Rural public health nurse.* Daughter of Robert Holman and Elizabeth Ann Holman. Never married. EDUCATION: 1895, graduate of Philadelphia General Hospital School of Nursing. CAREER: 1894, in charge of the emergency hospital at Mt. Carbon,

Pennsylvania, a facility for typhoid patients; 1895-1897, private duty nursing for the physicians of Pottsville, Pennsylvania; 1897, probably served as head nurse at the County Alms House Hospital, Schuylkill Haven, Pennsylvania; September-December 1898, served at John Blair Gibbs General Hospital, Lexington, Kentucky, then at Macon, Georgia, during the Spanish-American War; May 1901, nurse in the slums of Philadelphia; 1902-1903, nurse, Henry Street Settlement, New York City; December 1900-May 1901, and 1903 to her retirement due to illness in the 1950s, rural public health nurse in North Carolina; 1912, listed as superintendent, Holman Association, Altapass, North Carolina.
CONTRIBUTIONS: Lydia Holman was a pioneer in rural public health nursing. She was working in the slums of Philadelphia when she answered a call for a nurse to care for a typhoid fever victim in the mountains at Ledger, North Carolina. The patient was a well-educated woman of considerable means who was vacationing in her summer home. The woman's recovery amazed the people of the area, who were accustomed to many deaths from typhoid. As a result, Holman found herself caring for many persons who came for her assistance. After a brief return to Philadelphia in May of 1901 and a year at the nurses' settlement, Henry Street, in New York City, where she worked with Lillian Wald (q.v.), she made the mountains of North Carolina her home.

For more than forty years, she lived in a cabin and worked on her own, caring for herself and her horse, riding twenty-five and thirty miles over mountain trails, up stream beds, and fording rivers, travelling from one patient to another. Carolyn Van Blarcom (q.v.) wrote of Holman that at one home, she found the only receptacle to be an iron skillet, which she used to bathe the mother and baby after the delivery and then made supper for the husband in the same pan. Over the years, she attended several hundred deliveries. She had a tiny hospital on top of her mountain with doctors and nurses, although patients had to be brought in by wagon or on stretchers, sometimes carried as far as fifteen miles. She worked alone and accepted for pay whatever her patients could offer. She paid for her own cabin, horse, and food out of what patients gave her, and she often accepted produce or poultry in place of cash. In 1911, she moved to Altapass, North Carolina, where she established a temporary infirmary.

After eleven years on her own, she returned to Baltimore and told friends about her work. As a result, the Holman Association for the Promotion of Rural Nursing, Hygiene, and Social Service was founded and funded, with some of the aid coming from the faculty of the Johns Hopkins Medical School. In 1915, the Brooklyn Holman Association was founded as a voluntary organization which provided financial support for her work from that year to at least 1946. By the 1940s, she had extended her services into many of the surrounding counties of North Carolina, caring for the sick and teaching girls in the various communities how to care for their own sick. She kept a garden at Altapass, where her cabin was located, to demonstrate what could be done to improve nutrition. She also distributed cod liver oil to undernourished children, and nourishing food to those unable to get it any other way. She even established a small circulating library. At Christmas she would collect and distribute hundreds of toys through the schools and in person. She never received a salary for her work.

She served on the first board of directors of the National Organization for Public Health Nursing. In 1936, she was elected a member of the Mitchell County Board of Health (North Carolina). Holman was still carrying on her work in the 1950s, but the Holman Association was short-lived (1911-1912), being dissolved before the development of Red Cross rural nursing.

WRITINGS: Numerous articles in professional journals, including *American Journal of Nursing* (May 1903), pp. 664-665 and (May 1960), p. 634; reports of the Holman Association; unpublished records and notes.

REFERENCES: *American Journal of Nursing* (July 1914), pp. 864-865 and (May 1960), p. 634; Annie M. Brainard, *The Evolution of Public Health Nursing* (1922); *The Bulletin* published by the Alumnae Association of the Philadelphia General Hospital School of Nursing (June 1946), pp. 17-19; Lavinia L. Dock, Sarah E. Pickett, Clara D. Noyes, Fannie F. Clement, Elizabeth G. Fox, and Anna R. Van Meter, *History of American Red Cross Nursing* (1922); M. Louise Fitzpatrick, *The National Organization for Public Health Nursing, 1912-1952* (1975); Lydia Holman, "Visiting Nursing in the Mountains of Western North Carolina," *American Journal of Nursing* (1907), pp. 831-837; Portia B. Kernodle, *The Red Cross Nurse in Action 1882-1848* (1949); unpublished papers in the National Archives, Washington, D.C.; two letters from Lydia Holman, and typed ms. entitled "Pioneer Nurses of North Carolina," records of the North Carolina Board of Nurse Registration and Nurse Education, North Carolina State Archives, Raleigh; death certificate (dated March 8, 1960), in the Office of Vital Statistics, North Carolina State Board of Health, Raleigh; record dated January 7, 1890, when she was twenty-two years old, in Philadelphia General Hospital nurses' records, Philadelphia City Archives, City Hall; Philadelphia General Hospital School of Nursing Archives, Center for the Study of Nursing, University of Pennsylvania; Carolyn Conant Van Blarcom, *Obstetrical Nursing* (1923 and 2d ed., 1928); Yssabella Waters, *Visiting Nursing in the United States* (1909); Mary L. Wyche, *History of Nursing in North Carolina* (1938).

JOELLEN WATSON HAWKINS

HOWELL, MARION GERTRUDE (September 28, 1887, Freeport, Ohio--c. August 16, 1975, Beaver Falls, Pennsylvania). *Educator; public health nurse.* Daughter of John G. Howell, Quaker physician, and Mary Jane (Knox) Howell. Never married. EDUCATION: 1912, received Ph.B. from Wooster College, Wooster, Ohio; 1918, enrolled in the course to prepare college graduates for nursing, Vassar Training Camp, Poughkeepsie, New York; 1920, received diploma, Lakeside Hospital Training School for Nurses, Cleveland, Ohio; 1921, M.S. in social administration, Western Reserve University, Cleveland, Ohio; 1922, certificate in public health nursing, Western Reserve University. CAREER: 1912-1918, instructor of English and later assistant principal of the Minerva (Ohio) High School; 1921-1922, school nurse, Fairmont, West Virginia; 1922-1923, instructor, and public health nurse, University Nursing District, Cleveland, Ohio; 1923-1932, director, University Public Health Nursing District and instructor, Western Reserve University; 1924-1938, director of the course in public health nursing, Western Reserve University; 1932-1946, dean, Western Reserve University School of Nursing.

CONTRIBUTIONS: Marion Howell was a major influence in the evolution of nursing education in the third and fourth decades of the twentieth century. As dean of the Frances Payne Bolton School of Nursing at Western Reserve University (1932-1946), she changed the entrance requirement in the basic course in nursing to the bachelor's degree. She also reshaped the traditional program of nursing education to include nursing in relation to preventive medicine and emphasized the importance of public health nursing. She helped to organize the Association of Collegiate Schools of Nursing, which was to become a major force in advancing the cause of undergraduate and graduate nursing education.

She had a lifelong interest in public health, which she attributed to her two months' field experience in public health nursing when she was an undergraduate. Before becoming dean, she was the director of the University Public Health Nursing District, the laboratory for those in Western Reserve University's public health nursing course and staffed by instructors from the University. When she became dean, Howell expanded the course work in public health nursing, and the program was enlarged to include parent education and mental hygiene. She also must be credited with developing international exchanges with visitors from Europe, South America, and Asia and for securing a grant from the Rockefeller Foundation to strengthen the public health field education of foreign students. Her program was important in helping to meet the need for public health nurses and for providing field training to ensure that qualified public health nurses were available to staff the programs created under the Social Security Act (1935), which included services to handicapped children and prevention of premature births. She was especially aware of the needs of the preschool child. Her efforts directed to these needs included regular examinations of children, and supervision by the staff nurses of preschool-aged children as a routine part of their home visits and health education.

She held offices in several professional organizations, including president of the Lakeside School of Nursing Alumnae Association and president of the American Nurses' Association district organization of public health nurses. Her activity in professional organizations included attending the meetings and conferences from which she felt she gained so much, among them the International Congress of Nurses, which met in London and Paris, the American Public Health Association, the National Organization for Public Health Nursing, and the Association of Collegiate Schools of Nursing.

During World War II she served as chairperson of the nursing subcommittee of the National Nursing Council for War Service and on the advisory committee for the Cadet Nurse Corps. In summarizing her memories, she stated that her greatest satisfaction was helping prepare more than 200 college graduates for the field of nursing and then to see them serve overseas in World War II and later in positions of leadership all over the world. Over the course of her career, she received a number of awards, beginning with induction into Phi Beta Kappa and in 1921 receiving the Edward Fitch Cushing scholarship for further study in public health nursing. In 1942, she received an honorary doctor of laws degree from Wooster College (Ohio). In 1946, upon her retirement, she was given emeritus status as dean and professor emeritus of the Frances Payne Bolton School of Nursing. Two years later, she received an honorary L.H.D. degree from Western Reserve University.

REFERENCES: *American Women* (1935, 1940); *Cleveland Press* (August 17, 1975); Margene O. Faddis, *The History of the Frances Payne Bolton School of Nursing* (1948); Eleanor Farnham, *Pioneering in Public Health Nursing Education* (1964); Nursing Archives, Mugar Library, Boston University (the American Journal of Nursing Collection includes a personal summary by Howell and a monograph by Annie Goodrich entitled "Marion Gertrude Howell."

ALICE HOWELL FRIEDMAN

HUBBARD, RUTH WEAVER (1897, Brooklyn, New York--December 7, 1955, Rush, New York). *Public health nurse.* EDUCATION: 1921, graduated from the Army School of Nursing, Washington, D.C.; 1925,

B.S., Teachers College, Columbia University, New York City; post-graduate studies at Yale University, New Haven, Connecticut, and the University of Pennsylvania, Philadelphia. CAREER: 1922-1925, staff nurse, Brooklyn Visiting Nurse Association, Brooklyn, New York; 1925-1927, head nurse and instructor at Yale University hospital and nursing school, New Haven, Connecticut; 1927-1929, educational director, New Haven Visiting Nurse Association; c. 1929-1955, general director, Visiting Nurse Society of Philadelphia; 1933, she travelled through the Scandinavian countries on a Rockefeller foundation fellowship; 1936-1942, lecturer, University of Pennsylvania School of Nursing, Philadelphia, and the University of California, Berkeley; 1948, consultant on public health administration, University of Minnesota, Minneapolis.
CONTRIBUTIONS: Ruth Hubbard devoted her life to the field of public health nursing and was a fervent spokeswoman for its cause. Many nurses distinguished themselves in the area of public health, but Hubbard's added dimension was her ability to express in writing the philosophy of public health nursing and her beliefs about the ideal role of the nurse. She was a national leader in public health nursing, serving as president (1946-1950) of the National Organization for Public Health Nursing (NOPHN). She was president during the turbulent years of that organization when a financial crisis and changes in the numbers and structures of nursing organizations had a profound impact on the profession. Indeed, the NOPHN held its last meeting on June 19, 1952, and the *Public Health Nursing Journal* ceased publication at the end of that year. Meanwhile, the National League for Nursing held its first meeting on June 20, 1952, with a department of public health nursing. She was a board member of the Philadelphia Social Service Exchange and was active in the Pennsylvania Nurses' Association. She was one of the founders of the Philadelphia Home Care Plan for long-term illnesses.

She received many honors during her career. In 1949 the Pennsylvania Nurses' Association awarded her the bronze medal for distinguished service in nursing. In 1955, she received from a coalition of professional women's groups the Friendship Fete Award for outstanding service to humanity. In October of that same year she shared with Mamie Eisenhower the honor of being selected as one of Pennsylvania's Distinguished Daughters. In 1956, after her death, the Ruth Weaver Hubbard Foundation was established to enable nurses to prepare for positions of leadership in nursing through advanced education or special studies.
WRITINGS: Among many were "Working Together for Public Health," *The Canadian Nurse* (February 1952), pp. 111-114; "Public Health Nursing, 1900-1950," *American Journal of Nursing* (October 1950), pp.

608-611; "An Understanding of Health in Nursing," *Public Health Nursing* (January 1943), pp. 21-25.

REFERENCES: *American Journal of Nursing* (January 1956), pp. 218-219; Marlette Conde, *The Lamp and the Caduceus* (1975); M. Louise Fitzpatrick, *The National Organization for Public Health Nursing, 1912-1952* (1975); Cordelia W. Kelly, *Dimensions of Professional Nursing* (2d ed., 1968); *New York Times* (December 8, 1955), p. 37; *Nursing Outlook* (July 1955), p. 401 and (January 1956), p. 34; *Public Health Nursing* (May 1949), pp. 308-309; unpublished materials, nursing service archives, Veterans Administration, Washington, D.C.

LORETTA P. HIGGINS

J

JAMME, ANNA C. (1865, Poughkeepsie, New York--July 4, 1939, San Francisco). *Leader in nursing organizations.* Daughter of a mining engineer. Never married. EDUCATION: Attended a private French school at Bourbonnais near Chicago and the Convent of the Sacred Heart, Halifax; 1897, graduated from Johns Hopkins Training School for Nurses, Baltimore, Maryland (she was living in St. Paul, Minnesota when she applied for admission to the nursing program at Johns Hopkins). CAREER: 1897-1901, head nurse, out-patient department and maternity ward, Johns Hopkins Hospital, and private duty nursing; 1901-1905, superintendent, New England Hospital for Women and Children, Roxbury, Massachusetts; 1906-1911, superintendent, school of nursing, St. Mary's Hospital, Rochester, Minnesota; 1911-1912, cared for her mother; 1912, moved to California; 1913-1928, chief, Bureau of Registration for California; 1918, assistant director, Army School of Nursing; August 1, 1928-July 1, 1936, executive secretary, California State Nurses' Association; 1936, retired.

CONTRIBUTIONS: Anna Jamme played several important roles over her long career in nursing. She was a pioneer in prenatal care, developing prenatal visiting in the homes of expectant mothers. In her first administrative position, at the New England Hospital for Women and Children, she established the eight-hour day for nurses, improved the course of instruction for nursing students, and encouraged development of a strong and permanent alumnae association. Her second superintendent position was at St. Mary's Hospital, affiliated with the Mayo Clinic, where she helped to establish the school of nursing and a system of training nuns to be professional nurses. She was the first superintendent of the school. Moving to California in 1912, she was a major force in the passage of a nurse practice act. She then served as the chief of the

Bureau of Registration for its first fifteen years. For seven months in 1918, she took a leave of absence to serve as Annie Goodrich's (q.v.) assistant at the Army School of Nursing. In 1928, she became the executive secretary of the California State Nurses' Association and editor of the *Pacific Coast Journal of Nursing.* During her tenure, the association grew tremendously, as did the scope of nursing practice. She proved to be an able administrator for the large organization. At the time of her appointment, the headquarters of the association were newly established. On August 1, 1928, she became director of headquarters and editor of the *Pacific Coast Journal of Nurses.* On September 1, headquarters were formally established. The president at that time was Anne A. Williamson (q.v.), and the two worked closely to bring districts into harmony with the state association.

In addition to her contributions to nursing education and to the profession in the state of California, she was a leader in national professional organizations. She was a member of the board of directors of the American Journal of Nursing Company from 1917 to 1919, and from 1917 to 1920 she was the western representative on the board of the American Nurses' Association (ANA). From 1920 to 1922, she served as president of the National League of Nursing Education. She also served on the committee for the Florence Nightingale School and of the Jane Delano (q.v.) memorial. In 1936, she assumed responsibility for arrangements for the ANA biennial convention held in Los Angeles. She was also a member of the endowment fund committee for the Johns Hopkins Hospital School of Nursing (1915) and of a special committee of its alumnae association to examine the school and its affiliation with Johns Hopkins University (1926). For four years, she was a member of the national committee of the American Red Cross Nursing Service.

Jamme decided to be a nurse as a result of her own childhood illnesses. Although her father was reluctant to let his daughter go into nursing, she convinced him to take her to Johns Hopkins to meet with the head of the nursing school. There, the charming M. Adelaide Nutting (q.v.) won over yet another reluctant parent, and she was enrolled. Her education was once more interrupted by periods of illness, but these did nothing to lessen her determination to complete the course.

Accustomed to travel from her childhood when her father's profession took the family across the United States and to Canada and even to France, Jamme travelled around the world shortly before her retirement. After her retirement, she continued to serve as an advisor to leaders in nursing.

WRITING: *Textbook of Nursing Procedures* (1921); numerous articles and editorials in professional journals.

REFERENCES: Alan Mason Chesney Medical Archives, Johns Hopkins Medical Institutions, Baltimore, Maryland; *American Journal of Nursing* (September 1921), p. 885, (July 1927), p. 570, (August 1928), p. 808, (July 1930), p. 918, (August 1936), pp. 856-857, and (August 1939), pp. 939-940; archives of the California Nurses' Association, San Francisco; Lavinia L. Dock, Sarah E. Pickett, Clara D. Noyes, Fannie F. Clement, Elizabeth G. Fox, and Anna R. Van Meter, *History of American Red Cross Nursing* (1922); Minnie Goodnow, *Nursing History* (7th ed., 1943); Ethel Johns and Blanche Pfefferkorn, *The Johns Hopkins Hospital School of Nursing, 1889-1949* (1954); Cordelia W. Kelly, *Dimensions of Professional Nursing* (1962); Helen W. Munson, *The Story of the National League of Nursing Education* (1934); National League of Nursing Education, *Biographical Sketches of Nursing Leaders* (1940); Meta Rutter Pennock, *Makers of Nursing History* (1940); archives of St. Mary's Hospital and School of Nursing, Rochester, Minnesota; *Trained Nurse* (August 1939), pp. 147-148.

JOELLEN WATSON HAWKINS

JOHNSON, SALLY MAY (May 10, 1880, East Morris, Connecticut--March 24, 1957, Boston). *Nurse-administrator.* Daughter of Francis H. Johnson and Sophia (Judson) Johnson. Never married. EDUCATION: Graduate of Litchfield (Connecticut) High School; 1898, graduated from New Britain Normal School (now Central Connecticut State College); 1910, graduated from Massachusetts General Hospital School of Nursing, Boston; 1911, completed six-month post-graduate course in psychiatric nursing, McLean Hospital, Waverly, Massachusetts; 1932, B.S., Teachers College, Columbia University, New York City. CAREER: 1898-1907, taught fifth grade, Winsted, Connecticut, public schools; 1911, instructor of practical nursing, St. Luke's Hospital, New Bedford, Massachusetts; 1912, instructor of practical nursing, Peter Bent Brigham Hospital School of Nursing, Boston; 1913-1916, assistant superintendent of nurses, Peter Bent Brigham Hospital; 1917, superintendent of nurses and principal of the nursing school, Albany Hospital, Albany, New York; 1918, director, Army School of Nursing, Walter Reed Hospital, Washington, D.C.; 1919-1920, returned to her previous position at the Albany Hospital; 1920-1946, superintendent of nurses and principal of the nursing school, Massachusetts General Hospital.

CONTRIBUTIONS: Sally Johnson was best known for her contributions as superintendent of nurses and principal of the Massachusetts General Hospital (MGH) School of Nursing, one of the oldest nursing schools in the United States. Before she took that position, no director had remained at MGH for longer than ten years; Johnson served as director for twenty-six years. During her tenure in that position, more than 1,900 students graduated from the school. She was best known for her administrative abilities and for the creation of a stable but evolving nursing service in the hospital. Since she served during the Great Depression, when it was difficult to financially support an extensive nursing service, and World War II, when there were shortages of nurses at home as well as in the military, she had many more problems than most of her predecessors at MGH. She was known for her integrity, which was reflected in her ability to continue a high-quality nursing school program and to make the changes necessary to meet or surpass the standards which were established in 1927 by the National League of Nursing Education's (NLNE) *Curriculum for Schools of Nursing.* In addition, when she was in charge of the nursing program at MGH, nursing schools began to be studied nationwide by the grading committee of the American Nurses' Association, and at the time when *Nurses, Patients, and Pocketbooks* (1928) exposed questionable practices in nursing education and cast public attention on every nursing school in the country.

Johnson was noted for making needed changes in both nursing service and nursing education. Those she instituted at MGH included the introduction of the ward helper and the ward secretary, the staff nurse, and the assistant head nurse. She added a school librarian and a physical-social director, and appointed to the faculty a public health nurse and a supervisor of clinical instruction. She was a firm supporter of the eight-hour day for private duty nurses, at a time when others insisted that it was not possible. When she was at the Albany Hospital, prior to her move to MGH, Johnson was able to reduce the working day for special duty nurses from twenty-four hours to twelve, and at the MGH she reduced the twelve-hour day to eight. In addition, she fought to have the private duty nurse paid in full upon completion of each assignment, which was a great help in putting nurses on a sound financial basis. While director of the MGH School of Nursing, she faced many challenges, challenges which were perhaps more memorable than significant. These included her ban on bobbed hair and her insistance that nurses not smoke.

She was a strong advocate of a sound education for nurses, and she insisted that a high-school education was essential for admission to the nursing program at MGH at a time when many of the schools which had that as a requirement for admission did not adhere to it if it meant reducing the number of student nurses and the number of hospital employees. Johnson even encouraged prospective students to complete college before entering nursing school, and she encouraged graduates to complete a baccalaureate program as soon as possible after they received their diploma from the MGH School of Nursing. She was a leader in the plan which resulted in the creation of a coordinated diploma-baccalaureate program at Radcliffe College (c. 1945-1966), which was the culmination of what Johnson believed to be essential in a nurse: the combination of a well-educated woman with a high-quality training in nursing. Unfortunately, although the program was established, it had a very brief existence and disappeared shortly after her death.

Johnson was active in local, state, and national nursing organizations. While in Albany, she organized the nursing service of the American Red Cross Base Hospital of the Albany Hospital, and her outstanding administrative skills were recognized when she was chosen to direct the Army School of Nursing during World War I. She was a member of the board of directors of the NLNE (1928-1935), the American Journal of Nursing Company, and the American Nurses' Association (ANA). While in Albany she served on the legislative committee of the New York State Nurses' Association, and she was in constant attendance at hearings related to the licensing and status of nurses in the state. She was an active participant in the development of the state's registration bill for nurses as it was created. When she moved to Massachusetts, she became president of the Massachusetts League of Nursing Education and president of the New England division of the ANA. In 1929, while presiding over the annual meeting of the ANA, she delivered her famous address, "The Reminiscence of a Connecticut Yankee." For six years, she also was president of the Suffolk County (Massachusetts) Central Directory for Nurses.

Over the course of her career, she received several important honors in recognition of her achievements. Upon her retirement in 1946 she was named director emeritus of the MGH School of Nursing. In 1953, the Quota Club of Boston presented her with its Woman of Achievement Award. In 1956, the year before she died, she was given honorary membership in the MGH Nurses' Alumnae Association. In 1957, the *Quarterly Journal*, the magazine of the alumnae association, published a memorial issue in her memory.

WRITINGS: Several articles in nursing publications.

REFERENCES: *American Journal of Nursing* (1957), pp. 650-651; Carrie M. Hall, "Sally Johnson," *National League of Nursing Education Biographical Sketch* (n.d.); Massachusetts General Hospital School of Nursing archives, Francis E. Countway Library of Medicine, Boston; Sylvia Perkins, *A Centennial Review: 1873-1973 of the Massachusetts General Hospital School of Nursing* (1975).

ALICE HOWELL FRIEDMAN

JONES, ELIZABETH RINKER {KRATZ} (September 18, 1868, Hilltown, Pennsylvania--November 1937, Burbank, California). *Military nurse.* Daughter of Dr. and Mrs. Harvey Kratz. Married Theodore Everett Jones, February 21, 1911. No children. EDUCATION: December 5, 1893-June 1, 1895, attended Blockley Hospital (later Philadelphia General Hospital) School of Nursing, graduating 1895. CAREER: June-December 5, 1895, nurse at Blockley Hospital; 1896-1897, nurse, Dr. E. E. Montgomery's Private Hospital, Philadelphia; 1897, nursed elderly in Ohio; August 2, 1898-September 30, 1899, Spanish-American War nurse; January-August 1899, nurse on the U.S. Army transport *Manitoba*, serving off the coast of Cuba; 1901, head nurse, Delaware Hospital, Wilmington, Delaware, and Meadville Hospital, Pennsylvania; December 1901-March 1904, nurse, Municipal Hospital, Philadelphia; 1904, volunteer nurse, Russo-Japanese War; 1905-1908, head nurse of the men's medical department, Episcopal Hospital, Philadelphia; 1908, nurse during the construction of the Panama Canal; October 1909-1910, charge nurse of the hospital in Wenatchee, Washington; 1911, retired from nursing upon her marriage.

CONTRIBUTIONS: Elizabeth Kratz was one of the pioneers in military nursing during the Spanish-American War. She was recruited for service by the Daughters of the American Revolution and served as an army contract nurse. From August 2, 1898, to September 30, 1899, she was stationed at Fort Myer, Virginia, a 200-bed hospital in Riding Hall. On January 17, 1899, she left on the transport *Manitoba*, bound for Cuba. She served in Velado, Cuba, until August of that year. A contract for her services as a nurse listed her as being in Havana, Cuba, from March to July 31, 1899. A note appended gives August 5, 1899, as the date of annulment of the contract. In 1901, she attended the first annual Spanish-American War nurses' convention in Washington, D.C., and was present at the White House reception with President and Mrs. Theodore Roosevelt. In that same year, 1901, the letter authorizing her appointment to the Army Nurse Corps finally reached her, after a journey of two years.

In 1901, she became head nurse at Delaware Hospital, Wilmington, and then at Meadville Hospital, but on December 15, she received a call to return to Philadelphia to care for smallpox patients. For over two years, she nursed smallpox and scarlet fever victims; over 5,000 were cared for at Philadelphia's Municipal Hospital during that time. In 1904, she joined Dr. Anita Newcomb McGee's volunteers to nurse the Japanese wounded during the Russo-Japanese War. She also helped to educate Japanese women to nurse under the auspices of the Japanese Red Cross. She was not paid for this volunteer humanitarian work.

Returning to the United States in 1905, she took a position as head nurse of a men's medical department at Philadelphia's Episcopal Hospital, and she helped to care for 2,500 cases of typhoid fever. In April 1908, she travelled to Panama to nurse the ill workers who were constructing the Panama Canal (for sixty dollars a month), declining an offer to be head nurse at South California State Hospital to continue her humanitarian work. Her contract for that work is dated March 18, 1908, with the Isthmian Canal Commission contracting with her to provide nursing service.

When she returned to the United States, she went to Boise, Idaho, where she had family, and then she started a nursing home in Washington State with another nurse (around 1910). She was head nurse at Wenatchee Hospital in the state of Washington, and while there she applied for registration in Pennsylvania. She also met her future husband, and in 1911 she married Theodore Everett Jones of Ephrata, Washington; as was the custom of the day, she retired from nursing. Together, they operated a fishing boat until his death on July 4, 1929. They lived in Sequin, Washington.

After her husband's death, Elizabeth Kratz Jones moved to Burbank, California, where she died eight years later. She did maintain contact with friends and colleagues, however, as was evident from the fact that in 1935 she met with three of her friends from the Russo-Japanese War at the thirty-fifth encampment of the Spanish-American War veterans. For her service during the Russo-Japanese War and for her work in training Japanese nurses, she was made a life member of the Japanese Red Cross.

REFERENCES: Contracts from the Isthmian Canal Commission, Washington, D.C., office, March 18, 1908, and from the U.S. Army Medical Department, March 1, 1899; information provided by Irene Matthews, R.N., Holmes, Pennsylvania, and from Edith Nunan, Museum of Nursing History, Pennsylvania Hospital, Philadelphia; records of the Philadelphia General Hospital, City Hall, Philadelphia; information provided by Sara P. Trude, Boise, Idaho, niece of Elizabeth Kratz Jones.

JOELLEN WATSON HAWKINS

K

KEMBLE, ELIZABETH L. (c. 1907, Greenville, Ohio--November 30, 1981, Raleigh, North Carolina). *Educator*. EDUCATION: Graduated from the University of Cincinnati College of Nursing and Health; B.S. in nursing, New York University; M.Ed and D.Ed., Teachers College, Columbia University, New York City. CAREER: Various teaching and administrative positions in New Jersey, New York, and Ohio; 1941-1945, assistant and then associate director of the nurse testing division, Psychological Corporation; 1946-1950, director of the National League of Nursing Education department of measurement and guidance; 1950-1967, dean, University of North Carolina School of Nursing, Chapel Hill, continuing as a professor until her retirement in 1971.

CONTRIBUTIONS: As the first dean of the nursing school at the University of North Carolina, Elizabeth Kemble established the state's first master's degree program in nursing, and she also founded the university's continuing education program in nursing (1963). She had a rich background in teaching as well as in educational testing. Her work with the Psychological Corporation as assistant and associate director of the nurse testing division helped to prepare her for the position of director of the newly established department of measurement and guidance of the National League of Nursing Education. It was a busy time for this department and a time of transition; the volume of testing had increased immensely, necessitating the creation of her department. A national test pool was developed for the registration of nurses, in addition to the development of tests to indicate an applicant's aptitude for nursing. Under Kemble's leadership, a practical nurse test service was also created, along with a variety of other testing services.

On November 16, 1963, she was honored by the department of nursing education of New York University's School of Education, with an award for her outstanding contributions to the profession. After her death, the board of directors of the American Nurses' Association placed a tribute to her in the association's records.

WRITINGS: "Shopping for a School of Nursing," *American Journal of Nursing* (February 1942), pp. 166-167; "What Applicants Hope and Fear about Schools of Nursing," *American Journal of Nursing* (October 1945), pp. 829-830; "Shorter and Sharper Testing Tools," *American Journal of Nursing* (May 1947), pp. 327-330; "Studying Students or Testing Teachers?" *American Journal of Nursing* (July 1947), pp. 481-483; "State Board Test Pool Examinations," *American Journal of Nursing* (August 1947), pp. 552-555 (with Emma Spaney).

REFERENCES: *American Journal of Nursing* (March 1942), p. 298, (September 1946), p. 628, (April 1950), p. 247, (August 1950), p. 28 adv., and (February 1982), pp. 320-321; *Nursing Outlook* (January 1964), p. 8.

LORETTA P. HIGGINS

KENNEDY, CECILA ROSE (July 1885, Drifton, Luzerne County, Pennsylvania--January 9, 1981, St. Francis Country Home, Darby, Pennsylvania). *Red Cross nurse.* Daughter of a mining engineer and a music teacher. Never married. EDUCATION: Attended St. Mary's private academy, Scranton, Pennsylvania, and Atlantic City High School, New Jersey; 1906-1909, attended Philadelphia General Hospital School of Nursing, graduating May 11, 1909; 1909-1913, night courses in social work, University of Pennsylvania, Philadelphia; earned degree in social service from New York University. New York City. CAREER: 1909-1916, private duty nursing in Philadelphia and abroad; 1916-1919, social service worker, Red Cross, serving in England; 1918, nurse with the Red Cross in France; 1918-1934, service with the International Red Cross, in Europe; 1934-1959, service with the Red Cross in the United States.

CONTRIBUTIONS: Cecile (as she was known to her family and friends) Kennedy was a leader in Red Cross nursing, in both the United States and abroad. For over forty years, she served the Red Cross, combining her original career as a nurse with her preparation in social work. Because her father's occupation required frequent relocation, she travelled a great deal as a child. Before graduating from high school in New Jersey, she had lived in Canada, New York, West Virginia, and New Jersey. Her aunt and cousin were graduates of the nursing school at the Philadelphia General Hospital, and that influenced her decision to enter nursing, as well as her choice of a school. After graduating, she was a private duty nurse for a number of years, including time abroad with the families of her well-to-do patients. When in Philadelphia, however, she began to study social work through evening college courses.

Finally, in 1916, Kennedy engaged in what was to be her life work with the Red Cross. Before the United States had entered World War I, she went into social service work with the Red Cross in England. In 1918, three months before the armistice, she was transferred to France, where it was discovered that she was a nurse rather than a social worker. Since nurses were so desperately needed, for the remainder of the war she served as a nurse. After the war was over, however, she returned to her previous role as a social worker, appraising the needs created by the war and by other disasters, and working to provide support services for those in desperate need of assistance. For nine years, she remained in Europe with the Red Cross, spending seven years at the headquarters of the International Red Cross at Geneva, Switzerland.

In 1934, she returned to the United States, continuing her Red Cross work. Again she travelled extensively through the states and to Alaska, setting up courses for Grey Ladies, nurses' aides, home nursing, and disaster relief. Her Red Cross service continued through World War II and the reconstruction efforts after the war. During the war, she was the head of the Red Cross service in Pennsylvania. After her retirement, she served on President Dwight David Eisenhower's Peace Council.

Over the course of her long career, she received a number of honors in recognition of her service to humanity. She received honorary degrees from Villanova University and Duquesne University, both in Pennsylvania. On January 13, 1939, she received the Meritorious Service Medal of the State of Pennsylvania for her work during the Pennsylvania floods. In December 1945, she received the distinguished service medal of the American Red Cross, the only woman from Pennsylvania to receive it for service during World War II. On June 12, 1946, she received the Meritorious Service Medal of the Commonwealth of Pennsylvania for her work in civilian defense during World War II. Two years later, on August 1, 1948, she was recognized by the American Red Cross for her twenty-eight years of service to that organization.

REFERENCES: Copies of award citations from the archives of the American Red Cross, Philadelphia; oral history interviews with Cecile Kennedy, Edith Nunan, and Mary Rabenstein, all conducted by Irene Matthews, R.N., Holmes, Pennsylvania, 1959; records of the Pennsylvania General Hospital, City Hall, Philadelphia.

JOELLEN WATSON HAWKINS

KIMBER, DIANA CLIFFORD (August 12, 1857, Tracey, Oxfordshire, England--January 25, 1928, Powick Asylum, Worcestershire, England). *Nurse-educator; author.* Daughter of a well-known family of Oxfordshire, England. Never married. EDUCATION: Liberal education in England and Germany; 1884-1887, attended Bellevue Hospital Training School, New York City. CAREER: 1887, charge nurse in the surgical ward, and night superintendent, Bellevue Hospital; 1887, assistant superintendent, Illinois Training School, Chicago; January 1, 1888-February 1898, assistant superintendent, New York City Training School for Nurses, Old Charity Hospital at Blackwell's Island, and then February-May 1898, superintendent; after spending several years living at home in England, joined an Anglican sisterhood, the Community of the Holy Name, on November 8, 1906, and worked until 1926 among the poor in England; worked first from the Community Mission House at Wimbledon, near London; 1907-March 1908, worked in the Home of the Good Shepherd, a residential home in Malvern for moral welfare work with girls; March-October 1908, worked in the original parish of the order, St. Peter's, Vauxhall, London; May 27, 1909, was professed in life vows as Sister Diana Mary, C.H.N., and spent the remainder of her life working among the poor of the large manufacturing towns of England.
CONTRIBUTIONS: Diana Kimber's greatest contribution was the fact that she published one of the first scientific textbooks for nurses written by a nurse. As a teacher of nursing in Chicago and New York City, she recognized the need for textbooks with a focus not on the practice of medicine but on the practice of nursing. In 1894 she helped meet the need by the publication of her *Text-Book of Anatomy and Physiology*, the first on this topic written by a nurse. The book ran through six editions before her death, dominating the market for a third of a century. A former pupil of hers, Carolyn Gray (q.v.), revised the book, so in fact the book was used as a text in nursing schools for more than fifty years.

Kimber was an active supporter of professional organizations for nurses and in 1893 was among the nurses who met at the Chicago World's Fair and began the organization which would later become the National League for Nursing (NLN). She was one of the first members and an active participant in the American Society of Superintendents of Training Schools for Nurses, as the NLN was first named, and she remained so until her return to England. She also contributed important ideas about the need for district visiting nursing.

Shortly after graduating from the Bellevue Hospital Training School and after working for less than a year as night superintendent at Bellevue Hospital, she accepted a position as assistant superintendent of the Illinois Training School for Nurses which was affiliated with Cook County Hospital. Although her tenure in that position was very brief

(February-December of 1887), she is cited in the history of that institution for her contributions to its development.

Kimber left the Chicago school to assist her close friend, Louise Darche (q.v.). As classmates at the Bellevue Hospital Training School, they had become friends, and when Darche became superintendent of the newly approved New York City Training School on Blackwell's Island, Kimber became her assistant. Their first trip to the hospital was made in a small boat, negotiating their way through the ice of the East River, hardly an auspicious beginning for the nursing leaders of that institution. Although Darche was superintendent, Kimber planned the curriculum, taught all the classes, and assumed responsibility for the students on a day-to-day basis. In establishing the school, she and her classmate fought numerous political battles and endured conditions that were scarcely comfortable in the cold, gray stone buildings on a windy island on New York's East River. When Darche's health failed, Kimber assumed the position of superintendent (February 1898) until the end of that academic year, resigning to travel to England with her friend. Characteristic of the care and attention she gave to each of her positions, she examined the institution department by department before her departure, and she remained until after commencement.

In England, she lavished care on her ailing friend and colleague but to no avail. Darche's death was a severe blow, and for a number of years, Diana Kimber lived quietly at home with her family. Then she joined an Anglican sisterhood, becoming Sister Mary Diana, and she spent most of the remainder of her life working among the poor of England's large cities, providing care much like that of public health nurses in the United States. Two years before her death, failing health forced her to give up her work and she retired to the Convent of the Holy Name, Malvern, England. When she died, she was buried in the community plot at Malvern Wells Cemetery, England. An American nursing colleague who had visited her at the convent commented in the *American Journal of Nursing* that Sister Diana spent her last years surrounded by the roses she so loved and which she had struggled to nurture in the barren environment on Blackwell's Island during her tenure there. The class of 1916 established in her name (and that of Louise Darche) a scholarship fund at the New York City Training School (later known as City Hospital School of Nursing).

WRITINGS: *Text-Book of Anatomy and Physiology* (1893, 1902, 1909, 1914, 1918, 1923); many articles in nursing journals, including "Trained Nursing for People with Moderate Income," *Trained Nurse and Hospital Review* (March 1897), pp. 131-133, and "A New Field of Work for Nurses," *Trained Nurse and Hospital Review* (December 1895), pp. 292-293.

REFERENCES: *American Journal of Nursing* (October 1919), p. 40, and (May 1928), pp. 486-487; *The Community of the Holy Name* (brochure, 1983); correspondence with Sister Jane Cicely, C.H.M,. Convent of the Holy Name, Malvern Link, Worcestershire, England, March 11 and April 10, 1987; National League of Nursing Education, *Early Leaders of American Nursing* (undated); Meta Rutter Pennock, *Makers of Nursing History* (1928), pp. 80-81 and (1940), p. 109; Susan Reverby, *Annual Conventions, The American Society of Superintendents of Training Schools for Nurses* (1985); Grace Fay Schryver, *A History of the Illinois Training School for Nurses, 1880-1929* (1930).

JOELLEN WATSON HAWKINS

KINNEY, DITA (HOPKINS) (September 13, 1855, New York City--April 16, 1921, California). *First superintendent, Army Nurse Corps.* Married to Mark H. Kinney, 1874 (died 1878); one son. EDUCATION: Graduated from Mills Seminary (later Mills College), California; 1889 or 1890 to 1892, attended Massachusetts General Hospital Training School, Boston, graduating in 1892; 1909, post-graduate work, Massachusetts General Hospital. CAREER: 1892, lecturer on nursing subjects; 1893-1895, worked for the Massachusetts Emergency Hygienic Association of Boston, teaching hygiene to poor mothers and training young women as assistants to trained nurses; 1895-1898, private duty nursing, staff nurse at the Almshouse Hospital on Long Island, in Boston Harbor, and at the City and County Hospital, St. Paul, Minnesota; 1898, joined the Army Nurse Corps during the Spanish-American War: assigned to the army hospital at the Presidio; released to take charge of a convalescent hospital for soldiers which was established by the Red Cross in the foothills behind Oakland, California; c. 1899, nurse at French Hospital, San Francisco; 1900, chief nurse, Fort Bayard, New Mexico; December 1900-March 1901, assigned to the office of Surgeon-General George M. Sternberg, Washington, D.C. (January 1, 1901, assigned in charge of the Army Nurse Corps); March 15, 1901-July 31, 1909, superintendent of the Army Nurse Corps; 1910-1914, superintendent of a hospital in Gloucester, Massachusetts.

CONTRIBUTIONS: Dita Kinney's greatest contribution was the organization of the Army Nurse Corps during the Spanish-American War. Left a young widow with a child to support after the untimely death in 1878 of her husband, she probably stayed home for a number of years caring for her child and then enrolled in the training school at the Massachusetts General Hospital, graduating in 1892. For a number of years after graduation, she established a reputation as a lecturer on nursing subjects and lectured throughout New England. She also worked for the Massachusetts Emergency Hygienic Association of Boston where she taught hygiene and child care, trained nurses' aides, and lectured to associations of young women associated with churches.

After a brief period of employment in Massachusetts and Minnesota, she returned to California where she had been raised, and she joined the Army Nurse Corps at the outbreak of the Spanish-American War in 1898. She was appointed a contract nurse to the army on September 10, 1898, serving for one week. Her contract was renewed on October 18 of that same year, and she served for one month, until November 17, 1898. Among her assignments was service in the office of the surgeon-general, Washington, D.C., and where she obviously demonstrated sufficient competence and administrative ability to be offered the position of superintendent of the Army Nurse Corps (upon the resignation of Dr. Anita McGee). The eight years she spent as superintendent of the corps not only brought organization to army nurses serving across the country and in the Philippines but also provided a much-needed foundation for later development of the corps under her successors. She was able to institute improvements in the conditions under which nurses worked and lived, including a saloon mess for nurses at sea. She also insisted that corps nurses have a distinctive identity, and a green enamel badge was adopted.

At the first Congress of the International Council of Nurses in Buffalo (1901), Kinney spoke about the Army Nurse Corps, but interestingly she did not mention the contributions of either the American Red Cross or organized nursing in establishing the corps. Resigning in 1909 from the corps, she returned to school, enrolling in a post-graduate course at Massachusetts General Hospital, and then she became superintendent of a hospital in Gloucester, Massachusetts, until 1914 when failing health forced her to retire. She returned to California where she taught Red Cross classes in home nursing during World War I and also taught in a hospital in the town in which she lived.

WRITINGS: Numerous articles in professional journals, as well as unpublished speeches and reports.

REFERENCES: *American Journal of Nursing* (December 1900), pp. 403-404, (March 1901), pp. 403-404, and (July 1921), p. 764; Edith A. Aynes, *From Nightingale to Eagle* (1973); Massachusetts General Hospital Training School for Nurses Collection, 1896-1940, deposited in the Countway Library of Medicine, Harvard University Medical School, Boston; Dita A. Kinney, "Army Nursing," *Trained Nurse and Hospital Review* (1901), pp. 337-340, and "Dr. Anita Newcomb McGee and What She has Done for the Nursing Profession," *Trained Nurse and Hospital Review* (March 1901), pp. 129-134; *Pacific Coast Journal of Nursing* (August 1921), p. 458; Sara E. Parsons, *History of the Massachusetts*

General Hospital Training School for Nurses (1922); Julia C. Stimson, *History and Manual of the Army Nurse Corps* (1937).

JOELLEN WATSON HAWKINS

KNAPP, BERTHA L. (September 19, 1880, Dewitt, Michigan--August 1, 1965, Neillsville, Wisconsin). *Nurse-educator.* Married Dr. Richard A. Smith, geologist, July 24, 1958. No children. EDUCATION: 1903, graduated from University of Michigan's School of Nursing, University Hospital, Ann Arbor. CAREER: 1903-1907, supervisor of the children's and medical departments and then assistant superintendent of nurses, University Hospital, Ann Arbor, Michigan; 1907-1908, public health nursing supervisor, Chicago Visiting Nurses' Association; 1908-September 1, 1943, superintendent of the training school and the hospital nursing services, Wesley Hospital, Chicago.

CONTRIBUTIONS: Bertha Knapp was one of a number of leaders of nursing education in the early years of the twentieth century. She was unique among her peers because she had graduated from one of the early university-affiliated training schools (University Hospital, of the University of Michigan). Early in her career, she became superintendent of the training school and the hospital nursing services at Wesley Hospital, Chicago, a position she held from 1908 to 1943. Almost as soon as she arrived at Wesley Hospital, she began to make changes which served to shape and refocus the path of nursing. In her first two years, enrollment in the nursing school increased sharply, and she convinced the hospital administrators of the need to increase the nursing staff. By 1912, there was one full-time instructor for the school, two assistant superintendents, a night supervisor, one surgical and three floor head nurses, a dietitian, and a masseuse. Because enrollments increased, more living quarters for nurses were secured, but Knapp continued her fight for what became a long struggle to secure adequate and comfortable quarters for her nurses.

Convinced that care in hospitals had to improve, she helped to construct a philosophy for the school that espoused an approach to patient care that was more personal than had previously been the case. She also scheduled ward duties for students so there was time for specialized instruction, and she insisted that students have four years of high school at a time when the Illinois laws required only one year for nursing students. In 1917, teaching hours at Wesley Hospital's nursing school exceeded state requirements by more than one hundred hours. By the 1920s, coursework requirments exceeded those recommended by the National League of Nursing Education. By that time, affiliations were in place for clinical experience in the care of patients with communicable diseases, in psychopathic nursing, pediatric nursing, and community health nursing.

In addition to curriculum reforms, Knapp attended to the social and psychological development of her students. Students at Wesley Hospital's nursing school had two half-days off a week and four weeks of annual vacation time. Extracurricular events were an integral part of training school life at Wesley, and students were required to have both physical education and classes in personal hygiene. A school yearbook was instituted in the 1920s, as well as a chorus, and a volunteer group offering Bible study and the preliminaries for foreign missionary work was also organized. In 1925, a social director was hired, who also served as counselor, librarian, and advisor to the yearbook staff.

The Great Depression brought significant changes to the school, however, and in 1935 due to financial problems the three-year program was discontinued. During these dark times, Knapp continued her strong leadership, insisting that standards for the department of nursing remain at their previous high levels, refusing to compromise by hiring less than well-prepared nurses to supplement the dwindling staff. In 1935, she reinstituted the eight-hour workday. Staff meetings and lectures were held regularly to keep nurses aware of modern trends and developments in the field, and nurses at Wesley Hospital were encouraged to enroll in university courses. The long-awaited new building was completed and the move accomplished, all under Knapp's administration. In 1942, a merger was negotiated between Washington Boulevard Hospital and Wesley Memorial, and the issue of reopening the school and accepting students from Washington Boulevard's school became urgent. In the summer of 1942, the nursing school was reopened, and an affiliation with Northwestern University was re-established. In 1943, a five-year combination baccalaureate and diploma program was approved, with graduates received B.S. degrees from Northwestern University as well as a diploma from the hospital's training school.

Perhaps at this point, Knapp felt that her mission had been accomplished. Whatever the reason, after thirty-five years of service to Wesley Hospital, she announced her plans to retire effective on September 1, 1943. The trustees conferred on her the title of superintendent of nurses, emeritus, and she returned to her native Michigan and remained an active member of her alumnae association in Ann Arbor. In 1958 she married Dr. Richard A. Smith, who had first proposed to her while they were students at Michigan sixty years earlier. They were married at her summer home in Wisconsin, where she died just before her eighty-fifth birthday seven years later.

Knapp did not devote all her professional time to Wesley Hospital. She was the first chairperson of the Illinois Board of Nurse

Examiners when it was established in 1917. She also was a director of the Illinois League of Nursing Education, the Illinois State Nurses' Association, and the Central Council for Nursing Education. In 1943, the year in which she retired from Wesley Hospital, the Bertha L. Knapp Scholarship Fund was established by the alumnae association. The women's auxiliary held a tea in her honor, which was attended by a large number of guests, including several nursing leaders among them Nellie X. Hawkinson (q.v.). A portrait of Bertha L. Knapp Smith was commissioned by the Wesley Nurses' Alumnae Association in 1959.
WRITINGS: Numerous articles in professional journals.
REFERENCES: *American Journal of Nursing* (January 1924), pp. 303 and 323, (March 1939), p. 309, (August 1942), pp. 960-961; (July 1943), p. 687; Vernon K. Brown, *Cathedral of Healing: The Story of Wesley Memorial Hospital, 1888-1972* (1981); unpublished materials, Northwestern Memorial Hospital Archives, Chicago; Susan Sacharski, unpublished history of the Northwestern Memorial Hospital, Chicago, chapters entitled "The Chicago Training School for City, Home and Foreign Missions, The Chicago Deaconess Home, Wesley Memorial Training School for Nurses, 1888-1935" and "Wesley at War, 1935-1945," provided by Susan Sacharski, archivist, Northwestern Memorial Hospital Archives and Library, Chicago.

JOELLEN WATSON HAWKINS

KRATZ, ELIZABETH RINKER. See **JONES, ELIZABETH (KRATZ).**

L

LALLY, GRACE B. (1897, Ashland, Pennsylvania--June 21, 1983, Drexel Hill, Pennsylvania). *Leader in Navy Nurse Corps.* EDUCATION: Graduated from Merion Mercy Academy, Merion, Pennsylvania; 1917, graduated from St. Joseph's Hospital School of Nursing, Reading, Pennsylvania. CAREER: 1917, private duty nurse, Brooklyn, New York; 1918-1919, member of the Army Nurse Corps; 1919-1921, private duty nursing, as well as work as staff nurse at Bellevue Hospital and head nurse, St. Vincent's Hospital, both in New York City; 1921-1946, member of the Navy Nurse Corps.

CONTRIBUTIONS: Grace Lally had the distinction of serving the United States during two world wars and in two different branches of nurse corps. Shortly after her graduation from nursing school in 1917, she joined the Army Nurse Corps, serving at Camp Pike, Arkansas. Returning to the service after a brief stint of private duty and staff nursing, she joined the Navy Nurse Corps in 1921 for what was to be the remainder of her career. Her first duty station was at the League Island Hospital, Philadelphia. After six months, she was ordered to report for duty with the fleet aboard the "Mercy Ship" out of Guantanamo Bay, Cuba. After three months of shore duty at Annapolis, she returned to sea duty, this time aboard the U.S.S. *Relief.* Having received an outdoor uniform for her first stint on ship, she was reassigned to a ship because she had that uniform; it was one way the navy apparently saved money, for only nurses on sea duty were issued outdoor uniforms. After two years stationed in Boston and three in the hospital at Great Lakes, Illinois, she was sent by the navy to the University of Pennsylvania for a course in anesthesia, and then to duty in Washington, D.C. From there, she was shipped to Guam. While en route, her orders were changed to the Philippines at the request of a surgeon who had heard of her anesthesia experience and wanted her with him. From the Philippines, she went to China in 1938 aboard the U.S.S. *Canopus* to transport dependents to Japan. Then she returned to Washington, D.C., and from there she went to San Diego where she became chief nurse of the hospital. Brooklyn, New York, was her next stop, and she helped to outfit the U.S.S. *Solace* as a hospital ship. At that time, Lally had twenty years of service, and she held the Navy Nurse Corps record for sea duty. The *Solace* arrived in Hawaii in October 1941. Her time in the Pacific was marked by experiences in an event which was to shape the course of history.

On December 7, 1941, Lally was the chief nurse aboard the *Solace*, a 432-bed hospital ship which was one of only twelve such ships in the U.S. Navy and the only one present in Pearl Harbor on that day. According to her own account, she was getting dressed for church when she heard low-flying planes. Her first thoughts were that it was a drill and that the pilots were flying much too low and too near the ship. Stepping to the porthole of her cabin, she watched the beginning of the attack on the U.S. fleet by Japanese planes. Immediately, she realized that emergency wards had to be established and, as bombs continued to fall around the ship, she and her twelve nurses prepared for the large numbers of injured and wounded seamen who would require immediate medical attention. Of the ninety-six ships in the harbor when the attack occurred, the *Solace* alone was fully equipped to provide emergency medical and surgical care. It was anchored near the battleship row with the *Arizona*, the *Nevada*, and others which were disabled or destroyed in the attack. The *Solace* sustained little or no damage, while the ships all around it were sunk, burned, or crippled. When one of the nurses reported to Lally that a Japanese submarine was hiding under the ship, her reply was, "Nonsense, we have no time for that now; get busy in the operating room!" Sailors on the deck of a cruiser near the *Solace* thought they spotted the periscope of a submarine near the hospital ship, but it was only a tin can.

After Pearl Harbor, the ship made trips to the fighting front to transfer patients to New Zealand and elsewhere. When the war "quieted down," Lally and other nurses were sent to New Caledonia for rest and recreation; the island was famous as the site for the movie *South Pacific*. She then returned to duty in Bethesda, Maryland and she travelled through the United States on a public relations mission, an assignment she was not fond of, especially when she had to speak at Radio City Music Hall. In 1946, due to a heart condition Lally was given a medical discharge, having served for twenty-seven years and having attained the rank of lieutenant commander. She received the American Defense Medal, a navy unit commendation ribbon, and the World War II Victory Medal.

Interestingly, her original goal was not to be a nurse and certainly not to be in the military. While young, she entered a contest for a scholarship from a music school in Philadelphia, hoping to win and be able to study the piano. Although she won the contest and the scholarship, her mother refused to let her attend; instead, she was enrolled in the Mercy Sisters Academy. An attack of appendicitis changed the course of her life, as it did with a number of other women who were impressed by the quality of nursing care they received while ill. Her experience in the hospital sparked an interest in nursing, and a chance encounter on the street with a woman whose daughter was studying at St. Joseph's Hospital School of Nursing led her to enroll there.

When she retired in 1946, she returned to her native Pennsylvania. For almost twenty more years, she continued to be interested in her profession and to share her experiences with those who were interested in the history of the profession. She died in Delaware County Hospital, Upper Darby, Pennsylvania, at the age of eighty-six, and she was buried with full military honors in Saints Peter and Paul Cemetery, Marple, Pennsylvania.

REFERENCES: Unpublished recollections and oral history (1971) by Irene Matthews, R.N., Holmes, Pennsylvania; Wyatt Blassingame, *Combat Nurses of World War II* (1967); Walter Lord, *Day of Infamy* (1957); records of Merion Mercy Academy, Merion, Pennsylvania; Paul Stillwell, ed., *Air Raid: Pearl Harbor!* (1981); Helen Wright and Samuel Rapport, eds., *Great Adventures in Nursing* (1960).

JOELLEN WATSON HAWKINS

LEETE, HARRIET L. (c. 1875, Cleveland, Ohio--November 19, 1927, Brooklyn, New York). *Child health nurse; Red Cross nurse.* EDUCATION: March 23, 1902, graduated from Lakeside Training School for Nurses, Cleveland, Ohio. CAREER: 1902-1906, private duty nurse in sanatoriums in New York City, Rochester, Dansville, and elsewhere; supervisor of the men's surgical ward, Lakeside Hospital, Cleveland; 1906-1917, member of the nursing staff, Infant's Clinic, Cleveland, Ohio; May 1917-July 15, 1919, nurse, American Red Cross; c. 1920, field director, American Child Hygiene Association; 1920-c. 1925, director of the Brooklyn Maternity Center Association; c. 1925-1927, director of Wavecrest convalescent home, Far Rockaway, New York.

CONTRIBUTIONS: Harriet Leete was among the earliest pioneers in child health nursing. When the Babies Dispensary was opened in 1906, in the Friendly Inn in the Haymarket district of Cleveland, she served as superintendent for the nurses. The central dispensary provided care for sick infants; in the branch dispensaries, nurses taught mothers how to care for their infants and encouraged them to bring their infants in to be weighed and examined. In the process of her work, she established standards for infant health care that were later to be emulated across the United States.

Her work can be divided into two major segments: infant and child health nursing and Red Cross nursing. Although her work with infants began early in her career, in 1907 she volunteered to work for the Rochester chapter of the American Red Cross, being member 159 of the original enrollment of Red Cross nurses. From 1906 to 1917, however, she continued to work in child health in Cleveland. She served on the first board of directors of the National Organization for Public Health Nursing (1912), and she was a charter member of the National Committee on Red Cross Nursing Service, which examined the role of Red Cross nurses in the United States and when the American Red Cross served abroad.

With the need for nursing service overseas during World War I, Leete became a member of the nursing staff of U.S. Army Base Hospital Number 4 (Lakeside unit), assigned to the British Expeditionary Forces. That was the first hospital unit to sail for Europe (May 7, 1917). She then served with the Bureau of Tuberculosis of the Red Cross, coordinating efforts of the Rockefeller Commission for the Prevention of Tuberculosis to assist French sanatoriums and hospitals. On September 15, 1917, she transferred for duty as chief nurse with the American Red Cross Children's Bureau of the Department of Civil Affairs, Red Cross Commission for France, and she started training French women to serve as home visitors in Paris. She served until transferred once more to military duty, as chief nurse of American Red Cross Military Hospital Number 5, Auteuil Tent Hospital. On January 1, 1919, she was released by the army and assigned by the Red Cross to the Balkan Commission, being made chief nurse for northern Serbia and assigned to Palanba Hospital, Serbia. She was recognized by the government of Serbia for her wartime service. While in Serbia, she came down with typhus (April 1919) and returned to the United States on July 15, 1919.

One may surmise that the tour of duty as chief nurse with the Red Cross Children's Bureau in France had a major impact on her career, especially since her work with children was interrupted by service during wartime. Following her return to the United States, she again took up child health nursing and assumed a leadership role in that area. She accepted a position as field director for the American Child Hygiene Association, an assignment which entailed overseeing the implementation of the standards of child care she had developed in Cleveland. The American Child Hygiene Association later joined with the American

Child Health Association, a merger enabling her to serve an older group of children than she had served in Cleveland and in her early work with the child hygiene association.

Her next position was as director of the Brooklyn Maternity Center Association, which provided free clinics for prenatal and postnatal care. In the summer of 1924, she organized a Mothercraft Club through which women were provided prenatal care and instruction; it was the first club of its kind in the United States.

The typhus she had contracted in Europe permanently affected her health through her remaining years, however. Her health problems forced her to retire from the Maternity Center and to accept a less demanding position as director of a convalescent home for children in Far Rockaway, Long Island. When she died in Brooklyn of an acute mastoid infection following emergency surgery, she was buried at Hartfield, near Jamestown, New York, with full military honors. At the time of her death, she was planning to attend the annual meeting of the National Committee on Red Cross Nursing Service.

WRITINGS: Numerous articles in professional journals.

REFERENCES: *American Journal of Nursing* (January 1928), pp. 71-72, 95; Annie M. Brainard, *The Evolution of Public Health Nursing* (1922); Lavinia L. Dock, Sarah E. Pickett, Clara D. Noyes, Fannie F. Clement, Elizabeth G. Fox, and Anna R. Van Meter, *History of American Red Cross Nursing* (1922); M. Louise Fitzpatrick, *The National Organization for Public Health Nursing, 1912-1952* (1975); Portia B. Kernodle, *The Red Cross Nurse in Action, 1882-1948* (1949); Meta Rutter Pennock, ed., *Makers of Nursing History* (1928), pp. 62-63, and (1940), p. 99; James H. Rodabaugh and Mary Jane Rodabaugh, *Nursing in Ohio* (1951); Carolyn Conant Van Blarcom, *Obstetrical Nursing* (2d ed., rev., 1928).

JOELLEN WATSON HAWKINS

LIVERMORE, MARY {RICE} (December 19, 1820, Boston--May 23, 1905, possibly in Melrose, Massachusetts). *Civil War nurse.* Daughter of Timothy Rice and Zebiah Vose (Ashton) Rice. Married Daniel Parker Livermore, minister; number of children unknown. EDUCATION: Attended Miss Hall's private school and Hancock Grammar School, Boston; c. 1835, attended Charlestown Female Seminary, Charlestown, Massachusetts, completing the four-year course in two years. CAREER: c. 1836-1837, taught at Charlestown Female Seminary (while she was a student); 1838-1840, governess in Virginia; c. 1840, principal of Duxbury High School, Duxbury, Massachusetts; 1857, editor of a religious newspaper, *New Covenant*, Chicago; c. 1861-1865, active in the U.S.

Sanitary Commission; 1869-1870, established *The Agitator*, a women's suffrage newspaper; lectured and wrote during the remaining years of her life.

CONTRIBUTIONS: Although known as a feminist, abolitionist, author, lecturer, organizer, fund-raiser, and advocate for nursing, Mary Livermore is remembered most for her valiant efforts on behalf of the Northern soldiers during the Civil War. As a member of the U.S. Sanitary Commission, she inspected hospitals where the wounded were warehoused with no beds, blankets, food, or nursing care. She used her influence and her skills of oratory and writing to improve the conditions of those hospitals. She organized soldiers' aid societies and used her talents to organize great sanitary fairs which raised money and goods needed for the care of the soldiers. In addition to her important work as a fund-raiser and organizer working for the Sanitary Commission, she was responsible for assigning nurses to their posts, and she even escorted them there and helped them get started in their humanitarian responsibility. When soldiers were discharged from the hospital and from the service, she occasionally accompanied them to their homes. Simultaneously, she continued writing columns in her husband's anti-slavery newspaper and therefore gained even more support for all of her humanitarian activities. For the Sanitary Commission, she wrote numerous circulars, bulletins, and monthly reports.

She apparently became a staunch abolitionist as a result of her experiences as a governess for a Virginia family, when she came into direct personal contact with slavery and came to recognize its destructive influence. After her marriage to an ardent abolitionist minister, they found that many members of the congregation condoned slavery and rejected their ideas. In addition, they supported the temperance cause, and although the prohibition law won in Maine and Connecticut, they found that their temperance views further divided the congregation. Daniel Livermore resigned his position, and they moved to Weymouth, Massachusetts, apparently finding many of the same divisions among churchgoers in that town. While in Weymouth, their oldest daughter died at the age of five.

They decided to join a group going west in the 1850s, very likely intending to settle in Kansas and thereby support the free-soil cause in its conflict with slave staters who came from Missouri to support the expansion of slavery into the newly developed territory. The illness of their daughter, however, forced them to stop and settle in Chicago, which was to be their home for fifteen years, from 1857 to 1872. After the Civil War and her work for the Sanitary Commission, Livermore became involved in the women's rights movement, having become convinced during the war years of its necessity when she observed how poorly men were handling the nation's decision making. She arranged for a women's suffrage convention to meet in Chicago, and among those attending were suffragists Susan B. Anthony and Elizabeth Cady Stanton. The lectures that were delivered at the convention were the first she had ever heard on the topic, and they obviously stirred her to become actively involved in the movement. Soon afterward, the Illinois Woman Suffrage Association was founded, and Livermore was elected president.

In 1870, she merged her paper, *The Agitator*, with Lucy Stone's *Woman's Journal*. Soon after, the Livermores moved back east, settling in Melrose, Massachusetts. Because she had no particular fondness for household duties expected of a housewife, she allowed herself to be convinced to become a public lecturer, and her husband supported the idea. She became so popular on the lecture circuit that she was known as "Queen of the Platform." She became president of the Massachusetts Suffrage Association, the honorary president of the Women's Christian Temperance Union, the president of the Beneficent Society of the New England Conservatory of Music, a life member of the Boston Women's Educational and Industrial Union, and an active member of the Masachusetts Indian Association, the National Conference of Charities and Correction, the Woman's Relief Corps, and the aid society of the Massachusetts' Soldiers Home. Twice, she was a delegate to the Massachusetts state Republican convention.

Over the years, she received recognition for her humanitarian activity and for her accomplishments. In 1896, the year that Tufts University graduated its first class of women, Livermore was presented an honorary doctor of laws degree. In 1903 when the Associated Alumnae of the United States gathered in Boston for their sixth annual meeting, she was a featured speaker, expressing her joy at being among so many trained nurses.

On May 6, 1895, Daniel and Mary Livermore celebrated their fiftieth wedding anniversary, and sharing in the occasion were their children, grandchildren, a sister, nephews, and nieces, along with people from the town of Melrose and countless representatives of various committees, schools, and associations. Telegrams were received from many states, from coast to coast. A bust of Livermore was made by Annie Whitney and was presented to the Shurtleff School in Boston by the alumnae association of that school.

WRITINGS: *My Story of the War* (1899); *The Story of My Life* (1899); hundreds of newspaper articles and letters.

REFERENCES: Mary Ellen Doona, "Nursing Revisited. The 1903 Convention," *Massachusetts Nurse* (June 1984), p. 6; Phebe A. Hanaford, *Daughters of America* (1883); Edith Horton, *A Group of Famous Women:*

Stories of their Lives (1914); Mary Livermore, *My Story of the War* (1899) and *The Story of My Life* (1899).

LORETTA P. HIGGINS

LOGAN, LAURA R. (Amherst, Nova Scotia, Canada--July 18, 1974, Sackville, Canada). *Nursing leader; educator.* She was the only daughter in a family of five children. Never married. EDUCATION: Attended Amherst Academy, Nova Scotia; 1901, B.A., Acadia University, Wolfville, Nova Scotia; 1904, diploma, Mt. Sinai Hospital School of Nursing, New York City; 1908, B.S. and diploma in education and hospital economics, Teachers College, Columbia University, New York City. CAREER: 1904-1907, private duty nursing, New York City; 1908-1910, instructor and supervisor, Mt. Sinai Hospital, New York City; 1910-1914, superintendent of Hope Hospital and principal of the Hope Hospital School of Nursing, Fort Wayne, Indiana; 1914-1924, director of Cincinnati General Hospital and of the nursing service, director of the School of Nursing and Health and professor of nursing, University of Cincinnati, Cincinnati, Ohio; taught nursing education and administration at Marquette University and Leland Stanford University (summers); 1924-1932, head of the Illinois Training School for Nurses (ITSN), title changed to dean of ITSN and director of Cook County (Chicago) Hospital's nursing service; 1925, instructor of nursing education, administration, and supervision (summer program), University of Chicago; 1932, surveyed schools of nursing in Europe for the Rockefeller Foundation; 1936, principal, Flower-Fifth Avenue Hospital School of Nursing and nursing superintendent of the hospital, New York City; 1937-1940, director of the school of nursing and nursing service, Boston City Hospital, Boston; c. 1940-1953, director of St. Louis (Missouri) City Hospital; 1953, retired from active nursing.

CONTRIBUTIONS: Laura Logan established the University of Cincinnati School of Nursing and Health, the first five-year combined nursing and liberal arts course leading to the diploma in nursing and the bachelor of science degree. This was accomplished in 1916, the same year that she became professor of nursing at the university, making her the second nurse in the United States to become a university professor. The creation of this professional school within the university was an educational highlight in nursing for that time, when the standard of nursing education was quite low.

Logan was for five years the dean of the independent (financially and administratively) Illinois Training School for Nurses (ITSN). She was in charge of the school during the period when it merged with the University of Chicago, with the hospital-based diploma school becoming a collegiate-level undergraduate school of nursing. She directed the first summer course in nursing at the University of Chicago, remaining for three more years as the director of nursing services and dean of the Cook County School of Nursing, which was founded when the ITSN no longer provided the nursing service for that hospital.

As dean of these schools and several others that she directed, she was responsible for vast changes in the basic preparation of nurses. She was one of the few nurses to have completed a baccalaureate degree before 1910, and she implemented many of the new ideas about nursing education that she learned through the program in hospital economics at Teachers College. She brought about a closer correlation of teaching and practice and extended the pre-clinical course from four to six months, adding more basic courses in the biological and social sciences. She led the movement to extend the nursing program from thirty to thirty-six months. Her belief that admission practices in schools of nursing should include mental testing of students was adopted. She began the practice of requiring students to write case studies of typical patients. She believed that every nurse should have preparation in public health nursing, and in 1926 she introduced courses in public health nursing into the curriculum. These included such public health concepts as the prevention of disease, promotion and maintenance of health, and health education. She supported the idea that the undergraduate program should not rely upon nurses taking post-graduate courses to make up for deficits in the basic curriculum, and as a result she insisted that major courses in psychology, sociology, nutrition, and hygiene be included in the undergraduate curriculum. Logan improved the living conditions for nurses by upgrading the standards at nurses' residences. While at Chicago, she was responsible for a library established in the nurses' home. She also sought to reduce, for all hospital workers, the required work week from fifty-six to fifty hours. Finally, she was noted for her ability to recruit a faculty of strength and prominence.

During World War I, she recruited the nursing service for Base Hospital number 25 and was slated to be the chief nurse, but the national Red Cross headquarters asked all heads of nursing schools to remain at their posts. She then became chairperson of the state and local branch of the nursing section of the women's committee of the Council of National Defense while she continued as director of the University of Cincinnati School of Nursing. Logan was president of the Ohio State Nurses' Association and the Ohio State League of Nursing Education. She was secretary and then for three terms president of the National League of Nursing Education, serving as a member of its board for twelve years. For nine years, she chaired the department of nursing education for the

American Journal of Nursing. She was a member or chairman of various local, state, and national committees, including the National Organization for Public Health Nursing, the National Red Cross Nursing Service Committee, the Committee on the Grading of Nursing Schools, the committee on standards of the National League of Nursing Education, and the American Nurses' Association committee on the Florence Nightingale international foundation, and she assisted in the writing of the National League of Nursing Education's publication, *Essentials of a Good School of Nursing* (1936).

Over the course of her career, she received numerous honors. These included an honorary master of arts degree from her alma mater, Acadia University (1929), and an honorary doctor of science degree from the University of Cincinnati. A residence at the University of Cincinnati was named for her, and her portrait hangs at Cook County Hospital, Chicago.

WRITINGS: Many articles on nursing and health in such publications as the *American Journal of Nursing*, the *Lancet Clinic*, *Hospital Social Service*, *Modern Hospital Management*, and *Hospital Progress*; "Educational Obligations" speech in the *Proceeding of the Twenty-third Annual Convention of the National League of Nursing Education* (1917)

REFERENCES: *American Journal of Nursing* (1974); *Biography and Genealogy Master Index* (2d ed.), p. 566; Teresa Christy, *Cornerstone for Nursing Education* (1969), pp. 56, 99; Katherine J. Densford, "Laura R. Logan," *National League of Nursing Education Biographical Sketch* (n.d.); Meta Rutter Pennock, *Makers of Nursing History* (1940), pp. 90-91; Grace Fay Schryver, *A History of the Illinois Training School for Nurses, 1880-1929* (1930), pp. 152-154, 172-173.

ALICE HOWELL FRIEDMAN

LOUNSBERY, HARRIET {CAMP} (November 3, 1851, Indianapolis, Indiana--March 24, 1946, Huntington, West Virginia). *Pioneer nurse of West Virginia.* Parents were from Vermont and she moved back there with them as an infant. Married Dr. Lounsbery, 1893. EDUCATION: Graduated from Temple Grove Seminary, Saratoga Springs, New York (now Skidmore College); 1881, graduated from Brooklyn Homeopathic Hospital School for Nurses, Brooklyn, New York; 1920, post-graduate summer at Western Reserve University, Cleveland, Ohio; 1923, post-graduate summer courses, Columbia University, New York City. CAREER: 1881-1885, private duty nursing, Brooklyn, New York; 1885-1892, superintendent, Brooklyn Homeopathic Hospital School of Nursing; 1898, chief nurse, Sternberg Hospital, Chickamauga Park,

Georgia; 1907-1924, school nurse, Charleston, West Virginia (including four years as supervisor).

CONTRIBUTIONS: Harriet Camp Lounsbery contributed to the development of nursing through her organizational work in the state of West Virginia, her work as a pioneering school nurse, and her work during the Spanish-American War. Her organizational work included establishing in 1905 the West Virginia State Nurses' Association and in serving as its president from 1905 to 1918. One of the first acts of the association was to submit a bill to the legislature for the registration of nurses. Lounsbery prepared the bill, which was defeated in 1905 but passed in 1907. West Virginia presented an unusual problem for nurses in that its state constitution contained a little-known regulation that made it impossible for women to hold public office. That meant that the Board of Nurse Examiners could not include any women; therefore the first members were all male physicians, including Lounsbery's husband who served as its secretary. Possibly because professional nurses were unable to play a major role in determining state policy, it was many years before they recognized the need to require a uniform curriculum for the West Virginia schools of nursing.

In addition to her work on behalf of the profession, she also contributed a great deal to public health nursing in West Virginia. In 1907, when she became a school nurse in Charleston, West Virginia, it was only five years after the first nurse to be employed by a school system started this work in 1902 in New York City. She also was a pioneer in including health education as part of the school program, following the example of Isabel Hampton Robb (q.v.) by giving lectures on practical hygiene. During the 1918 influenza epidemic, she was in charge of an emergency hospital in West Virginia. Later, when nurses were being recruited for World War I, she certified those who entered government service from West Virginia.

Almost a decade before she was to influence the evolution of nursing in West Virginia, she achieved recognition for her service to the nation. During the Spanish-American War she volunteered her services, and she succeeded Anna C. Maxwell (q.v.) as chief nurse of the army hospital at Chickamauga Park, Georgia. The Sternberg Hospital was the largest facility for Northern enrollees, with 70,000 soldiers in the summer of 1898. Because of inadequate sanitary facilities, typhoid fever, malaria, and dysentery caused many soldiers to become ill, and Lounsbery and her staff of 160 nurses provided the desperately needed nursing care. She also kept careful records of the progress of each case of typhoid fever among both the soldiers and the nurses. These statistics were valuable in establishing the epidemiology of the disease and were of use in the investigations into the prevalence of typhoid fever in the military camps of the day.

Lounsbery was an early member of the nursing service of the Red Cross, and she proudly displayed her badge number 1,050. It was as a result of the extensive experience in hospital nursing during the Spanish-American War that the Red Cross, which previously had not been involved with nursing, actively sought a role. After the war, she became president and then secretary of the Organization of Spanish-American War Nurses. She also was chairperson of the West Virginia Red Cross Nursing Service, as well as a founder and director of the Charleston (West Virginia) Public Library.

Lounsbery was a pioneer nurse-author. One of her earliest publications, under her maiden name of Harriet Camp and written while she was superintendent of a nursing school, was a text on ethics (*A Reference Book for Trained Nurses*, 1889) which is considered one of the first of its type. In 1912, she also published *Making Good on Private Duty: Practical Hints to Graduate Nurses*.

WRITINGS: *A Reference Book for Trained Nurses* (1889); *Making Good on Private Duty: Practical Hints to Graduate Nurses* (1912); "Some Reminiscences of Sternberg Hospital," *American Journal of Nursing* (October 1902), pp. 1-5, and (November 1902), pp. 81-84; in addition articles on private duty nursing published in the early issues of *Trained Nurse* and the *American Journal of Nursing*.

REFERENCES: *American Journal of Nursing* (1927), p. 197, (1936), p. 11, and (June 1946), p. 431; personal summary by Mrs. Lounsbery, American Journal of Nursing Collection, Nursing Archives, Mugar Library, Boston University; Lavinia Dock, *A History of Nursing* (1912); Philip Kalisch, "Heroine of '98," *Nursing Research* (1975), pp. 411-429.

ALICE HOWELL FRIEDMAN

M

MAASS, CLARA LOUISE (June 28, 1876, East Orange, New Jersey--August 24, 1901, Cuba). *Public health nurse.* Daughter of Robert E. Maass, mill worker, and Hedwig Maass. Never married. EDUCATION: Attended public schools of East Orange, including high school; 1893-1895, attended the Christina Trefz Training School for Nurses, Newark German Hospital, Newark, New Jersey, graduating in 1895. CAREER: 1892, worker in Newark Orphan Asylum; 1895-c. 1898, private duty nurse and staff nurse while awaiting approval of enlistment as an army nurse; October 1898-February 5, 1899, army nurse at field hospitals in Jacksonville, Florida, Savannah, Georgia, and Santiago, Cuba; November 20, 1899-May 7, 1900, served at the Field Reserve Hospital, Manila, the Philippines; 1901, returned to Cuba, employed by the sanitary department of Havana, which was then part of Cuba's military government, assigned to Las Animas Hospital.

CONTRIBUTIONS: A heroine in the war against yellow fever, Clara Maass volunteered to take part in experiments in Cuba which would prove conclusively that yellow fever was transmitted by mosquitoes. Prior to that experiment, Maass had acquired a reputation for courage in caring for patients with a variety of infectious diseases and for disregarding any risks to her own health to perform her duties. While in the Philippines, for example, she contracted dengue and was near death for several days. When she recovered, she was sent home to convalesce. As soon as she had regained her strength, she returned to duty and assumed her post in Cuba. The first time she was bitten by an infected mosquito as part of the Cuba yellow fever experimentation, the resulting fever was too mild to render her immune; therefore, she agreed to let herself be bitten again, this time in August 1901. A virulent fever ensued, causing her death ten days later. She was the only woman and the only American to die during the experiments which demonstrated conclusively that yellow fever was transmitted through mosquito bites. In 1902, her body was returned to the United States, and she was buried with full military honors at Fairmont Cemetery, Newark, New Jersey.

A flurry of newspaper stories appeared after her death, but soon her name and her deeds were all but forgotten except in the Newark area. In 1912, the Clara L. Maass Memorial Room was dedicated at the Newark Memorial Hospital. Few outside the Newark area knew of her sacrifice until 1923, when another nurse, Leopoldine Guinther, became curious about the portrait of Clara Maass and the Clara L. Maass Memorial Room at the hospital. She investigated the details of Maass' story, travelled to Cuba to gather information, and publicized the story of the brave, young nurse. In 1930, a new grave memorial with a bronze plaque bearing Maass' likeness was placed on her grave. In 1941, a stained glass window called the Clara L. Maass Memorial Window was dedicated at the Community Church, Mountain View, New Jersey. Her mother was granted a pension from the U.S. government, which recognized the importance of her sacrifice even though at the time of the experiment she was employed by the Cuban government and not by the U.S. Army. In 1951, Cuba issued a commemorative stamp honoring her, as did the United States on August 18, 1976, making Maass the first nurse to be so honored. The Franklin Mint struck a medal in memory of her birth, and on August 11, 1957, the Clara Maass Memorial Hospital, Belleville, New Jersey, was dedicated. In 1976, she was inducted into the Hall of Fame of the American Nurses' Association.

REFERENCES: *American Journal of Nursing* (February 1932), pp. 172-173, and (June 1950), p. 343; John T. Cunningham, *Clara Maass: A Nurse, a Hospital, a Spirit* (1968); M. Patricia Donahue, *Nursing: The Finest Art* (1985); Leopoldine Guinther, "A Nurse among the Heroes of the Yellow-Fever Conquest," *American Journal of Nursing* (February 1932), pp. 173-176; newspaper files, New Jersey Historical Society, Newark; *New York Times* (July 18, 1976); *Trained Nurse and Hospital Review* (August 1942), pp. 94-97, and (September 1948), p. 170.

LORETTA P. HIGGINS

McCLEERY, ADA BELLE (?, Americus, Kansas--?). *Leader in nursing administration.* Daughter of James Martin McCleery and Sarah Agnes (French) McCleery, pioneer farmers. Never married. EDUCATION: One-room country school, then in a larger school in rural Kansas; graduated from White City High School, Kansas; prepared for a teaching career, with private tutors and at the School of Civics and Philanthropy,

Chicago; 1907-1910, enrolled in Wesley Hospital Training School for Nursing, Chicago, graduating April 20, 1910. CAREER: Nurse for Camp Goodwill (fresh-air camp for needy children), Evanston, Illinois; business manager, Cook County Tuberculosis Hospital, Dunning, Illinois; business manager, tuberculosis division of Cook County Institution, Oak Forest, Illinois; May 1, 1915-1921, superintendent of nurses, Evanston Hospital, Illinois, and 1921-retirement in 1941, administrator of the hospital; 1931, lecturer in hospital administration, Teachers College, Columbia University, New York City; beginning in 1931, lecturer on hospital administration, University of Chicago.

CONTRIBUTION: Ada Belle McCleery's talent for administration led her to a leadership position not only of a training school but also of a hospital. At her first position after graduation, at a fresh-air camp for needy children from Chicago's tenement districts, she recognized the need for public health services and the role nurses could play in the administration of such services. She then developed her organizational abilities by serving as the business manager of two tuberculosis hospitals, the first an institution housing 220 male patients with advanced cases of the disease and the second with over 600 patients. Leaving that work in 1915, she became superintendent of the Evanston Hospital School of Nursing. In 1916, she proposed to Philip R. Shumway, trustee of the hospital, that through special arrangements with Northwestern University students in the training school be given special courses in anatomy, physiology, chemistry, and bacteriology; "since it is necessary to give a high grade professional training to a physician, it is becoming more important that we give a higher grade professional training to our nurses," she said. Such an affiliation was developed in 1919, providing student nurses with a liberal arts component in addition to the traditional hospital-based nursing program.

Since World War I had begun in Europe when McCleery assumed control of the hospital's training school, there was a nationwide shortage of nurses, with so many enlisting for military service. As a result, McCleery's most important responsibility was in recruiting more students and increasing enrollment at the school. She was able to do so without any reduction in standards; she rigidly enforced the high-school graduation requirement, changed the pattern of admission from individual to group, increased the probationary period from two to three months, and in spite of the pressures of the war, she worked out a classroom program totalling 600 hours, which represented a substantial increase. In 1919, she worked out an affiliation with Northwestern University, thereby adding a liberal arts component to the traditional nursing course. Students could earn a bachelor of science degree if they had completed two years of work at an approved college and took additional courses during their diploma program. It was the first degree program for nurses in Illinois.

In 1921, when the hospital's superintendent resigned, McCleery accepted the challenge of that position, relinquishing her position with the nursing school in order to devote full time to her new job as the hospital's superintendent. During her administration, the hospital more than doubled in size, changing from a modest neighborhood institution to a modern medical center with medical, surgical, obstetrical, pediatric, and communicable disease services. During that period, fund-raising resulted in the tripling of the hospital's endowment, with a large number of persons contributing to its support. Among her innovations were the use of cash payments rather than free meals for employees, establishment of an "inclusive rate" system of charging patients, development of medical and nursing education programs, and extending the benefits of the Chicago Plan for Hospital Care to the whole hospital family, including the nursing students. The Chicago Plan for Hospital Care was an early experiment in pre-paid medical and hospitalization insurance, and it was quite progressive for a hospital to offer it to all employees and students at that early date.

McCleery also contributed to the profession through her participation in numerous organizations. She was a member of the board of directors of the Illinois State Nurses' Association and its president for two years. She was treasurer of the Illinois State League of Nursing Education and a member of the examining committee of the state's Department of Registration and Education. She served also as a member of the executive committee of the Central Council for Nursing Education and chaired the credentials committee for several years. In 1924, she was elected secretary of the National League of Nursing Education, remaining in the office for five years and then serving a term on the league's board of directors. She was a trustee of the American Hospital Association, as well as second vice-president, representative on the committee on the grading of nursing schools, member of the administrative council, and the council on association development, and she was the first woman to chair the administrative section of the association. She was also the only woman on the board of directors of the Chicago Hospital Council. In addition to her professional contributions, she was active in community affairs as president of the Zonta Club and as a member of the Evanston Woman's Club and the University Guild.

WRITINGS: Numerous articles in professional journals.

REFERENCES: *American Journal of Nursing* (November 1923), p. 115; Vernon K. Brown, *Cathedral of Healing: The Story of Wesley Memorial Hospital, 1888-1972* (1981); Ada Belle McCleery to Philip R. Shumway, April 1, 1916, Thomas Franklin Holgate Papers, Northwestern University

Archives, Evanston, Illinois; Northwestern Memorial Hospital Archives, Chicago; Elizabeth W. Odell, *National League of Nursing Education Biographical Sketches, 1937-1940* (1940); Clare Louise Smith, *The Evanston Hospital School of Nursing, 1898-1948* (1948); *Trained Nurse and Hospital Review* (April 1938), pp. 410-417.

JOELLEN WATSON HAWKINS

McCLELLAND, HELEN GRACE (July 25, 1887, Austinburg, Ohio--December 20, 1984, Columbus, Ohio). *Leader in nursing education.* Daughter of Rev. Raymond G. McClelland, Presbyterian minister, and Harriet Lee (Cooper) McClelland. Never married. EDUCATION: Attended Shepardson Preparatory School, Granville, Ohio; 1907, attended Denison University, Granville, Ohio (left school in March 1908 due to attack of appendicitis, which led to her interest in nursing); October 30, 1908-May 1912, attended Pennsylvania Hospital School of Nursing, Philadelphia. CAREER: July 1, 1912-1913, graduate nurse, Weiser Hospital, Weiser, Idaho; 1913-1915, head nurse of the operating room, Norfolk (Virginia) General Hospital; 1915 (for six months), operating room nurse and nurse-anesthetist, American Ambulance Hospital, Neuilly, France; 1916 (for three months), returned to position in Norfolk, Virginia; November 1916-May 1917, nurse, Easton (Maryland) Hospital; May 7, 1917-May 25, 1919, nurse, Base Hospital Number 16, British Expeditionary Force, Le Treport, France; 1919-1926, nurse, Easton Hospital; 1926-July 1, 1956, nursing staff, Pennsylvania Hospital, including 1937-1956, director of nursing.

CONTRIBUTIONS: Helen Grace McClelland made significant contributions to the profession as director of nursing at Pennsylvania Hospital. During her tenure, she instituted changes and innovations that profoundly affected the development of the profession. She instituted a shorter workday, comparable to that in other fields, and she encouraged faculty and staff members to seek additional education and experience, offering them leaves of absence and encouraging friends to endow scholarships. After World War II, she responded to the nursing shortage by implementing a two-year program to prepare nurses for bedside care, and by designing a four-year collegiate course. In addition, she was instrumental in bringing American Indian girls to the Pennsylvania Hospital for training as nurses. These young women were sponsored by the Colonial Dames, and they came from Indian reservations all over the United States, including some from Alaska and Hawaii. McClelland was also instrumental in bringing the Cadet Nurse Program to the hospital during World War II.

She served in both World Wars I and II. During World War I, she served in the American Ambulance Hospital (1915), and when the United States entered the war, she joined the Army Nurse Corps, serving for two full years. During an air raid on a front-line British surgical unit (August 1917), she saved the life of her tentmate, Beatrice Mary MacDonald. During World War II, she organized the nursing component of the Pennsylvania Hospital's Fifty-second Evacuation Hospital.

As was the case with a number of other early nurses, she became a nurse as a result of her own experience with illness. She had an acute attack of appendicitis, and she was so impressed with the two nurses who cared for her at Newark's City Hospital that she abandoned her plans to attend Denison University and instead enrolled in the Pennsylvania Hospital School of Nursing, the alma mater of the two nurses who had cared for her in Newark. She reported on October 30, 1908, with four blue uniforms, twelve aprons, six collars, and a silver napkin ring engraved with her name. In spite of contracting typhoid during her second year, she completed the program in May 1912.

After retirement on June 30, 1956, she settled on an eighty-three acre farm near Reading where she enjoyed hunting, fishing, and gardening. In her eighties, she moved to Fredericktown, Ohio, near her birthplace. She received several important honors in recognition of her service. For her wartime contributions, she received America's Distinguished Service Cross, and she was inducted into the Legion of Valor. She was mentioned in a dispatch from Field Marshall Sir Douglas Haig, dated November 7, 1917, for gallant and distinguished service with the British Expeditionary Force, and it was signed by Winston Churchill, then the British secretary of war. Around 1930, she was featured with Captain Eddie Rickenbacker on the "Chevrolet Chronicles," a popular radio program of the time. On December 31, 1977, a CBS news special, "Women in Combat: The Battle Ahead," featured McClelland, along with General William Westmoreland, Senator William Proxmire, and Senator Barry Goldwater. She was given honorary membership in the British Royal Red Cross and in 1978 was inducted into Ohio's Women's Hall of Fame. The Helen McClelland Nurses' Conference Center of the Pennsylvania Hospital was named in her honor and dedicated on June 15, 1987.

REFERENCES: Transcript of "Chevrolet Chronicles," a radio program with Captain Eddie Rickenbacker, c. 1930; "Reminiscences of Helen Grace McClelland," typed manuscript (1987) provided by Irene Matthews, R.N., Holmes, Pennsylvania; correspondence with Irene Matthews, June 16, 1987; "In Memory Helen Grace McClelland," printed program from memorial service held January 11, 1985, Pennsylvania Hospital.

JOELLEN WATSON HAWKINS

McCRAE, ANNABELLA (1863, Quebec, Canada--February 1948, Boston). *Nurse-educator.* Daughter of John McCrae, a farmer, and Anne (McCallum) McCrae. Never married. EDUCATION: 1892, graduated from McLean Hospital nursing school, Somerville, Massachusetts; post-graduate studies in a private school in Montreal; 1895, graduated from Massachusetts General Hospital Training School for Nurses, Boston; summer 1916, attended Teachers College, Columbia University, New York City. CAREER: 1895, assistant superintendent, Quincy Hospital, Quincy, Massachusetts; 1902, second assistant and then first assistant with teaching responsibilities, Massachusetts General Hospital; 1912-1934, full-time instructor of nursing practice, Massachusetts General Hospital nursing school; summer of 1918, teacher of nursing practice, army school of nursing, Fort Devens, Massachusetts.

CONTRIBUTIONS: One of the earliest American nurses to achieve distinction as a teacher, Annabella McCrae is remembered for her continuous efforts to improve nursing education. Her first ten years at the Massachusetts General Hospital (MGH) were served in several administrative capacities before she became a full-time teacher. When she was able to devote all of her time and attention to education, she was responsible for teaching the introductory basic course in nursing procedures. Her teaching skills were reflected in the improved quality of nursing care provided by her students. McCrae was a full-time teacher for twenty-two years (1912-1934), and it has been estimated that she taught more than 2,000 students at the MGH. Many of her students went on to become teachers of nursing, and they modelled their commitment to the art of teaching after McCrae.

In addition to her work as a nurse-educator, McCrae was a well-known author. Her textbook, *Procedures in Nursing: Preliminary and Advanced*, was originally published in two volumes (volume 1 in 1923, volume 2 in 1925). She began to write this book in 1918, and it was completed seven years later. In the days when there were very few nursing textbooks and almost none that focused on the correct way to give care, McCrae's *Procedures in Nursing* was very well received. Indeed, it went through nine editions, from 1923 to 1934. Previous to the publication of this book, the student nurse had to watch the instructor and take notes on what the instructor was doing. For review, or in preparation for patient care, the student had only her notes to consult, and it was often the case that the notes were incomplete or even incorrect. The book could be available in each unit of a hospital, serving as an invaluable reference for not only student nurses but also for information about procedures which were not frequently followed but may have been necessary for individual patients. Examples might be how to prepare a slush bath, usually for patients suffering from typhoid fever, how to place a patient in Fowler's position, probably for either pneumonia or abdominal infection, or how to do a Dakins-Carrol irrigation for wound infections. At a time when nursing procedures were not at all standardized, this textbook served an essential role in helping to standardize procedures and to improve patient care in the process. Eventually the two volumes were combined into a single volume, and it was also translated into Chinese and Turkish and used in nursing schools abroad.

In addition to her work as an educator and author, McCrae was active in the early years of various nursing organizations. She was one of the nurses who in 1903 attended the meeting at Boston's Faneuil Hall to organize the Massachusetts State Nurses' Association. She was also chairperson of the census committee which examined the credentials of the nurses who applied for membership in the association, and she evaluated the quality of preparation provided by various training schools. She was an early member of the National League of Nursing Education and served as secretary-treasurer. She was one of the five nurses who formed the original committee to establish a county Central Registry, which provided professional leadership for private duty nurses who wanted to register their availability for nursing positions. Previously, private duty nurses had to rely upon word of mouth, a doctor's recommendation, or a good word from a local druggist. For many years, McCrae was president of the MGH sick relief association, which has through the years provided assistance to graduates in need.

In 1934, her contributions to nursing education were recognized when she was presented the Walter Burns Saunders Medal for distinguished service in the cause of nursing. In June 1948, during the progam to commemorate the seventy-fifth anniversary of the MGH School of Nursing, a special tribute service was held in honor of McCrae.

WRITINGS: *Procedures in Nursing: Prelimary and Advanced* (first published in 1923-1925).

REFERENCES: Papers of Annabelle McCrae, Massachusetts General Hospital School of Nursing Collection, Francis Countway Medical Library, Boston; Sara E. Parsons, "Annabelle McCrae," *National League of Nursing Education* (n.d.); Sylvia Perkins, *A Centennial Review: the Massachusetts General Hospital School of Nursing* (1975); Mary M. Roberts, *American Nursing: History and Interpretation* (1954).

ALICE HOWELL FRIEDMAN

McISAAC, ISABEL (January 9, 1858, Waterloo, Iowa--September 21, 1914, Washington, D.C.). *Nurse educator; administrator.* Never married.

EDUCATION: 1888, graduated from Illinois Training School for Nurses, Chicago. CAREER: 1888-1891, second assistant to the superintendent, Illinois Training School for Nurses; 1891-1893, first assistant to the superintendent, Illinois Training School; 1893-1895, assistant superintendent of the Illinois Training School, in charge of nursing at Presbyterian Hospital, Chicago; 1895-1904, superintendent, Illinois Training School for Nurses; 1904-1909, took time off to write nursing textbooks; 1910-1912, interstate secretary, Society of Superintendents of Training Schools for Nurses and the American Nurses' Association; 1912-1914, superintendent, Army Nurse Corps.

CONTRIBUTIONS: Isabel McIsaac was a superlative teacher and competent administrator who played major roles in the pioneer years of the nursing profession. She was probably the first to institute clinical demonstrations as a way to instruct pupils about nursing procedures and patient care (c. 1895). This was not only a revolutionary method of teaching for schools of nursing but also for medical schools, which had for generations tried to train physicians through lectures in large amphitheaters. The medical as well as nursing student had been left alone to make clinical applications of what they had learned through lectures and through reading of textbooks. In addition to her contributions to clinical teaching, McIsaac also was known for having designed methods of continuing education of graduate nurses. She did not believe that the completion of a course in a nurse-training school was sufficient education for the graduate nurse, seeing also the need to supplement the education for those graduate nurses whose formative training had been inadequate. She opened post-graduate clinical experiences at the Illinois Training School to a broad spectrum of nurses, thereby providing advanced training to a large number of nurses in the Midwest. McIsaac recognized that nursing conventions had to play an educational role as well as foster discussions about legislation and educational policies. As a result, she urged that practical nursing sessions be scheduled at annual conventions, an idea which clearly played a major role in the continuing education of many graduate nurses.

She believed that a proper system of nurse education had to teach students how to "nurse" patients rather than simply to carry out the doctor's orders. She asked, "are we preparing nurses or assistants to surgeons?" At the turn of the century, she made the radical observation that as medical education progressed, nursing education would deteriorate because students were being asked to provide more hospital service at the expense of education. She was blunt in insisting that the sources of many nursing problems were with the substandard schools which were being established in large numbers in order to staff the newly developing hospitals in an inexpensive manner.

It has been suggested that her professional development was influenced greatly by her mentors at the Illinois Training School, Isabel Hampton Robb (q.v.), Lavinia Dock (q.v.), and Edith Draper (q.v.). McIsaac had served as assistant to some of the pioneering nurse-educators, and she clearly had learned from the best. Yet she was innovative, always analyzing the situation to determine whether problems still existed and how best to resolve them. When she became superintendent at the Illinois Training School, she extended the length of the program from two to three years; that was one of the first schools which adopted this policy. In addition, she planned and developed clinical experiences for students, giving them grades based on their clinical practice as well as on their textbook knowledge. She believed that clinical work must reinforce the idea that students were in the hospital setting not only to provide patient care, but also as pupils whose training was basic to the advancement of the profession. She added courses in hygiene and bacteriology for the probationers, as the beginning students were called; the reason was not merely because the trained nurse needed a knowledge of those areas, but also because of her recognition of the problem of illness among her own students. She demanded that all student illnesses be promptly reported, and she insisted that proper care be provided to students who were recuperating. She also contributed to nursing education by writing several important textbooks. Indeed, she took almost six years off in order to have sufficient time for her writing. Her texts, *Primary Nursing Technique*, *Hygiene for Nurses*, and *Hygiene for Use of Public Schools*, were aimed at the beginning nursing student.

McIsaac was a charter member of the Illinois Training School for Nurses Alumnae Association, serving as its first vice-president. This association was one of the first in the country. At the first meeting of nurse-educators, held at the Chicago World's Fair of 1893, McIsaac was one of the speakers who endorsed the expansion of nurse alumnae associations. She was a convincing speaker who urged other superintendents of nurse-training schools to create their own alumnae associations, associations which would soon unite into what would become the American Nurses' Association (ANA).

In 1912, she presented a report to the convention of the major nursing organizations, a report which probably contained the first reference to the status of nursing education in the entire United States. McIsaac had been chosen to be the interstate secretary of a joint committee established by the ANA and the National League of Nursing Education. In that position, she travelled across the country, helping groups of nurses with their organizational problems. She visited a substantial cross-section of nursing schools and saw first-hand the conditions at those institutions. For a two-year period, she travelled across the country, speaking to state, county, city, and alumnae groups, as well as to groups of student nurses.

She also was one of the founders of the *American Journal of Nursing*, and she served for two terms as president of the American Journal of Nursing Company. She was one of the seven editors who assisted Sophia Palmer (q.v.) prepare the early editions of the *Journal*. McIsaac's department was "Practical Points on Private Nursing." At a time when very few nurses wrote about their experiences, she had the difficult task of collecting articles for that department.

In addition to her contributions to nursing education and to the *American Journal of Nursing*, McIsaac was keenly interested in the nursing profession around the world. She gave the opening address before the Third International Congress of Nurses, held in Buffalo, New York, in 1901. As presiding officer, she described what she saw as problems shared by nurses in all countries as they tried to upgrade nursing education and nursing service. She believed that their problems were the need for uniform admission standards to schools of nursing, a uniform curriculum, clearer definition of the term "nurse," state registration and licensure, local and national organizations to speak for the needs of nurses, and an awareness of the need for professional ethics.

In 1913, she became the acting president of the ANA when the elected president, Sarah Sly, resigned due to illness. As acting president, McIsaac addressed the sixteenth convention of the ANA, which was held in June 1913 at Atlantic City, New Jersey. At that time, she was superintendent of the Army Nurse Corps. While she was superintendent of the corps, a brief war with Mexico began, and one of her final official tasks was to send the list of nurses who were being assigned to Vera Cruz, Mexico. She was suffering from pernicious anemia, and in spite of failing health she remained in her position with the Army Nurse Corps until her replacement was not only selected but arrived to assume her important role. McIsaac's resignation was to take effect on October 1, 1914, but three weeks before that date, she died at Walter Reed Hospital, Washington, D.C. After her death, a national loan fund for nurses was named after her, as the Isabel McIsaac Fund (1914).

WRITINGS: *Primary Nursing Technique* (1907); *Hygiene for Nurses* (1908); *Bacteriology for Nurses* (1909); "Illinois School for Nurses, Chicago, U.S.A.," *Nursing Mirror* (England, 1900), p. 261.

REFERENCES: *American Journal of Nursing* (1914), pp. 85-86, and 91-102; National League of Nursing Education, *Some Early Leaders of American Nursing: Isabel McIsaac* (1922); Mary M. Roberts, *American Nursing: History and Interpretation* (1954); Grace Fay Schryver, *A History of the Illinois Training School for Nurses, 1880-1929* (1930).

ALICE HOWELL FRIEDMAN

McIVER, PEARL (June 23, 1893, Lowry, Minnesota--June 3, 1976). *Public health nurse; researcher.* Daughter of Hugh McIver and Anna (Erickson) McIver. Never married. EDUCATION: 1912, graduated from Minnesota State Teachers College, St. Cloud, Minnesota; 1919, graduated from University of Minnesota School of Nursing, Minneapolis, Minnesota; 1930, B.S., and 1932, M.A., Teachers College, Columbia University, New York City. CAREER: 1912-1926, teacher, elementary schools of Hatton and Webster, North Dakota; 1919, visiting nurse, University of Minnesota Student Health Service; 1922-1932, director of public health nursing, Missouri State Board of Health; 1933, nursing analyst, U.S. Public Health Service research division; 1936-1944, senior nurse consultant, U.S. Public Health Service; 1944-1957, chief, office of public health nursing, U.S. Public Health Service; 1957-1959, executive director, American Journal of Nursing Company.

CONTRIBUTIONS: Under the leadership of Pearl McIver, public health nursing in the U.S. Public Health Service expanded into a modern and extensive agency serving the needs of the American public. For more than twenty-five years, she was employed in the field of public health nursing administration, first with the Missouri State Board of Health and then with the U.S. Public Health Service. In 1933, she became the first public health nurse on the staff of the U.S. Public Health Service. In that position, she served as a public health nursing analyst, collecting data and analyzing it as to the need for more public health nurses in the agency. Until then, there had been no centralized office responsible for studying the public health nursing services in the country and determining precisely where there was a need for more or better service. Believing that higher standards for professional performance would result from planning based on accurate annual information on the status and numbers of public health nurses, she initiated *The Census of Public Health Nurses* which became an annual publication of the federal government. She also organized the consultation service through the U.S. Public Health Service which was intended to assist local nursing agencies, especially those in rural districts which did not have access to expert consultants. She provided the leadership in numerous studies which demonstrated the effect of public health measures and evaluated techniques as well as methods of administering nursing services.

Her research began to take a coherent shape when she was working on her master's thesis at Columbia University's Teachers College. Her thesis consisted of an analysis of first-level public health nursing in ten selected public health organizations. That study of the tasks expected of public health nurses eventually became the foundation for much of her later research, research which began the year after she received her master's degree (1933) and joined the U.S. Public Health Service. In addition, her thesis provided the basis for a most useful document, "Functions, Standards, and Qualifications," which was developed by the public health nurses' section of the American Nurses' Association (ANA).

McIver was a pioneer in the improvement of civil service standards for the nursing service. From 1941 to 1943, she administered the nurse education program of the U.S. Public Health Service, which later evolved into the U.S. Cadet Nurse Corps program, a program by which the federal government stimulated an increase in the student nurse population during World War II. After the war, McIver was chairperson of the National Nursing Planning Committee, and her influence extended to other countries when the United States established technical assistance programs which included public health missions to more than thirty other countries. In implementing the public health mission program, she travelled extensively to those countries which received assistance, as well as to other countries which were prime candidates for technical assistance. In 1949, she was an American delegate to the meetings of the Royal Sanitary Institute (Brighton, England), and delegate to the International Council of Nurses convention in Sweden. In 1954, she was chosen to serve as a special consultant in preparing for the technical sessions which were part of the 1955 World Health Organization assembly.

She was president of the ANA from 1948 to 1950, and in that position she was active in raising the professional and economic standards of nursing. She was the first public health nurse who was elected as ANA president and she chaired the joint structure committee which investigated the possibility of combining six national nurse organizations into two. In 1948, she helped to organize the celebration of the diamond jubilee of nursing, an occasion which served to focus public attention on a three-point program intended to solve national nursing problems, most notably the shortage of trained nurses. The three-point program consisted of economic security for the individual nurse, uniform license laws in the various states, and more effective counseling and placement of graduate nurses where they could be most effectively utilized. Under her leadership, the ANA took a census of all professional nurses for the National Security Board, which was examining the country's resources. It was found that the demand for nurses far outstripped the supply, even through the number of newly-trained nurses was rapidly increasing. McIver launched a recruitment goal of 40,000 additional student nurses to meet the needs of the future. At the same time, the ANA began a drive for better wage-hour contracts. This was clearly an attempt not only to improve the economic condition of America's nurses, but also to discourage nurses from seeking alternate positions which were less demanding and financially more rewarding.

She was president of the board of directors of the American Journal of Nursing Company, and after her retirement from federal service, she became its executive director. In addition to her active role in federal service and in the ANA, McIver was one of the first nurses to become a vice-president of the American Public Health Association. She also was an active member of the National Organization for Public Health Nursing, as well as the National League of Nursing Education, the National Red Cross Nursing Committee, the American Academy of Political and Social Science, and the American Association for the Advancement of Science.

Over her career she received numerous awards in recognition of her contribution to humanity and to the profession. The American Public Health Association gave her a public health nurse citation as well as a statuette of Florence Nightingale. In 1951, she received from the University of Minnesota an outstanding achievement award; the citation described her as "a celebrated nurse and pioneer in the federal health service." That description was certainly accurate, although it was far too brief for such an illustrious career. In 1955 she received the Albert Lasker Group Award of the American Public Health Association (along with Margaret Arnstein {q.v.} and Lucille Petry. The following year, the ANA bestowed upon her its public health nurse award, which in 1957 was renamed the Pearl McIver Public Health Nurse Award of the ANA. In 1957 she received an honorary degree from Western Reserve University (Cleveland, Ohio), and in 1961 she was the eighteenth recipient of the Florence Nightingale Medal of the International Council of Nurses. She was also an honorary member of Sigma Theta Tau, the national honor society of nursing.

WRITINGS: "Census of Public Health Nursing," *Public Health Nursing* (1941), pp. 21-23, 473-474, (1942), pp. 32-38, and (1944), pp. 498-501; "National Survey of Registered Nurses," *Public Health Nursing* (1941), pp. 472-473, (1942), pp. 154-156; "Preliminary Report," *Public Health Nursing* (1943), p. 340; "Our Nursing Resources," *Public Health Nursing* (1942), pp. 32-38; "Registered Nurses in the U.S.A.," *American Journal of Nursing* (1942), p. 769; "Analysis of the Present Qualifications of Public Health Nurses in the United States," *American Journal of Public Health* (1941), p. 151; "Trends in Public Health Nursing," *American Journal of Public Health* (1935), p. 551; "Federal Aid for Nursing Education and Student War Nursing Reserve," *Hospitals* (1943), p. 21.

REFERENCES: *American Journal of Nursing* (1948), p. 360; *Current Biography* (1949), pp. 378-380; Lyndia Flanagan, *One Strong Voice: The Story of the American Nurses' Association* (1976); James Gray, *Education for Nursing: A History of the University of Minnesota School* (1960); Pearl McIver, personal papers, Nursing Archives, Mugar Memorial Library,

Boston University; Mary M. Roberts, *American Nursing: History and Interpretation* (1954); *Starbuck Times* (Starbuck, Minnesota), October 25, 1951.

ALICE HOWELL FRIEDMAN

MACLEOD, CHARLOTTE (November 10, 1852, New Brunswick, Canada--October 21, 1950). *Leader in nursing education.* She was left an orphan and raised by an uncle. Never married. EDUCATION: 1891, graduated from Waltham Training School for Nurses, Waltham, Massachusetts; post-graduate courses at McLean Insane Hospital, Belmont, Massachusetts; Newport Hospital, Newport, Rhode Island; Presbyterian Hospital, New York City; and Long Island College Hospital, Brooklyn, New York. CAREER: Schoolteacher for over fifteen years before attending nursing school; May 1892-c. 1897, superintendent, Waltham Training School for Nurses; January 1898-c. summer 1904, superintendent of the Royal Victorian Order of Nurses, Ottawa, Canada; October 1906-end of 1908, superintendent and teacher, Training School for District Nurses, Boston District Nursing Association; January 1909-February 1912, superintendent of training school for attendants, Brattleboro Mutual Aid Association, Brattleboro, Vermont; January-c. September 1913, superintendent of nurses, Miradero Sanitarium, Santa Barbara, California; fall 1913, superintendent of nurses, Waltham Training School; 1914, acting matron, Roxbury House of Mercy, Roxbury, Massachusetts; 1915-1917, parish and social work for Christ Church Parish, New York City; March 1917-1921, returned to Waltham Hospital Training School.

CONTRIBUTIONS: Charlotte Macleod made her most significant contributions in organizing some of the early training schools for nurses. Following her post-graduate studies, she accepted the position as principal of the Waltham Training School, very likely due to the fact that she already had fifteen years of teaching experience prior to her nursing education and that she was undoubtedly familiar with the educational theories and techniques of the time. As principal, she played a significant role in improving the school and its small cottage hospital. Among the major innovations credited to her leadership were the expansion of the preliminary course to six months and the inclusion of instruction in homemaking. Before establishing a course on homemaking, she conducted a survey of all the training schools in the United States and Great Britain, requesting information about the role of homemaking in the curriculum. Since many of the early training school graduates became private duty nurses, going into the patient's home and providing for their health care as well as doing cooking, cleaning, and other household chores, a homemaking course, she believed, would be useful to the beginning nurse. Her survey indicated that the only institution which had a homemaking course as part of the nursing program was the Old Royal Infirmary, in Glasgow, Scotland. She planned such a course, and it was offered for the first time in 1895, at the Waltham Training School for Nurses. The course included instruction in sewing, cooking, and housekeeping, and during the probationary period, students practiced the household arts they had learned by caring for the nurses' home while they were enrolled in classes in anatomy and physiology, general chemistry, personal hygiene, nursery hygiene, record-keeping, reading, and note-taking. The students were also provided with experiences in district nursing of convalescent and chronic-disease patients.

In December 1896, she was able to travel to England, beginning a five-month leave of absence which enabled her to study the schools there and to spend six weeks with Rebecca Strong, the superintendent of the Old Royal Infirmary. She also visited various London hospitals, spent time with the Queen Victoria Jubilee Institute Nurses in the slums of Liverpool and London, and consulted with Florence Nightingale.

In January 1898, she assumed the position of chief superintendent of the Victorian Order of Nurses, which was founded in Ottawa, Canada, by Lady Aberdeen, wife of the governor-general. It was a district nursing program, similar to that of the Queen's Jubilee Nurses in Great Britain, and it was named as a tribute by the women of Canada on the occasion of the sixtieth anniversary of Queen Victoria's accession to the throne. Lady Aberdeen had learned that the Waltham Training School was unique in offering a district nursing program, and as a result Macleod was recruited to play a leadership role in the order. There were two training homes connected with the Victorian Order of Nurses, one in Montreal and the other in Toronto. Both of them offered four-month post-graduate courses in district nursing. Macleod was responsible for overseeing the schools, as well as the work of the order. She remained in Canada for the next six and a half years, resigning due to ill health. While she was recovering, she travelled in Great Britain during 1904 and 1905, and while there she was urged to accept the position of general secretary of the Queen Victoria Jubilee Institute Nurses. In addition, she was invited to take charge of a nursing program being initiated in India, but she declined both offers and chose to return to the United States.

In 1906, she organized and planned the Training School for Visiting Nurses (which later merged with the School of Public Health of Simmons College) of the Boston Instructive Visiting Nurse Association. Because of her experiences with district nursing in Waltham, Canada, and England, she was the most appropriate choice for this innovative program, the first of its kind in the United States. By going on the rounds with her students, she personally taught them the difference between hospital and home nursing. From Boston, she went to Vermont to serve as superintendent of the training school for attendants established by the Brattleboro Mutual Aid Association. This school was also innovative, the first of its kind. It also could have been used as a model for nurses wishing to extend their professional services, as it was a cooperative plan through which individuals could prepay for nursing services.

In 1921, after having served in positions in Santa Barbara, California, in Waltham, and Roxbury, Massachusetts, and in New York City, she served as director of the Waltham Hospital's two-month course in home nursing for attendants; the program included lessons and practice in cleanliness and care of the home, as well as hygiene of the sick room. Graduates of the two-month course could register to serve in homes requiring unskilled nursing service. When the registry, previously run by the Graduate Nurses' Alumnae, was turned back to the school, Macleod also took charge of that.

Living her last years in retirement, ill health prevented her from participating actively in nursing activities. Yet she continued to be interested in the development of the profession and to inspire those who followed her in providing leadership.

WRITINGS: Articles in professional journals; numerous unpublished letters and reports.

REFERENCES: *American Journal of Nursing* (February 1901), pp. 381-382, and (September 1901), pp. 875-876; Annette Fiske, *First Fifty Years of the Waltham Training School for Nurses* (1949); *A History of the Graduates of the Waltham Training School for Nurses* (1937); Meta Rutter Pennock, *Makers of Nursing History* (1928, 1940); Alfred Worcester, *Nurses for Our Neighbors* (1914).

JOELLEN WATSON HAWKINS

McNAUGHT, ROSE MADELINE (March 6, 1893, Holyoke, Massachusetts--August 1978). *Nurse-midwife.* Daughter of William McNaught, papermaker, and Mary (Hurley) McNaught. Never married. EDUCATION: Graduated from Holyoke High School; 1912-1913, attended Westfield Normal School, Westfield, Massachusetts, graduating in 1913 with a teaching certificate; c. 1920, graduated from the Army School of Nursing, Washington, D.C.; 1928, certificate in nurse-midwifery, York Road Lying-In Hospital, London, England. CAREER: 1913-c. 1917, taught elementary grades in the public schools of Holyoke and Whately, Massachusetts; c. 1920-1922, head nurse, Holyoke Hospital; 1922-1926, staff nurse, then supervisor, Henry Street Settlement, New York City; 1926-1927, nurse, Frontier Nursing Service, Leslie County, Kentucky; 1928-1931, nurse-midwife, Frontier Nursing Service; 1931-1945, supervisor, Lobenstine Clinic (for midwifery), New York City; 1942-1945, teacher of nurse-midwifery, Maternity Center Association, New York City; 1945-1957, supervisor, John E. Berwin Clinic, New York City; 1957-c. 1962, consultant to the Maternity Center Association, New York City.

CONTRIBUTIONS: Rose McNaught was the first American-born nurse-midwife to practice her profession in New York City. For many years, she was the only nurse-midwife to practice outside the hills of Kentucky. After serving several years as a midwife with the Frontier Nursing Service (FNS) in Kentucky, she went to New York City where she organized the Lobenstine Clinic on the city's West Side. From 1931, when the clinic was established, it paralleled in an urban setting what had been developed in Leslie County, Kentucky. In the beginning, she was supervisor of the clinic; she set up the nurse-midwifery service and a school of midwifery. The clinic served the poor of one part of New York City, while medical students managed home deliveries of the poor in the East Side. Prior to her development of a school of nurse-midwifery, all trained nurse-midwives, such as those serving with the FNS, had gone abroad for their training. Self-taught midwives served most of the immigrant population of the various cities, and one of McNaught's responsibilities was to win the respect of the lay midwives in order to help them improve their skills and knowledge. She also was responsible for introducing the idea of nurse-midwifery to the skeptical medical profession of the city.

Perhaps McNaught's greatest contribution was through her work as a teacher of nurse-midwives. Through her students, she made a great impact on the specialty of nurse-midwifery, helping make it a recognized area of nursing. She opened up opportunities for many nurses who wanted a greater role in the care of mothers and infants than that offered to obstetrical nurses. Her influence continued through the careers of the nurse-midwives she knew in their student days, and many went on to leadership positions in the profession after having become skillful practitioners.

Interestingly, Rose McNaught's introduction to midwifery came when she became head nurse of the obstetrical unit of the Holyoke, Massachusetts, hospital, where she began to serve the immigrant mill workers of that papermaking city. She then moved to the Henry Street Settlement, New York City, having secured the position through her former teacher at the Army School of Nursing, Annie Goodrich (q.v.). While at Henry Street (1922-1926), McNaught assisted physicians with the delivery of infants in the crowded tenements of New York City. She became critical of the local physicians who accepted the fee for a home delivery but who often relied upon the visiting nurse to conduct an emergency delivery without him. She came to recognize that nurses needed specialized training before they could be expected to manage home births reliably. While at Henry Street, she became aware of the magnitude of services that nurse-midwives could offer, and she came into contact with the director of the Maternity Center Association and met two nurse-midwives from the FNS who were doing advanced work at Columbia University Teachers College (including Mary Willeford {q.v.}).

After serving at Henry Street for five years, she moved to Kentucky as a nurse-midwife with the FNS. She recognized her own inadequacy, however, and in 1928 she decided to return to school for specialized training in midwifery. Since there were no training schools for nurse-midwives in the United States, she followed the lead of Willeford by going to London where she studied at the York Road Lying-In Hospital. After serving several more years with the FNS, Mary Breckinridge (q.v.), director of the FNS, encouraged her to go to New York City and open the Lobenstine Clinic. Later, McNaught assumed the supervisory position with the Berwin Clinic, and she continued her practice and teaching there. Finally, in 1958, the home delivery service ended because of the decreased demand for service; the first-generation immigrant population no longer needed home deliveries, and the second and third generations preferred to rely upon hospitals and physicians. At that point, nurse-midwifery education moved into an academic setting.

McNaught was given life membership in the American College of Nurse-Midwives (ACNM), and in 1977 she was presented with the Hattie Hemschemeyer Award at the twenty-second annual meeting of the ACNM.

REFERENCES: *Briefs* (March 1979), pp. 35-36 (official publication of the Maternity Center Association); Sally A. Tom, "Rose McNaught: American Nurse-Midwifery's Own 'Sister Tuto,'" *Journal of Nurse-Midwifery* (1979), pp. 3-8, and "The Evolution of Nurse-Midwifery," *Journal of Nurse Midwifery* (1982), pp. 4-13; information from the archives, Westfield State College, Westfield, Massachusetts.

ALICE HOWELL FRIEDMAN

MAHER, MARY ANN (March 12, 1902, Exeter, New Hampshire--February 11, 1982, Amherst, Massachusetts). *Nurse-educator; public health nurse.* Daughter of William Maher and Ellen (Sheehan) Maher. Never married. EDUCATION: 1920, graduated from Robinson's

Seminary, Exeter, New Hampshire; 1930, received diploma, Rhode Island Hospital School of Nursing, Providence, Rhode Island; 1936, received certificate in public health nursing, Simmons College, Boston; 1941, B.S., and 1949, M.A., Teachers College, Columbia University, New York City.
CAREER: 1930-1931, teacher and supervisor, School of Nursing, Strong Memorial Hospital, Rochester, New York; 1931-1936, instructor, Rhode Island School of Nursing; 1936-1938, staff nurse and special project director, Visiting Nurse Association of Boston; 1938-1940 and 1941-1943, public health nursing instructor, Massachusetts General Hospital School of Nursing, Boston; 1943-1946, supervisor of schools of nursing, Commonwealth of Massachusetts Board of Registration in Nursing; 1946-1947, regional public health nursing consultant, U.S. Childrens' Bureau, New York City; 1947-1948, dean, Boston College School of Nursing; 1950-1953, associate professor, Boston University School of Nursing; 1953-1970, dean, University of Massachusetts School of Nursing, Amherst.
CONTRIBUTIONS: Mary Ann Maher was the first to serve as dean of two schools of nursing in the commonwealth of Massachusetts. She became the founding dean of the Boston College School of Nursing and later the founding dean of the University of Massachusetts School of Nursing, where she served for seventeen years. In a state noted for private education, she was a pioneer in forming a state-supported school for basic nursing education and later for graduate-level nursing education.

Always an advocate of high-quality education for nurses, Maher was concerned about the importance of adequately prepared faculty in all nursing schools in higher education. To assist this process, she was able to secure federal funding for a successful seven years of summer workshops for the continuing education of nursing faculty from a variety of schools in New England, with the focus on the arts, sciences, and humanities.

She had a profound interest in the family as a unit of public health nursing, an approach which apparently was developed through her early employment in Rochester's Strong Memorial Hospital, where she participated in a multi disciplinary approach to health. That interest is reflected in the preface of the text (1951) by the well-known pioneering psychiatric nurse, Hildegarde Peplau, who credited Maher as one of those who had been of assistance in her work. In 1951, there were relatively few who saw mental hygiene (and the family's influence) as having any relation to nursing practice, but Maher was instrumental in having these concepts included in the curriculum of university schools of nursing.

In addition, she believed that students should learn to work with other health professionals, and when she was an instructor at Massachusetts General Hospital, she was instrumental in ensuring that students learned about and worked with social workers, nutritionists, early childhood educators, and so forth. She was one of the first to require student nurses to visit nursery schools, for instance, to have the opportunity to see healthy children, not just the sick who were hospitalized.

Through her research, she documented the needs of persons in urban, high-rise, low-income housing who had little access to health care. With federal funding, she and her faculty demonstrated that services could be brought successfully to the residents of housing projects.

In 1960-1961, she was president of the Massachusetts League for Nursing. She was a member of the state Board of Registration in Nursing, as well as a number of other professional and health related organizations, including the executive committee of the Massachusetts Committee on Children and Youth and the Governor's Advisory Committee for Planning for Mental Health. During its founding years, she was on the executive committee of the New England Council on Higher Education for Nurses, and she was active in the department of baccalaureate and higher-degree programs of the National League for Nursing.

Maher received an honorary doctor of science degree from Boston University in September 1969 in recognition of her role as a "distinguished nursing educator." A scholarship fund in her name was set up at the University of Massachusetts at the time of her retirement. She is mentioned in the bicentennial publication of the Massachusetts Nurses' Association as one of the nurses of the commonwealth whose achievements helped to develop the profession. On June 16, 1973, Maher received from the Nurses' Alumnae Association of the Rhode Island Hospital School of Nursing the Award of Honor for her outstanding contribution to the nursing profession. That group also recognized her as an outstanding graduate on November 6, 1980, which marked her fifty years as a graduate of that school.

REFERENCES: *American Journal of Nursing* (June 1982), p. 998; *Daily Hampshire Gazette* (Northampton, Massachusetts, February 11, 1982); Alice H. Friedman, "Nursing Revisited: Oral History and Mary A. Maher," *Massachusetts Nurse* (May 19, 1984); Nursing Archives, Mugar Library, Boston University; Sylvia Perkins, *A Centennial Review: 1873-1973, of the Massachusetts General Hospital School of Nursing* (1975).

ALICE HOWELL FRIEDMAN

MAHONEY, MARY ELIZA P. (May 7, 1845, Dorchester, Massachusetts--January 4, 1926, Roxbury, Massachusetts). *First black graduate nurse.* Daughter of Peter Mahoney and Mary Jane (Stewart) Mahoney. Never married. EDUCATION: May have attended Phillips Street School, Boston; 1878-1879, attended nursing classes at the New England Hospital for Women and Children, graduating on August 1, 1879. CAREER: 1879-c. 1910, private duty nursing.

CONTRIBUTIONS: Mary Mahoney was the first black woman to enroll in and graduate from a formal training program for nurses that granted a diploma. Little is known of her life until the age of thirty-three, nor do we know how she came to be enrolled in the program at the New England Hospital for Women and Children just five years after Linda Richards (q.v.) became America's first trained nurse. Her course in nursing was sixteen months in length and included medical, surgical, night, and confinement nursing. Although she was quite small, under five feet tall and weighing about ninety pounds, she evidently had the stamina to endure the rigorous nursing course of that time period. After graduation, she practiced private duty nursing, caring for patients in their homes, as did most other graduate nurses of her day. She is listed in the registry of the Boston Medical Library's Directory and probably was listed in other directories and known to Boston's physicians.

One source states that for a time she cared for a patient in New Jersey, being called there since the individual had been one of the babies she cared for as a private duty nurse. Another time, she was called to Washington, D.C., to care for an army surgeon, the husband of a friend, who was suffering from tuberculosis. For most of her life, however, she lived in a small apartment on Warwick Street in Roxbury, Massachusetts.

Her contributions were not confined to her patients. Recognizing the need for nurses to work together for the profession and especially for black nurses to unite to promote their rights, she became a member of the National Association of Colored Graduate Nurses, and at its first conference (in Boston in 1909), she gave the welcoming address and was elected chaplain and a life member. She also arranged for a demonstration at the New England Hospital for Women and Children, as well as a tour of the wards and tea on the lawn. Through 1921, she attended conferences of this organization and was active in recruiting new members. At the 1921 meeting in Washington, D.C., she and other nurses who attended the conference were received at the White House by President Warren G. Harding.

After her retirement from the practice of nursing, she continued to support various professional organizations. She was one of the first black nurses to join the American Nurses' Association, joining through the Alumnae Association of the New England Hospital for Women and Children.

She was seventy-six years old when the Nineteenth Amendment was ratified and went into effect, and she registered for the vote in order to take advantage of that important opportunity for political equality. In 1923, she developed breast cancer and was admitted on December 7, 1925, to the New England Hospital for Women and Children, where she died less than one month later. She was buried at Woodlawn Cemetery, Everett, Massachusetts. In 1973, the gravesite was restored, and a granite monument was erected by Chi Eta Phi, a national black nurses' sorority, and by the American Nurses' Association. The first "national pilgrimage" to the gravesite was held in September 1984, when the four winners of the Mary Eliza Mahoney Award and other members of the American Nurses' Association and Chi Eta Phi gathered to pay homage to the pioneer black nursing leader.

The Mary Mahoney Medal was named in her honor. First given by the National Association of Colored Graduate Nurses in 1936, it is now given at biennial conventions of the American Nurses' Association. Several local affiliates of the National Association of Colored Graduate Nurses were named in her honor: for many years, the Mary Mahoney Nurses Local in Boston memorialized her through its name. The recreation hall at Camp Livingstone, Louisiana, was named in her honor in 1944. The seventy-fifth anniversary of her graduation was celebrated at the American Nurses' Association convention in 1954, and she was honored in the April issue of the *American Journal of Nursing*. In 1970, the Area 2 Family Life Center in Roxbury, Massachusetts, was named the Mary Eliza Mahoney Family Life Center. When the American Nurses' Association Hall of Fame was initiated in 1976, Mary Mahoney was among the fifteen nurses chosen as charter members.

REFERENCES: *The American Nurse* (October 1984), p. 14; American Nurses' Association, *Heritage Hall/Hall of Fame* (1976); Mary Elizabeth Carnegie, *The Path We Tread: Blacks in Nursing, 1854-1984* (1986); Mary Ella Chayer, "Mary Eliza Mahoney," *American Journal of Nursing* (April 1954), pp. 429-431; Antionette M. Ricks Demby, "The Future of the Colored Nurse," *Nursing World* (September 1928), pp. 320-321; Mary Ellen Doona, "Glimpses of Mary Eliza Mahoney," *Journal of Nursing History* (April 1986), pp. 20-34, and "Mary Eliza Mahoney (1845-1926)," *The Massachusetts Nurse* (November 1984), pp. 7-8; Darlene Clark Hine, ed., *Black Women in the Nursing Profession: A Documentary History* (1985); Cordelia W. Kelly, *Dimensions of Professional Nursing* (2d ed., 1968); *Notable American Women*, pp. 486-487; Mabel Staupers, *No Time for Prejudice* (1961); Adah B. Thoms, *Pathfinders: A History of the Progress of Colored Graduate Nurses* (1929).

Dictionary of American Nursing Biography

JOELLEN WATSON HAWKINS

MARKOLF, ADA MAYO {STEWART} (December 2, 1870, North Braintree, Massachusetts--April 26, 1945, Vermont Eastern Star Home, Randolph, Vermont). *Industrial nurse.* Daughter of William Henry Stewart, a navy chaplain, and Roline (Mayo) Stewart. Married Henry J. Markolf, March 14, 1918 (died September 14, 1934); no children. EDUCATION: 1893, graduated from Waltham Training School for Nurses, Waltham, Massachusetts; received diploma for having passed a course in massage taught by Dr. Douglas Graham, Boston. CAREER: 1893-1895, private duty nursing, Waltham, Massachusetts; 1895, industrial nurse, Vermont Marble Company, Proctor, Vermont; 1896-1898, matron, Proctor Hospital, Proctor, Vermont; 1898-1900, surgical nurse for Drs. Field and Duringer, Fort Worth, Texas; 1900, assistant superintendent, Rutland Hospital, Rutland, Vermont; served five years in Troy, New York, doing massage and teaching massage to nurses at Samaritan Hospital Training School; private duty nursing, Seattle, Washington, St. Augustine, Florida, and Lake Placid, New York (to c. 1918 when she apparently retired from nursing upon marriage to Henry J. Markolf).

CONTRIBUTIONS: Ada Stewart is best remembered as the first industrial nurse hired by an employer in the United States. When officials of the Vermont Marble Company decided to hire a nurse to provide care to their employees, they contacted the superintendent of the Waltham Training School for Nurses, which was unique among training schools of its day because it not only prepared young women for hospital nursing but also for visiting nursing in the homes of patients requiring specialized care. The superintendent selected Stewart, who had graduated in 1893 and who had spent the next two years as a private duty nurse in that city.

The residents of Proctor, Vermont, many of whom were employees of the Vermont Marble Company, welcomed Stewart and the visiting nurses who followed her in her pioneering work. (Ada's sister, Harriet Stewart Ross, also a Waltham graduate, was soon engaged to do visiting nursing in West Rutland and Center Rutland, near Proctor and also populated by employees of the marble company). When officials of the company recognized the need for a hospital to serve employees and their families, the Proctor Hospital was opened on August 6, 1896, in a private home which was transformed into a hospital. Stewart was the first matron of the hospital. Within ten years, the number of patients outgrew the facilities, and a new, modern building was opened on April 1, 1904. By that time, however, Stewart had gone on to other work. Having taken a course in massage, she added it to her nursing skills and soon was not only providing massage to her patients, but also teaching the art of massage to other nurses.

After her pioneering work as an industrial nurse in Vermont, Stewart devoted twenty years to a variety of positions in a number of states. At the age of forty-seven, she retired from nursing to marry Henry Markolf, and since the marriage was performed in West Rutland, Vermont, where her sister lived and where Ada and Henry Markolf purchased a home, it can be surmised that she met her future husband during a visit to her sister in Vermont. During the 1940s she spent some time writing about industrial nursing. Stewart continued to reside in West Rutland for six years after her husband died in 1934, and little information is available on the remaining years of her life. She eventually entered an Eastern Star Home in Randolph, Vermont, where she died.

WRITINGS: Numerous articles in professional journals, including "Industrial Nursing Begins in Vermont," *Public Health Nursing* (March 1945), pp. 125-129, and the section entitled "The Proctor Hospital" in *We Who Serve: A Story of Nursing in Vermont* (1941).

REFERENCES: Copy of death record, Public Records Division, Montpelier, Vermont; unpublished materials, Proctor Historical Society, Proctor, Vermont, and recollections of members of the society; information provided by Harriet Mead Ross, daughter-in-law of Harriet Stewart Ross (Ada Markolf's sister), West Rutland, Vermont; Vermont State Nurses' Association, *We Who Serve: A Story of Nursing in Vermont* (1941); Waltham Graduate Nurses' Association, *A History of the Graduates of the Waltham Training School for Nurses* (1937); Yssabella Waters, "Industrial Nursing," *Public Health Nurse* (September 1919), pp. 728-731; West Rutland, Vermont, town records, town clerk's office.

JOELLEN WATSON HAWKINS

MAXWELL, ANNA CAROLINE (March 14, 1851, Bristol, New York--January 3, 1929, New York City). *Educator; hospital administrator; Spanish-American War nurse.* Daughter of John Eglinton Maxwell, ordained clergyman, and Diantha Caroline (Brown) Maxwell. Never married. EDUCATION: Tutored at home; attended Ripley boarding school, Middleport, New York; 1876, attended three-month course in obstetrics at the New England Hospital for Women and Children, Boston; 1876-1880, attended Boston City Hospital Training School for Nurses, graduating in 1880. CAREER: 1874-1876, assistant matron at the New England Hospital for Women and Children, after which she attended the Boston City Hospital Training School for Nurses; 1880, spent six months attempting to establish a nursing school at Montreal General Hospital; 1881, visited various European hospitals; 1881-1889, director of Boston Training School for Nurses, Massachusetts General Hospital; 1889-1891, completed organization of the Training School for Nurses, St. Luke's Hospital, New York City; 1891-1921, director of the School of Nursing at Presbyterian Hospital, New York City; 1898, served as a nurse during the Spanish-American War.

CONTRIBUTIONS: As director of the Boston Training School for Nurses at the Massachusetts General Hospital (1881-1889), Anna Maxwell made remarkable changes considering the fact that the hospital was mired in tradition. Among the improvements she made were a nurses' residence on the hospital grounds, with private bedrooms, a reception room, and a library. She also introduced nurses into the operating rooms of the hospital, added a night superintendent of nurses, and established lessons in massage and cooking. As a result of her work, the attitudes of the house staff toward the nurses substantially improved.

After serving at the Massachusetts General Hospital, she accepted the challenge of completing the organization of the nursing school at St. Luke's Hospital, New York City, and although her stay at St. Luke's was relatively short (1889-1891), she was successful in improving the situation of the nurses in her charge. For example, she abolished the practice of twenty-four-hour duty which had required that a nurse remain with her patient day and night, sleeping on a narrow cot in the patient's room. Upon her resignation, the excellent quality of her work at St. Luke's was set down in the minutes of the Executive Committee of the Board of Managers, she was credited with the success of the training school, and her resignation was accepted with regret.

While director of the nursing school at Presbyterian Hospital (1891-1921) and in her months of service during the Spanish-American War, Maxwell earned the title of "The American Florence Nightingale." She recruited women of high caliber into nursing, and as a result the nursing school at Presbyterian Hospital boasted of an exceptionally-high-quality student body. With strong support from the administrators and medical staff, the school was built upon high educational standards. She became known for standardizing nursing techniques and procedures.

During the Spanish-American War, Maxwell and other superintendents of nursing schools were involved in selecting candidates for the Red Cross Auxiliary Number 3, which was to provide nurses to care for the sick and wounded soldiers. She and twenty other graduate nurses went to Chickamauga Park to take charge of a tent hospital for 1,000 patients, and in primitive conditions, they cared for patients who had been transported for several miles in crowded ambulances under the hot summer sun. She was so successful in organizing supplies and nursing care that attitudes of male army officers changed from one of skepticism about nurses in camps to one of appreciation of their service.

After the war, Maxwell was a member of a committee which was established to encourage Congress to establish a corps of nurses that would be ready to care for ill and wounded soldiers during future wars, and through these efforts the Army Nurse Corps was finally established. During World War I, she held the position of chief nurse of the Presbyterian Hospital Unit, and although considered too old for active duty, in 1916 she visited hospitals in the European war zones in order to learn more about nurses' work as part of a military organization. She headed a committee of New York chief nurses to choose a uniform for the nurses in military service. In 1918, she visited the Presbyterian Unit at Etretat, France, and while she was there American nurses were invited to join a parade in Paris; although sixty-seven years old at the time, she marched, carrying the Red Cross banner. During her busy years as director of the nursing school at Presbyterian Hospital and involvement in two wars, she found time to co-author *Practical Nursing: A Text-Book for Nurses* (with Amy Elizabeth Pope), which went through four editions.

In 1917 she was granted an honorary master of arts degree from Columbia University. Upon her retirement, a banquet was held in 1922, attended by over 500 friends and colleagues. In 1928, she received (at her bedside because she was seriously ill at the time) a Public Health Medal of Honor from the French government, awarded in appreciation of her work during World War I. After her retirement she continued to be active, travelling in Europe and attending the 1925 meeting of the International Council of Nurses, in Finland. She was the honorary chairwoman of a campaign committee to raise money for a nurses' residence at Columbia-Presbyterian Medical Center, which was named the Anna C. Maxwell Hall. She was described as having a zest for life, an excellent sense of humor, and a great amount of energy. She died of a heart condition, and after services in New York, she was buried with full military honors in the Arlington National Cemetery.

WRITINGS: *Practical Nursing: A Text-Book for Nurses* (with Amy Elizabeth Pope, 1st ed., 1907).

REFERENCES: Elizabeth Ashe, "As I Knew Miss Maxwell," *Pacific Coast Journal of Nursing* (February 1929), p. 70; *American Journal of Nursing* (June 1921), pp. 688-697, (June 1923), p. 766, and (February 1929), pp. 187-194; *British Journal of Nursing* (February 4, 1922), p. 71; Annie Warburton Goodrich, *The Social and Ethical Significance of Nursing: A Series of Addresses* (1932); *National League for Nursing Education Calendar* (1922); *Notable American Women*, II: 511-513; *Pacific Coast Journal of Nursing* (November 1915), pp. 526-529, and (February 1929), pp. 69-72; Sara E. Parsons, *History of the Massachusetts General Training*

School for Nurses (1922); Meta Rutter Pennock, *Makers of Nursing History* (1928); Anna A. Williamson, "With Miss Maxwell in the Spanish-American War," *Pacific Coast Journal of Nursing* (February 29, 1929), pp. 70-71.

LORETTA P. HIGGINS

MINNIGERODE, LUCY (February 8, 1871, near Leesburg, Virginia--March 24, 1935, Alexandria, Virginia). *Administrator.* Daughter of Charles Minnigerode and Virginia Cuthbert (Powell) Minnigerode. Never married. EDUCATION: Attended private schools; 1898, received diploma from Bellevue Hospital Training School for Nurses, New York City. CAREER: 1899-1914 and 1915-1917, private duty nursing, then superintendent of the Episcopal Eye and Ear Hospital, Washington, D.C., City Hospital, Savannah, Georgia, and Columbia Hospital for Women and Children, Washington, D.C.; 1914-1915, led a contingent of Red Cross nurses, Unit C, on the "Mercy Ship," and was stationed in Kiev, Russia; 1917-1918, assisted with the organization of special units as a staff nurse with the American Red Cross Nursing Service, Washington, D.C.; fall 1918, during the influenza epidemic, helped organize F Street Hospital, Washington, D.C., for the Red Cross and the U.S. Public Health Service; 1919, while still with the Red Cross, made an inspection tour of the U.S. Public Health Service hospitals at the agency's request; 1919-1935, superintendent of nurses, U.S. Public Health Service; died suddenly after spending the morning in her office and the afternoon gardening.

CONTRIBUTIONS: Lucy Minnigerode's major contribution came as superintendent of nurses for the U.S. Public Health Service (USPHS). At the same time of her appointment as superintendent (1919), an act of Congress placed beneficiaries of war risk insurance under the care of the USPHS. As a result, she had to build a huge nursing force to handle the care of those who came under the provisions of the new law. Since that included World War I veterans, the nursing staff grew to almost 1,800, thereby ensuring that veterans received the care they needed. In 1922, the Veterans Bureau assumed the responsibility for caring for veterans, and the USPHS was relieved of that major undertaking. That reduced the need for such a large number of USPHS nurses, and allowed nurses to concentrate on preventive work through education on diet, venereal disease prevention and treatment, and occupational safety. With the reduction of the responsibility of the USPHS, the number of its nurses was reduced from 1,800 to about 600, and many began working for the Veterans Bureau. Minnigerode eventually became a member of the advisory committee of the medical council of the Veterans

Administration. Her concern was with quality of nursing care as well as quantity of health providers, as reflected in the courses she established to improve the level of care in USPHS hospitals.

She was active in various professional organizations, and she was creative in her approach to them. For instance, because of her efforts the superintendents of nurses in the government nursing services became members of the advisory council of the American Nurses' Association (ANA). She then helped to establish a new section in the ANA for nurses who were in government service. In these ways, she helped make the profession aware of the needs of those who were in government service. She was a representative of the ANA, and from 1923 to 1928 she served as chairperson of its committee on federal legislation. She also served as a member of the Women's Joint Congressional Committee. During the same period, she chaired the Delano Memorial Committeee.

In 1919, she became a member of the National Committee on American Red Cross Nursing Service, and she was also a member of the executive committee of the District of Columbia chapter. In 1925, she was awarded the prestigious Florence Nightingale Medal by the International Red Cross Committee. Her most exciting years were probably during World War I, when she led a contingent of Red Cross nurses to Kiev, Russia, where they were stationed at a hospital in the aftermath of both the war and the Russian Revolution. For her service, Czar Nicholas II awarded her the Cross of Saint Anne. When she died, the honorary pallbearers were the directors of the government and Red Cross nursing services, and six officers of the USPHS, including the surgeon-general.

WRITINGS: "Instructions on Hygienic Methods," which was translated into several languages; several papers on the work of the USPHS nursing staff.

REFERENCES: *American Journal of Nursing* (September 1924), p. 964 and (May 1935), pp. 499-500; *Dictionary of American Biography*, XXI, supp. 1, p. 555; Jane E. Mottus, *New York Nightingales: The Emergence of the Nursing Profession at Bellevue and New York Hospital, 1850-1920* (1980); *New York Times* (March 25, 1935); Meta Rutter Pennock, *Makers of Nursing History* (1928, 1940); *Who Was Who in America*, I: 848.

LORETTA P. HIGGINS

MINOR, NANNIE JACQUELIN (June 15, 1871, Charlottesville, Virginia--January 30, 1934, Lewisburg, West Virginia). *Public health nurse.* Daughter of John B. Minor, professor of law at the University of Virginia, and Ann Fisher (Colstan) Minor. Never married. EDUCATION: 1900, graduated from the nursing school of Old Dominion

Hospital, Richmond, Virginia; post-graduate studies at Johns Hopkins, Baltimore, Maryland, and at the Thomas Wilson Sanitarium, Pikesville, Maryland. CAREER: 1900-1902, private duty nursing; 1902-1922, nurse, then head of the nursing staff, Instructive Visiting Nurse Association, Richmond; 1922-1932, director of public health nursing, bureau of child welfare, Virginia State Board of Health.

CONTRIBUTIONS: Nannie Minor is regarded as the "Mother of Public Health Nursing in Virginia." She was one of a group of nurses who, after graduating from the training school of Old Dominion Hospital, founded a nurses' settlement and devoted their off-duty hours to providing services to the lower classes of Richmond. The settlement led to the founding in 1902 of the Instructive Visiting Nurse Association, which began to organize the care of the sick in the city. Tuberculosis patients received services through the dispensary or were cared for at the Pine Camp Sanitarium, which was available to the indigent. These developments preceded the founding of a permanent health department of the city, and the visiting nurse association was the only organized source of social and health services during its first six years of existence.

After having served the city of Richmond for a twenty-year period, Minor moved from the local to the state level, where she organized public health nursing services of the Virginia State Department of Health. Her energetic work gave birth to forty-five public health nursing services throughout the state, a major contribution to preserving the public health of the citizens of Virginia, and especially to those in rural areas, which had no nursing service until it was provided by the state during the years in which Minor provided the leadership. It has been said that she was courageous to enter the field of nursing, for upper-class Southern women were not expected to serve humanity, but instead were supposed to be catered to by their own servants. She exhibited that same courage when she brought nursing services to previously unserved communities.

In addition to improving the lives of countless people through her work in public health, Minor helped to secure the nurses' registration law in Virginia, and for ten years she served on the board of nurse examiners. She was honored when a resolution memorializing her was prepared by the nursing section of the Medical College of Virginia alumni association and sent by that group to the *American Journal of Nursing*, and *Public Health Nursing Journal*, as well as to her family.

WRITINGS: "The Status of the Colored Public Health Nurse in Virginia," *Public Health Nurse* (May 1924), pp. 243-244.

REFERENCES: *American Journal of Nursing* (February 1925), p. 116, (March 1934), pp. 303-304; *Bulletin of the Medical College of Virginia* (Fall 1963); Jessie Wetzel Faris, "Two Hundred Years of Nursing in

Richmond," *American Journal of Nursing* (August 1937), pp. 847-849; unpublished material, American Journal of Nursing Collection, Nursing Archives, Mugar Memorial Library, Boston University.

LORETTA P. HIGGINS

MUSE, MAUDE BLANCHE (?--December 19, 1962, Savannah, Georgia). *Nurse educator; author.* Daughter of Mr. Muse and Mrs. ? (MacAusland) Muse. Never married. EDUCATION: Attended schools in California, Kansas, Nebraska, and Washington State; 1912, received diploma, Lakeside School of Nursing, Cleveland, Ohio; 1921, B.S., Teachers College, Columbia University, New York City (she began her studies at Columbia with scholarship aid from her home town in 1914); c. 1926, M.S., Teachers College. CAREER: c. 1906-1909, taught for three years in a small country school before entering nursing school; 1912, private duty nursing; 1915, nursing instructor, St. Luke's Hospital School of Nursing, New York City, and Lane Hospital School of Nursing, Leland Stanford University, San Francisco; summer 1918, instructor of materia medica, Vassar (nurse) Training Camp, Poughkeepsie, New York; 1921, part-time teacher; 1927-1947, member of the faculty at Teachers College, Columbia University, promoted to full professor in 1937.

CONTRIBUTIONS: Maude Muse stimulated interest in progressive educational philosophy and changes in methods of teaching nursing. She did much to raise the standards of teaching in nursing schools toward a professional level. She introduced the concept of group dynamics and adult education methods to nursing schools. She taught thousands of undergraduate registered nurses and graduate nurses. Soon after becoming a full-time instructor at Teachers College, she took over the entire supervision of graduate nurse students who were doing practice teaching in schools connected with several New York hospitals. Many of these became highly successful teachers and remembered her as a gifted teacher.

Her creative ability continued into her retirement, when she produced her most successful text, *Guided Learning Experience* (1950), on learning and its application to teaching in schools of nursing. She was a member of the National League of Nursing Education and of the committee which produced the educationally influential *A Curriculum Guide for Schools of Nursing* (1937).

WRITINGS: *A Textbook of Psychology for Nurses* (1925; 5th ed., 1945); *Syllabus of Psychology*; *An Introduction to Efficient Study Habits* (1929); *Materia Medica, Pharmacology and Therapeutics* (1936); *Guided Learning*

Experience (1950); numerous articles for nursing journals, including "Habits and Skills," *American Journal of Nursing* (October 1922), p. 1.
REFERENCES: *American Journal of Nursing* (December 1963), pp. 130-132; Bess V. Cunningham and Isabel Stewart, "Maude B. Muse--Nurse, Educator, Author, and Creative Thinker," *American Journal of Nursing* (November 1956), pp. 1434-1436; Meta Rutter Pennock, *Makers of Nursing History* (1940).

ALICE HOWELL FRIEDMAN

N

NELSON, SOPHIE CAROLINE (September 4, 1886, Denmark--February 10, 1964, Boston). *Public health nurse; insurance company home nursing administrator.* Never married. EDUCATION: 1912, graduated from Waltham Training School for Nurses, Waltham, Massachusetts; 1924, post-graduate course in public health nursing, Teachers College, Columbia University, New York City; post-graduate studies in public health administration, social and health problems, and business administration. CAREER: 1912-1915, private duty nursing; 1915, assistant matron, Thrall Hospital, Middletown, New York; c. 1915-1916, infant welfare nurse, Cambridge Board of Health, Cambridge, Massachusetts; 1917-1918, pediatric nursing service, American Red Cross, serving in Belgium and France; 1919-1921, superintendent, Babies' Milk Fund Association of the District Nurse Association, Louisville, Kentucky; 1921, assistant director of Red Cross work for Central Europe and the Balkans; 1922, acting director of European nursing service, Red Cross; 1923, director of nursing, Boston Health League; 1924, director, St. Louis (Missouri) Visiting Nurse Association; 1925-1953, director of the visiting nurse service, John Hancock Mutual Life Insurance Company, Boston.
CONTRIBUTIONS: Sophie Nelson is best remembered for her twenty-five years as director of the visiting nurse service of the John Hancock Life Insurance Company. Under her direction, a unique home-nursing service was made available to industrial holders of the John Hancock Company. Under this program, thousands of visits were made by registered nurses to policyholders. During her twenty-five years of supervision of the program, there was increasing growth of the service and recognition of its value and importance in hundreds of communities. Assistance was given to new mothers, babies, small children, older people, and others who were ill or disabled. These services were given free of

charge to those who were policyholders of industrial policies of the company, before the time when prepaid health insurance was developed on a large scale. In 1950, she was appointed assistant secretary of the John Hancock Life Insurance Company, the first woman to be given this distinction in the history of the company.

Nelson also had a distinguished career as a nurse and administrator for the American Red Cross during and following World War I. She developed hospitals for refugee children, who were dying by the thousands following the war. She developed nursing services in Montenegro and Albania, areas which were especially hard hit in the aftermath of the conflict. She helped establish camp hospitals, first-aid stations, camps of exchange fpr prisoners of war, and camps for those on leave from military service. As field director for the nursing service of the American Red Cross European relief program, she was responsible for the feeding of starving people and for setting up small hospitals for their care. At the same time, she was able to assist in the formation of a public health nursing course at the American Hospital at Constantinople. She was assigned by the Red Cross to assist in the Smyrna disaster of 1922, which rescued starving Greeks who had been driven to the sea by the Turks.

Nelson was also active in organizational work, particularly in those organizations associated with community health. She was president of the National Organization for Public Health Nursing from 1930 to 1934, the time when the organization was being called upon nationally to provide information regarding the provision of public health nursing services so desperately needed in the early years of the Great Depression. Many studies of public health nursing administration were conducted by Nelson, who in 1931 was called for four months to Washington, D.C., as a special consultant to the surgeon-general of the U.S. Public Health Service. She was instrumental in developing greater cooperation between the social agencies involved in public health work and various nursing organizations. She believed that the economics of nursing agencies required careful auditing, and that the effectiveness of services ought to be examined. She was one of five nurses ever appointed to the committee on administrative health practices of the American Public Health Association. This major committee influenced the establishment of administrative practices in public health units throughout the United States.

She was a member of the International Council of Nurses, and in 1937 she served as chairperson of its public health nursing section. She was president of the Massachusetts Central Health Council, vice-president of the Massachusetts Organization of Public Health Nursing, and president of the Greater Boston Nursing Council. She served on the executive committee of the Boston Health League.

In June 1951, she was given the Florence Nightingale Medal of the Red Cross. She also received the Lemuel Shattuck Award of the Massachusetts Public Health Association for her major contributions to the advancement of public health in the state.

WRITINGS: Many articles in the nursing literature, especially regarding the organization and delivery of public health nursing services; *Public Health Nursing* contains many of her articles about public health nursing administration and about the National Organization for Public Health Nursing.

REFERENCES: *A History of the Graduates of the Waltham Training School* (1937); Stella Goostray, "Sophie Nelson: Public Health Statesman," *American Journal of Nursing* (September 1960), pp. 1268-1269; Ella E. McNeil, "A History of the Public Health Nursing Section of the American Public Health Association" (1972); *Nursing Outlook* (1964), p. 16; *Daily Home Office News* (John Hancock Life Insurance Company, 1950 and 1951); personal papers, Nursing Archives, Mugar Library, Boston University.

ALICE HOWELL FRIEDMAN

NEWSOM, ELLA {KING} (Brandon, Rankin County, Mississippi--?). *Civil war nurse.* Daughter of Rev. T.S.N. King, a Baptist clergyman. Married Dr. Frank Newsom (died just before Civil War); married Colonel Trader after the war. EDUCATION: Trained under medical staff and Sisters of Mercy, Memphis City Hospital, Memphis, Tennessee. CAREER: 1861-1865, Civil War nurse.

CONTRIBUTIONS: For her work during the Civil War, chiefly on behalf of the Army of Tennessee, Ella Newsom became known as the "Florence Nightingale of the Southern Army." When the war began, she was a widow living in Winchester, Tennessee, and supervising the education of her younger sisters. She returned her sisters to their parents in Arkansas and went to Memphis, accompanied by several of her own servants. Being left with considerable means, she was able to obtain supplies needed to treat the wounded and ill Confederate soldiers. Desperate for volunteer nurses, the officers in the Confederate Army soon knew of the good work being done by Newsom, and they did all they could to facilitate her work. She labored in Memphis until December 1861, when she headed for Bowling Green, Kentucky, believing she could be of greater service there. She remained there until the surrender of Forts Donalson and Henry, when she went to Nashville where she apparently worked with the Howard Association, a benevolent society which provided humanitarian assistance during time of epidemic, to develop a hospital.

When the Confederate troops were forced to withdraw from Nashville, she moved the wounded to Winchester, Tennessee, where she oversaw the conversion of the local schools and churches into hospitals. When the Confederate forces moved toward what was to be the Battle of Shiloh, on April 6 and 7, 1862, she accompanied the troops. After the battle, she established a hospital at Corinth, Mississippi, where the Tishomingo Hotel was used as a hospital. Later that same year, she was in charge of the hospital established at the Crutchfield House at Chattanooga. After an inspection trip to military hospitals at Okolona, Columbus, and Meridian, Mississippi, she went to southwestern Virginia. In the summer of 1862, she was in Abington, where she helped convert Emery and Henry College into a hospital, making a brief trip to Richmond to extend her knowledge of and experience in hospital matters. The invasion of Kentucky in the summer of 1862 led her to Marietta, Georgia, where she took possession of the buildings around the public square and organized hospitals in them.

Her activities in 1863 and 1864 are difficult to trace, but it seems clear that she continued to serve the needs of the Confederate soldiers. During the winter of 1865, she journeyed to Arkansas to see her family. Braving a lack of supplies and perilous travel conditions, she journeyed from Marietta to Altanta and then west to Pine Bluff, Arkansas; from there she went to the place where her parents had fled upon the arrival of the Union soldiers. After visiting with her parents, she made her way back to Atlanta, intending to return to her hospital duties. Meanwhile, however, General Robert E. Lee had surrendered at the Appomattox Court House, in Virginia, signaling the end of the Civil War.

After the war, she married Colonel Trader, a Confederate officer who lived for a number of years. At his death, however, she was left not only in financial difficulties but with substantial physical impairments: she had lost the sight of one eye and was almost deaf. Her friends sought to help her, and in 1885, in Asheville, North Carolina, subscriptions were sought to provide her a home, but the appeal failed to raise sufficient funds for that purpose. In 1908, her case was presented before the Association of Medical Officers of the Army and Navy of the Confederacy at their reunion on June 9, and they passed a resolution recognizing her considerable contribution to the Confederacy. As a result of the publicity given to that event and in order to give her an honored place in American history, J. Fraise Richard published the story of her work.

WRITINGS: Articles in popular magazines and newspapers of the times.
REFERENCES: H. H. Cunningham, *Doctors in Gray: The Confederate Medical Service* (1958); Lavinia L. Dock et al., *History of Red Cross Nursing* (1922); J. Fraise Richard, *The Florence Nightingale of the Southern Army* (1914); Victor Robinson, *White Caps: The Story of Nursing* (1946).

JOELLEN WATSON HAWKINS

NORTHAM, ANNIE ETHEL (December 9, 1894, Atlantic Virginia--November 23, 1968, Snow Hill, Maryland). *Obstetrical nurse; nurse-researcher.* Never married. EDUCATION: 1909-1913, attended high school in Snow Hill, Maryland, graduating in 1913; 1918-1921, attended Johns Hopkins Hospital School of Nursing, Baltimore, Maryland, graduating in 1921; 1931-1941, occasional post-graduate studies at Johns Hopkins. CAREER: 1913-1918, substitute teacher, Worcester County, Maryland; January-May 1917, principal of primary school, Snow Hill, Maryland; 1921-1923, head nurse, medical and obstetrical wards, Johns Hopkins Hospital; 1923, head nurse, Mountainside Hospital, Montclair, New Jersey; 1923-1926, head nurse of a medical ward, then in the delivery room, Johns Hopkins Hospital; 1926-1929, instructor of obstetrical nursing, Johns Hopkins Hospital School of Nursing; 1929-1938, director of practical nursing, Johns Hopkins School of Nursing; 1938-1944, superintendent of nurses, Hospital for Women, Baltimore, Maryland; 1944-1945, superintendent of nurses, Sydenham Hospital, Baltimore; 1946-1961, superintendent of nurses, Frederick City Hospital, Frederick, Maryland.
CONTRIBUTIONS: Annie Northam's greatest contribution to the profession was in the evolution of nursing theory, a contribution which brought her little recognition during her lifetime. Only within the past two decades has her work been reexamined as interest in nursing theory has increased. Ethel Northam and her colleague Hester Frederick (q.v.) wrote *Textbook of Nursing Practice*, published in 1928. In that text, they espouse a sound theoretical basis for practice and describe the recipients of nursing services as care agents. According to this theory, nursing activities focus on the promotion of the care agent. It is possible from the perspective of the 1980s to trace the evolution of ideas from the work of Northam and Frederick to contemporary models and theories.

In addition to her textbook on nursing practice, she conducted an early time study in obstetrical nursing, which was an important pioneering work in nursing research (*American Journal of Nursing*, July 1927, p. 543). The study, conducted at the Woman's Clinic at the Johns

Hopkins Hospital, illustrates nursing time required for care of the mother and infant and what the nurse does in caring for each. The research was conducted with Chelly Wasserberg, R.N.

Throughout her life, Northam apparently remained an active alumna of Johns Hopkins Hospital School of Nursing. In 1958, she was photographed at an alumnae event with some of her classmates. Her professional activities were not confined to her alma mater, however. She was an active member of the American Nurses' Association and the National League of Nursing Education, and she was enrolled as a Red Cross nurse. In 1961, she retired to Snow Hill, Maryland, to live with her sister and brother, and seven years later she died and was buried in a cemetery in Snow Hill.

WRITINGS: *Textbook of Nursing Practice* (with Hester Frederick, 1928, 1938); "Temperature of Fluids for Infusion," *American Journal of Nursing* (February 1931); numerous articles in professional journals.

REFERENCES: Hester Frederick and Ethel Northam, *Textbook of Nursing Practice* (2d ed., 1938); *Johns Hopkins Nurses Alumnae Magazine* (July 1958); unpublished student and school records, Alan Mason Chesney Medical Archives, Johns Hopkins Medical Institutions, including a manuscript biography located with the records of the Johns Hopkins Alumni Association.

LORETTA P. HIGGINS

NOYES, CLARA DUTTON (October 3, 1869, Port Deposit, Maryland--June 3, 1936, Washington, D.C.). *Educator; administrator.* Daughter of Enoch Dutton Noyes, gentleman farmer, and Laura Lay (Banning) Noyes. Never married. EDUCATION: Attended private schools in Maryland and Connecticut; 1896, graduated from Johns Hopkins Hospital School of Nursing, Baltimore, Maryland. CAREER: 1896-1897, head nurse, Johns Hopkins Hospital; 1897-1901, superintendent of training school for nurses at the New England Hospital for Women and Children, Boston; 1901-1910, superintendent of the Hospital and Training School for Nurses, St. Luke's Hospital, New Bedford, Massachusetts; 1910-1916, general superintendent of training schools, Bellevue and Allied Hospitals, New York City; 1916-1918, director of the Bureau of Nursing Service of the American Red Cross; 1919-1921, director of the American Red Cross Department of Nursing; 1921-1936, director of Red Cross Nursing Service.

CONTRIBUTIONS: Clara Noyes' major contribution was in Red Cross nursing during and after World War I. During the war, she standardized surgical dressings and courses of instruction for nurses. As the head of the Red Cross Department of Nursing, she was responsible for designing and equipping all Red Cross Army nurses. Under her leadership, over 50,000 nurses were enrolled in the American Red Cross. Although much of that success was related to feelings of patriotism during the war and to the desperate need for assistance in war-torn Europe following the conflict, some of that success can be directly attributed to Noyes' personal appeals. In 1917 and again in 1920, she went on speaking tours to encourage nurses to sign up for overseas duty with the Red Cross. In addition, she was editor of the Red Cross department of the *American Journal of Nursing*, which undoubtedly helped influence many nurses to volunteer their services for international work.

After the war Red Cross nursing services were visible in a variety of areas, from caring for typhus patients in Poland to developing public health nursing in Italy. Noyes insisted that local European communities become involved in the nursing services, so the programs would continue when the American Red Cross left. She was influential in the establishment of schools of nursing in foreign countries, especially in Eastern Europe. She was known for her exacting standards, which occasionally took precedence over tact and diplomacy. In 1920, she toured Europe inspecting Red Cross nursing units and made recommendations that had far-reaching implications. She was firm in her belief that the work of the Red Cross in Europe would fall below its potential unless means were instituted to ensure its perpetuation after it withdrew. She recommended, therefore, involving local community leaders, as well as local physicians and other health care workers, in the work. The American Red Cross made that commitment, even granting subsidies to countries when it withdrew, enabling the work to continue.

In addition to her contributions to Red Cross nursing and to world health following World War I, she served the profession by her activity as a nurse-educator and as an officer of a variety of organizations. In 1911, while she was at Bellevue Hospital, a school for midwives was established, the first of its kind in the United States. From 1913 to 1916, she was president of the National League of Nursing Education; from 1913 to 1918, she was president of the board of directors of the American Journal of Nursing Company; from 1918 to 1922, she assumed the presidency of the American Nurses' Association; in 1925, 1929, and 1933, she was elected to the position of first vice-president of the International Council of Nurses. Through her leadership, she helped to unify the thoughts and purposes of the major nursing organizations in the United States. She was a guardian of the nursing profession, warning that the term *nurse* must be zealously protected and applied only to professional nurses and not to hastily trained nurses' aides. Although she appeared to be cold and aloof, her close associates and friends were more familiar with a sensitive, warm, caring personality that was not evident to her more casual acquaintances. She died from a heart attack suffered while driving to work.

During her lifetime, she received numerous honors and decorations in recognition of her important service to humanity. She was awarded the Florence Nightingale Medal of the International Committee of the Red Cross, and she also received the American Red Cross service medal, the Bulgarian Red Cross, the Latvian Red Cross, and from the French government the Medaille d'honneur d'hygiene publique and the Medaille de la reconnaissance. She was made an honorary member of the Red Cross societies of Costa Rica and Poland. In 1933, she received the Walter Burns Saunders Medal, and in 1935 she received a pin from the Florence Nightingale School of Bordeaux, France, at the same time as she was made an honorary graduate of that school.

WRITINGS: Editor of the Red Cross Department of the *American Journal of Nursing* and chair of the editorial committee that authored *History of the American Red Cross Nursing Service.*

REFERENCES: *American Journal of Nursing* (September 1916), pp. 1167-1168, (July 1936), pp. 701-702, 750-752; *British Journal of Nursing* (June 1936), p. 154, and (August 1936), p 212; Alice Fitzgerald, "Clara D. Noyes-An Appreciation," *The Trained Nurse and Hospital Review* (July 1936), pp. 19-21; *International Nursing Review* (August 1936), pp. 235-237; Portia B. Kernodle, *The Red Cross Nurse in Action* (1949); *Notable American Women*, p. 495; *National Cyclopedia of American Biography*, vol. B (1927): 181; *Pacific Coast Nursing Journal* (September 1916), p. 545 (November 1935), p. 622, (July 1936), pp. 400-410; Meta Rutter Pennock, *Makers of Nursing History* (1928); *Who Was Who in America*, I (1897-1942): 907.

LORETTA P. HIGGINS

NUTTING, M{ARY} ADELAIDE (November 1, 1858, Frost Village, Quebec, Canada--October 3, 1948, White Plains, New York). *Nurse-educator.* Daughter of Vespasion Nutting, clerk of the circuit court, and Harriet Sophia (Peasley) Nutting, seamstress. Never married. EDUCATION: c. 1863-1873, Shefford Academy, Waterloo, Quebec; 1873, studied French and music at a convent school in a nearby town; attended Bute House, a private school in Montreal; 1874, studied at an art school in Lowell, Massachusetts, and took private music lessons; 1889-1891, student at Johns Hopkins Hospital Training School for Nurses, Baltimore, Maryland, under the tutelage of Isabel Hampton (q.v.), graduating in 1891. CAREER: 1882-1883, taught music with her sister, Armine

(Minnie), at her sister's school in St. John's, Newfoundland; 1891-1893, graduate nurse and then head nurse on Dr. William Osler's medical ward at Johns Hopkins; 1893, took on some teaching duties at Johns Hopkins and was appointed assistant superintendent of nurses; spring 1894, named acting superintendent, and on December 13, 1894, received full appointment as superintendent of nurses and principal of the training school, effective September 1, 1895; held that position until April 1907; 1899-1907, part-time lecturer on special subjects in the experimental one-year program in hospital economics for graduate nurses, Teachers College, Columbia University, New York City; September 25, 1907, began her professorship at Teachers College, first as professor of domestic administration, then (in February 1910) to professor of nurses education; also served as chairperson of the department of institutional administration; 1910-retirement in 1925, chairperson, department of nursing and health, Teachers College; 1925-1948, professor emeritus.

CONTRIBUTIONS: M. Adelaide Nutting was a pioneering professional nurse who became the first professor of nursing in an American university (Columbia), and occupied the first endowed chair in nursing (endowed for $200,000 by Helen Hartly Jenkins). Her influence and importance ranged from the reform of nursing education at Johns Hopkins and at Columbia University, to the beginning of reform on the national scene. As superintendent of nurses and the training school at Johns Hopkins Hospital, she lengthened the course to three years (1895), sought to reduce the student's day to eight hours, and established the first course of training (preparatory course) preliminary to ward practice in the United States (1901).

She began her career at Columbia (1899-1925) as a member of the committee (chaired by Isabel Hampton Robb, {q.v.}), that persuaded Dean James E. Russell to introduce courses for graduate nurses at Teachers College. As chairperson of the education committee (1903-1920) of the National League of Nursing Education (NLNE), she led in the effort to produce the NLNE's *Standard Curriculum for Schools of Nursing* (1917). In 1917, she contracted with the Bureau of Education, Department of the Interior, to revise *Educational Status of Nursing*, which she first prepared in 1912. She was a member of the Committee for the Study of Nursing Education in the United States, from 1919-1923, whose findings were published as the Winslow-Goldmark report, *Nursing and Nursing Education in the United States* (1923).

Nutting was active in the development of professional organizations, during the early years of what later became the National League for Nursing and the American Nurses' Association. She served as vice-president (1897) and president (1896, 1909-1910) of the American Society of Superintendents of Training Schools for Nurses (which later became the NLNE and then the National League for Nursing). She was a founding member (1896) of the Nurses' Associated Alumnae of the United States and Canada (later the American Nurses' Association). She served as chairperson of a subcommittee of the Nurses' Associated Alumnae which was established to organize nurses in various states to lobby for an organized army nurse corps (December 1898), and also served (1900) as a member of the committee on periodicals, which established the *American Journal of Nursing* (its first issue appeared in October 1900). She served as president of the American Federation of Nurses (1901 to 1913), which represented an affiliation of the Nurses' Associated Alumnae and the American Society of Superintendents, for the purpose of applying for membership in the National Council of Women. In 1905, the organization withdrew from the National Council of Women and accepted an invitation to join the International Council of Nurses. In 1913, the American Federation of Nurses dissolved and the American Nurses' Association became the official representative to the International Council of Nurses. She was active in the International Council of Nurses and chaired the Education Committee from 1910 to 1925 as well as the Committee on International Standards in Nursing (1922).

Nutting was active in the struggle to receive professional recognition from military and governmental officials. She sponsored the bill for the establishment of an Army Nurse Corps (passed in 1901), and served on the national committee to secure rank for army nurses (1918-1920). During World War I, she organized and chaired the National Emergency Committee on Nursing and also served as chairperson of the Committee on Nursing, General Medical Board, Council for Defense (1917). With Isabel Stewart, of the National League for Nursing, and Jane A. Delano (q.v.), director of the Red Cross Department of Nursing, she helped to found the Vassar Training Camp for Nurses, which opened on June 24, 1918, in Poughkeepsie, New York. After the war, she was a member of the Committee on Devastated France and chairperson of a special committee to draft a plan for establishing a nursing school in Paris (1922-1924).

She organized and served as first president of the Maryland State Association of Graduate Nurses (1903), and helped to draft Maryland's first nurse practice (registration) act of 1904. She worked closely with officials of the American Red Cross, helping to secure nursing affiliation with the American Red Cross and then outlining courses in home nursing (1912). She also inaugurated a four-month post-graduate course in rural nursing at Teachers' College (1913).

She was a supporter of public health nursing, through her long friendship with Lillian Wald (q.v.) and Lavinia Dock (q.v.), serving on the board of the Henry Street Settlement, speaking and writing on public health nursing, and introducing public health experiences at Johns Hopkins (beginning as early as 1896) and an eight-month course at Teachers College (1917).

In addition to her contributions to nursing, she was a founder of the American Home Economics Association (1906), serving on its by-laws committee and on the committee which developed the *Journal of Home Economics*, which began publication in February 1909.

She promoted the collection of books, pamphlets, prints, and records related to nursing and nursing history, and she began the historical nursing library at Teachers College. The library was named after her, as the M. Adelaide Nutting Historical Nursing Collections. She founded the first historical society in nursing (1905). In 1922, she received an honorary M.A. degree from Yale University, being the first nurse and only the eighth woman so honored. The National League of Nursing Education established the M. Adelaide Nutting Medal to recognize outstanding leadership in nursing education, and awarded it for the first time to Nutting on May 5, 1944. In 1976, she was elected to the American Nurses' Association Hall of Fame.

WRITINGS: *History of Nursing* (with Lavinia L. Dock), vols. 1 and 2 (1907), vols. 3 and 4 (1912); *Standard Curriculum for Schools of Nursing* (1917); *Nursing and Nursing Education in the United States* (1923); *A Sound Economic Basis for Schools of Nursing* (1926); "The Education of Nurses," *American Journal of Nursing* (March 1902), pp. 799-804; "The Preliminary Education of Nurses," *American Journal of Nursing* (March 1901), pp. 416-424; numerous other articles, pamphlets, and reports.

REFERENCES: *American Journal of Nursing* (June 1925), pp. 444-454, (August 1943), p. 762, (June 1944), p. 587, and (November 1948), p. 625; Daisy Caroline Bridges, *History of the International Council of Nurses, 1899-1964* (1967); Teresa E. Christy, "Portrait of a Leader: M. Adelaide Nutting," *Nursing Outlook* (January 1969); *Dictionary of American Biography*, supp. 4: 631-33; Lyndia Flanagan, *One Strong Voice: The Story of the American Nurses Association* (1976); Stella Goostray, "Mary Adelaide Nutting," *American Journal of Nursing* (November 1958), pp. 1524-1529; Ethel Johns and Blanche Pfefferkorn, *The Johns Hopkins Hospital School of Nursing, 1889-1949* (1954); Helen E. Marshall, *Mary Adelaide Nutting* (1972); *Notable American Women*, 2:642-44.

JOELLEN WATSON HAWKINS

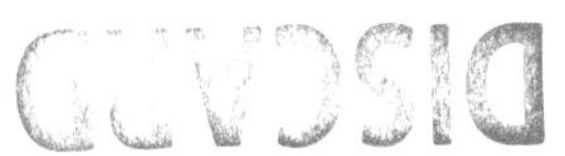

O

OSBORNE, ESTELLE GENEVA {MASSEY} RIDDLE (May 3, 1901, Palestine, Texas--December 12, 1981, Oakland, California). *Nurse-educator; black nursing leader.* Daughter of a man who was a janitor, general laborer, and trucker, and a woman who was a domestic and a seamstress. Married Dr. Bedford N. Riddle, physician, c. 1935, and a Mr. Osborne, c. 1945. EDUCATION: Attended two-year course at Prairie View State College, Prairie View, Texas, graduating at the age of sixteen; October 1920-1923, attended nursing school at City Hospital Number 2, St. Louis, Missouri, graduating in 1923; summers 1927-1929 and fulltime, 1929-1930, attended Teachers College, Columbia University, New York City, receiving a B.S. in 1930 and an M.A. in 1931. CAREER: c. 1917-1919, rural schoolteacher; 1923-1926, head nurse, City Hospital Number 2, St. Louis; 1926, visiting nurse, St. Louis Municipal Nursing Service; 1927-1929, faculty member, central nursing school of Kansas City, also teaching hygiene and physiology in the junior college program, Lincoln School; 1931-1934, education director, Freedmen's Hospital, Washington, D.C.; 1934-1936, investigator for Julius Rosenwald Fund; 1936, community nursing, Akron, Ohio; 1940-1943, superintendent of City Hospital Number 2 Training School (Homer G. Phillips Hospital School of Nursing); 1943, consultant for National Nursing Council for War Service; 1946-1954, faculty member, New York University, New York City; 1954-1966, staff member, National League for Nursing, serving as director of services to state leagues.

CONTRIBUTIONS: Estelle Osborne was one of the great nursing leaders, in both nursing education and the development of nursing organizations. She was raised by parents who helped her to believe that although she was a black woman living in the segregated South, she could achieve her goals in life. She experienced prejudice in her early education and in nursing school, both of which were in segregated schools, and she faced discrimination as a graduate nurse and as a student at Columbia University's Teachers College. The nursing profession reflected the ideology of the society, and as a result black nurses such as Osborne had to fight for the recognition of equal rights. Osborne made great strides for herself and as a role model for future black nurses, certainly a tribute to her ability as well as her courage.

Her nursing career began after she had graduated from a normal school (Prairie View State College), and after she had taught in a segregated rural school. She decided to enter nursing and enrolled at the segregated nursing school of St. Louis' City Hospital Number 2 (Number 1 was for white patients and for white nursing students). After graduating, she passed the Missouri State Board examinations with the highest score for that year. Her first position was as a head nurse in City Hospital Number 2, and then she accepted a position as a visiting nurse for the St. Louis Municipal Nursing Service. She resigned from the latter position, discouraged by the prejudice she encountered.

With the help of a friend, in 1927 she became an instructor in the so-called "central nursing school," a joint effort of Lincoln High School, Lincoln Junior College, and two hospitals (City Hospital Number 2 and Wheatley Provident Hospital). That same summer she began part-time study at Columbia University's Teachers College, financing her studies with a loan her principal helped her secure. A scholarship from the Julius Rosenwald Fund enabled her to have a year of full-time study to complete her bachelor's and another for her master's. She was the first black nurse to receive that scholarship as well as the first to earn a master's degree at Teachers College. During her studies, she was a part-time instructor, first at New York's Lincoln Hospital and then at Harlem Hospital's Training School.

After receiving her degrees from Teachers College, she became the first director of nursing education at Freedmen's Hospital (Washington, D.C.), where she developed extracurricular activities for the students and established a closer relationship with Howard University. She resigned from Freedmen's Hospital when she was invited by the Julius Rosenward Fund to make a study of rural schools and rural life in one county of Louisiana.

After that study was completed, she and her husband moved to Akron, Ohio, where she devoted her efforts to her role as the eleventh president of the National Association of Colored Graduate Nurses, having been elected in 1934. Prior to her election, she spent two years as chairperson of the institute committee of that organization, which was responsible for institutes held during the 1932, 1933, and 1934 conventions, as well as for the regional conferences in 1934. During her five years as president, she helped to establish the association's new headquarters in New York City.

Returning to St. Louis in 1940, she became the first black director of the Homer G. Phillips Hospital School of Nursing and its nursing service. She responded to a call in 1943 to serve as a consultant to the National Nursing Council for War Service, working in New York City. Under her leadership, black nurses were given more opportunities for service in the armed forces. After the war, in 1946, she became an assistant professor at New York University, remaining until 1954, when her service at the National League of Nursing began.

Many organizations were the beneficiaries of her talents. In 1932, she and Mabel Staupers were the first black nurses ever appointed to committees of the National Organization for Public Health Nursing; Osborne became a member of the organization's education committee. In 1948, she was the first black nurse elected for a four-year term to the board of directors of the American Nurses' Association, and in 1949, she was one of the four U.S. representatives to the International Council of Nurses meeting in Stockholm, Sweden. In 1954, she became assistant director of the National League for Nursing, becoming in 1959 its director of services for all state branches of the league, and then the League's associate general director. In 1967, she retired from nursing intending to travel extensively. Her committee work did not end with her retirement, however, and she devoted a great deal of time and energy to professional and community organizations.

Osborne contributed to various professional organizations not only as an officer and a committee member, but also as a speaker. Most important, she made a point of representing the needs and interests of the black nurses, speaking, for example, on the role of black nurses at the National League of Nursing Education convention in Washington, D.C. She also helped to desegregate nursing organizations; for instance on April 5, 1935, she was a featured speaker and the first black nurse to address the Southern division of the American Nurses' Association which convened in Louisville, Kentucky. For many years, Osborne devoted her energy to opening the American Nurses' Association to all nurses, and quite often she was one of a handful of black nurses who attended professional meetings which had always been attended exclusively by whites. She often encountered discrimination, such as being denied a place to sit at a banquet or having no one speak to her. At last, at the Atlantic City convention of the American Nurses' Association which was held in 1946, she and her black colleagues won membership for all qualified nurses, regardless of race. Then came the fight for the right to vote and to hold office, a struggle which took another six months of effort.

Osborne also gave much time to community service. She served on the legal defense fund of the National Association for the Advancement of Colored People, the health and welfare committee of the National Urban League, the advisory committee to the U.S. Surgeon-General and the U.S. Public Health Service, as a member of the federal citizens' committee to the U.S. Office of Education, and as vice-president of the national health project of Alpha Kappa Alpha sorority.

She received recognition for her work in many ways. In 1946, she was given the Mary Mahoney Award of the National Association of Colored Graduate Nurses. In 1959, she won the Nurse of the Year Award, presented by New York University. She was the first black nurse to be inducted as an honorary fellow of the American Academy of Nursing (1978). Finally, in 1984 she was inducted into the American Nurses' Association Hall of Fame.

WRITINGS: Numerous articles in professional journals including "The National Association of Colored Graduate Nurses," *American Journal of Nursing* (June 1933), pp. 534-536; "The Training and Placement of Negro Nurses," *Journal of Negro Education* (1935), pp. 42-48; "Negro Nurses: The Supply and Demand," *Opportunity: Journal of Negro Life* (November 1937), pp. 327-329; "Integration in Professional Nursing," *International Nursing Review* (August 1962), pp. 47-50 (with Mary Elizabeth Carnegie).

REFERENCES: Mary Elizabeth Carnegie, *The Path We Tread: Blacks in Nursing 1854-1984* (1986); Alma C. Haupt, "A Pioneer in Negro Nursing," *American Journal of Nursing* (September 1935), pp. 857-859; Darlene Clark Hine, ed., *Black Women in the Nursing Profession: A Documentary History* (1985); *Nursing Outlook* (February 1982), p. 78; Gwendolyn Safier, *Contemporary American Leaders in Nursing* (1977); Mabel Keaton Staupers, *No Time for Prejudice* (1961); Adah Thoms, *Pathfinders: A History of the Progress of Colored Graduate Nurses* (1929); Edna Yost, *American Women of Nursing* (1965).

JOELLEN WATSON HAWKINS

P

PALMER, SOPHIA FRENCH (May 2, 1853, Milton, Massachusetts--April 27, 1920, Forest Lawn, New York). *Nurse-leader; editor.* Daughter of Simeon Palmer and Maria Burdell (Spenser) Palmer, a descendant of some of the first settlers of New England. Never married; 1906, adopted a daughter named Elizabeth. EDUCATION: 1878, graduated from Boston Training School for Nurses (later called the Massachusetts General Hospital School of Nursing); c. 1900, studied journalism. CAREER: 1878-1884, private duty nursing in Pennsylvania and California; 1884-1886, superintendent, St. Luke's Hospital, New Bedford, Massachusetts; 1886-1888, charge nurse, Massachusetts General Hospital, Boston; 1889-1894, superintendent, Garfield Memorial Hospital, and director of the Training School for Nurses, Washington, D.C.; 1894-1896, editor, *Trained Nurse and Hospital Review*; 1896-1901, superintendent of the Rochester City Hospital and Training School (New York); 1900-1920, editor-in-chief, *American Journal of Nursing*.

CONTRIBUTIONS: Sophia Palmer was the first editor of the *American Journal of Nursing*. She had been an early advocate of the need for a magazine for nurses which would be owned and operated by trained nurses. She believed that the journal must reflect the issues facing the entire profession and not be limited to issues concerning nursing education. She was a member of the Associated Alumnae when it decided to start a professional magazine, and very likely because of her experience as editor of the *Trained Nurse and Hospital Review*, she became the guiding force behind the implementation of that decision (along with M.E.P. Davis {q.v.}). Palmer and Davis assumed the personal legal responsibility for the earliest issues of the *Journal*, which made it possible for the postal authorities to allow the organization to send them through the mail. Palmer and Davis developed the creative idea of selling stock to finance the publication; the stock was sold to individual nurses as well as to alumnae associations, all of whom recognized the desperate need for such a publication. It was not until 1912 that the American Nurses' Association, which evolved out of the Associated Alumnae, assumed ownership of the *American Journal of Nursing*.

As editor, Palmer was noted for her clear and forceful editorials in the *Journal*. She was said to write with a "trenchant pen." In many respects, the editorials provide the basis for a history of American nursing since 1900, but also a history of the disputes and differing ideas of the pioneers of the profession. Palmer was committed to the "ordinary woman, the isolated nurse--those who form the greater part of the army of nurses." Her articles and editorials clearly reflected her concern for the needs of the private duty nurse and the hospital nurse, as well as for those involved in leading the profession through organizational work, administration, or nursing education.

She was an ardent supporter of state registration and licensure of nurses, and she believed that the *American Journal of Nursing* could become a mechanism for advancing the profession and for providing a successful future for the American nurse. Indeed, she helped to frame many of the early nurse registration laws. One of the first steps toward state registration came in 1899 when Palmer read a paper before the New York State Federation of Women's Clubs, urging support for a law which would require every nurse training school to improve their standards and for the state to become involved in licensing those nurses who could meet the highest educational and professional standards. Palmer not only advocated passage of nurse registration and licensure legislation, but she became the first president of the New York State Board of Nurse Examiners (1903) and has been credited with developing the idea of putting teeth into such laws by requiring state inspectors to oversee the implementation of the state law.

Palmer was also an early leader of the movement to develop a national association of trained nurses. The first step toward such a goal came with the organization of the Society of Superintendents of Training Schools for Nurses, which would provide the leadership necessary for an organization which would have to appeal to graduates of the various training schools. Palmer was on the seven-person membership committee which outlined the goals of that organization. The second step toward a national association of trained nurses came with the creation of alumnae associations of the various schools of nursing. At the second annual convention of the Society of Superintendents of Training Schools for Nurses (February 1895), she spoke in support of this first step, urging the various superintendents to work toward the establishment of alumnae associations, which eventually would be able to work together toward the advancement of the entire nursing profession. She and Davis were instrumental in the formation of the alumnae association of the Massachusetts General Hospital School of Nursing, which was established in that same year, 1895. The next step was creation of the Associated Alumnae, an organization which brought together the alumnae associations of all the nurse training schools, and it was the Associated Alumnae which became the American Nurses' Association. Clearly, Palmer deserves a great deal of credit for the movement towards these important developments in the history of the American nursing profession.

Over the course of her career, she received many awards in recognition of her service to the profession. In 1939, the library of the Massachusetts General Hospital School of Nursing was named the Palmer-Davis Library in recognition of the important contributions of the two early leaders of that school and of the American nursing profession. In 1953, the American Journal of Nursing Company named its own library the Sophia Palmer Memorial Library. A tribute to Palmer appeared in *Landmarks in Nursing*, a bicentennial publication of the Massachusetts Nurses' Association. In 1976, Palmer was elected to the Nursing Hall of Fame which was in that year established by the American Nurses' Association.

WRITINGS: Numerous editorials and articles in the *Trained Nurse and Hospital Review* and the *American Journal of Nursing*.

REFERENCES: *American Journal of Nursing* (vols. 1-20) contain numerous articles and editorials by Sophia Palmer; Teresa E. Christy, "Portrait of a Leader: Sophia F. Palmer," *Nursing Outlook* (December 1975); Katharine DeWitt, "The Journal's First Fifty Years," *American Journal of Nursing* (October 1950); Lavinia Dock, *A History of Nursing* (1912), III: 142-153; *Notable American Women*, pp. 14-15; Meta Rutter Pennock, *Makers of Nursing History* (1940), p. 112; Sylvia Perkins, *A Centennial Review of the Massachusetts General Hospital School of Nursing, 1873-1973* (1975); Mary M. Roberts, *American Nursing: History and Interpretation* (1954).

ALICE HOWELL FRIEDMAN

PARSONS, MARION GEMETH (August 28, 1871, Fort Fairfield, Maine--August 29, 1968, Norway, Maine). *World War I nurse; educator*. Daughter of Horatio M. and Mary (Humphrey) Parsons. Never married. EDUCATION: Schools of Fort Fairfield, Maine; 1902-1905, attended Boston City Hospital Training School for Nurses, graduating in 1905; attended Teachers College, Columbia University, New York City.

CAREER: 1905-1909, head nurse, Boston City Hospital; 1909-1913, superintendent of the old City and County Hospital (later the San Francisco Hospital); 1913, instructor, New York Hospital, New York City; 1914-1917, overseas duty with the Harvard Unit of Boston; 1917-1919, service with Base Hospital Number 7, Tours, France; 1919, set up, and 1919-1923, director of the Czechoslovakia State School of Nursing, Prague; 1923-1940, instructor, Boston City Hospital; retired to Fryeburg, Maine.

CONTRIBUTIONS: Marion Parsons was well known for her service during World War I, both with the British Army before the United States entered the conflict and then with the Boston City Hospital unit at Base Hospital Number 7, Tours, France. Shortly after the beginning of the war, she volunteered for overseas duty with the Harvard unit, and she served for one year at a British base hospital at Camiers, France. When the United States entered the war and the Boston City Hospital formed a unit for duty in France, she transferred to that unit, and she saw most of her army service with it at Tours. In 1919, she established a nursing school in Czechoslovakia and served as its director until 1923, when she returned to teaching at the Boston City Hospital.

She received many awards for her service, including a decoration at Buckingham Palace, in which King George V of Great Britain honored her for her contributions to the British Expeditionary Force in France. In 1923, the Czechoslovakian government decorated her with the Order of the White Lion, along with a citation personally presented by President Thomas Masaryk. That honor was rarely bestowed upon a woman. She also received awards from the American Red Cross nursing service, and a badge from London's Committee of the Czechoslovakia State School of Nursing. In 1965, the *Portland* (Maine) *Sunday Telegram* featured her life in an article which cited her record of accomplishments and service to humanity.

REFERENCES: *Portland* (Maine) *Press Herald* (August 31, 1968).

ALICE HOWELL FRIEDMAN

PARSONS, SARA E. (c. 1864, Northboro, Massachusetts--October 25, 1949, Jamaica Plain, Massachusetts). *Educator; author.* Never married.

EDUCATION: 1893, graduated from the Boston Training School for Nurses (later the Massachusetts General Hospital School of Nursing); one-year course in psychiatric nursing at McLean Asylum, Somerville, Massachusetts (now McLean Hospital, Belmont, Massachusetts); 1905, studied at Teachers College, Columbia University, New York City; 1909, post-graduate course in administration at Massachusetts General Hospital.

CAREER: 1893-1894, head nurse, Massachusetts General Hospital; 1895, supervisor, McLean Hospital; 1896-1898, organized the school for nurses at the Butler Hospital for the Insane, Providence, Rhode Island; 1899, sailed to Cuba on the hospital ship *Bay State* for service during the Spanish-American War; c. 1900, travelled and studied abroad; c. 1901-c. 1904, superintendent of nurses, Adams Nervine Hospital, Jamaica Plain, Massachusetts; c. 1905, travelled abroad; 1906-1909, organized school of nursing at Sheppard and Enoch Pratt Hospital for the Insane, Towson, Maryland; 1909-1910, organized, equipped, and opened Griffin Hospital, Derby, Connecticut; 1910-1920, superintendent of nurses, Massachusetts General Hospital Training School; 1917-1919 (while on leave of absence from Massachusetts General Hospital), served as chief nurse of Base Hospital Number 6, a Massachusetts General Hospital Unit, established near Bordeaux, France; 1920-1924, after retirement from her position at the Massachusetts General Hospital, surveyed schools of nursing in Oklahoma and Missouri, was a lobbyist for nursing legislation in Washington, D.C., and wrote a history of the Massachusetts General Hospital Training School for Nurses; 1924-1926, assistant registrar and registrar of the Central Directory of Nurses, Boston; 1927-1936, travelled extensively, and lived abroad for a number of these years; 1937, took up residence at the Mount Pleasant home in Jamaica Plain, Massachusetts, dying there in 1949.

CONTRIBUTIONS: Sara Parsons is best known as one of the early superintendents of the prestigious Massachusetts General Hospital Training School for Nurses. While superintendent, she appointed the first two full-time instructors, and she improved the quality of the school in many ways. She improved the quality of its applicants by tireless recruitment efforts which included visits to women's colleges as well as to outstanding high schools. Always devoted to the welfare of her students, Parsons strongly supported student activities, such as the glee club, which was begun during her tenure. She believed in student participation in decision making, and while she was superintendent of nurses at the Massachusetts General Hospital Training School, student government was established. Also interested in the alumnae association, she lent her support to the establishment of an alumnae magazine, *The Quarterly Record*, and to the creation of the alumnae association endowment fund.

Another important legacy was her belief that the mentally ill had the right to skilled nursing care and that nurses in mental hospitals had to have specialized training to do justice to their patients. To that end, she established the training school for nurses at the Butler Hospital for the Insane. Prior to the founding of that school, nursing care there had been carried out by poorly trained attendants, all of whom were given an opportunity to enroll in the new school. Its first year was a trying one, with criticisms about the changes she had instituted, with resignations of members of the staff, and with a number of first-year nursing students (probationers) leaving school. One major problem that was not resolved during her tenure at the hospital was her lack of jurisdiction over the training of the male nurses. The most important attribute she looked for in applicants to the program was good character. She improved the living situation for the nurses by providing better quarters and more palatable food, while improving work conditions by hiring maids to do the domestic chores that had previously been done by the members of the nursing staff. Although working with the mentally ill was not popular among nurses in her day, Parsons clearly did wonders in providing high-quality education in the nursing school and in improving the quality of nursing at the asylum.

She lent her support to the fight for registration laws for nurses and the inspection of schools of nursing. She served her country during the Spanish-American War and World War I. In 1899, with other doctors and nurses, she went to Cuba to bring home sick and wounded U.S. soldiers. During World War I, she led the nurse contingent at Base Hospital Number 6, in Talence, near Bordeaux, France. At its peak, the hospital served over 4,000, including those with battle wounds, infections, as well as those who contracted influenza. She was also a contributor to the National League of Nursing Education, serving as its secretary, vice-president, and president. She was the author of two books, including *Nursing Problems and Obligations*, which provided nurses with an understanding of the ethical and moral problems facing nurses in their day-to-day work.

WRITINGS: *Nursing Problems and Obligations* (1916, with numerous reprintings); *History of the Massachusetts General Hospital Training School for Nurses* (1922); many articles in journals, including "Personal Experience in Training-School Organization," *American Journal of Nursing* (June 1903), pp. 673-677, and "Educational Standards for Nurses, State Registraton and Training School Inspection," *Boston Medical and Surgical Journal* (April 9, 1914), pp. 574-575.

REFERENCES: *American Journal of Nursing* (June 1903), pp. 673-677, (September 1916), p. 1171, (March 1924), p. 460, and (December 1949), pp. 818-819; *Boston Globe* (October 16, 1949); *Boston Medical and Surgical Journal* (April 9, 1914), pp. 574-575, 600; Mary Ellen Doona, "Nursing Revisited: The Massachusetts General Hospital Base Hospital No. 6," *The Massachusetts Nurse* (April 1984), p. 9; Mary Ellen Doona, Clare Sullivan, and Jan Read, *Psychiatric Nursing: Origins and Evolution at Butler Hospital* (n.d.); *New York Times* (October 26, 1949), p. 27; Sylvia Perkins, *A Centennial Review: The Massachusetts General Hospital School of Nursing, 1873-1973* (1975).

LORETTA P. HIGGINS

PEMBER, PHOEBE YATES {LEVY} (August 18, 1823, Charleston, South Carolina--March 4, 1913, Pittsburgh, Pennsylvania). *Confederate Civil War hospital matron.* Daughter of Jacob Clavius Levy and Fanny (Yates) Levy, prosperous and cultured Jews who moved to Savannah, Georgia, in 1850. Married Thomas Pember of Boston prior to the Civil War; he died of tuberculosis in 1861 at the age of thirty-six; no children. EDUCATION: Nothing is known about her education, although she probably studied under private tutors and may have attended a Northern finishing school as was the custom of upper-class Southerners before the Civil War; her wartime letters and reminiscences indicate that she was well-educated. CAREER: November 1862-1865, matron, Chimborazo Hospital, a Confederate military hospital outside Richmond, Virginia.

CONTRIBUTIONS: Phoebe Pember has been credited with providing exceptional nursing service to the Confederate soldiers during the Civil War. She was the first matron of Chimborazo Hospital, having been offered the position through her friendship with Mrs. George Randolph, wife of the Confederate secretary of war. Chimborazo was considered the largest hospital in the world, larger than Scutari in the Crimea or Lincoln Hospital in Washington, D.C. At peak capacity, there were five divisions within the hospital, and 150 wards were under her supervision. It has been estimated that at least 15,000 soldiers came under her care during the course of the Civil War. The functions of matron were listed in an act of the Confederate Congress, specifying that the matron see that the orders of surgeons were carried out, supervise the sanitary and commissary arrangements of the hospital, and satisfy the needs of the patients.

Like other women who undertook the nursing of soldiers during the Civil War, she encountered considerable opposition. It was not considered respectable for a woman to go into a hospital, especially one filled with men. Being a widow, however, she was able to overcome some of the prejudices against women. Nurses often were treated with disrespect by the male members of the hospital staff, and some of the patients subjected the women to "unusual and embarrassing experiences." For example, Pember complained that one of the patients at Chimborazo insisted on "pulling off all his clothes" whenever she entered his ward. She ignored the opposition as based on prejudice, and attacked the more tangible problems like procuring adequate food for the patients and supplies for those who required special diets. She had a great deal of difficulty securing the whiskey appropriations for the patients under her care. As matron, she was responsible for dispensing the whiskey prescribed for the patients, but many hospital employees tried to take it for their own use; on occasion she had to guard the supply with a gun. She was especially upset when a drunken surgeon treating a patient with a crushed ankle put the wrong leg in splints and "contributed to the soldier's death." She concluded that "there were some doubts afloat as to whether the benefit conferred upon the patients by the use of stimulants counterbalanced the evil effects they produced on the surgeons." She was a strong advocate of her patients' well-being and refused to allow the transfer of patients who in her opinion were too ill to travel. Even when the war officially ended, she stayed at her post during the transition from Confederate to Union control of the hospital, ensuring that her patients received the care they needed. In her letters, she left behind a colorful description of life in the Confederacy, writing about slow and dangerous railroad trips, about the eagerness of southern women for factory-made clothing, and about her own difficulties in securing proper clothing during Reconstruction.

She returned to Georgia after the conclusion of the hostilities, and little is known about her except that she did considerable travelling.

WRITINGS: *A Southern Woman's Story* (1879); a new edition of this book, edited by Bell I. Wiley and containing a biographical sketch and nine of her wartime letters, was published in 1959.

REFERENCES: Alfred H. Bill, *The Beleaguered City, Richmond, 1861-1865* (1946); H. H. Cunningham, *Doctors in Gray: The Confederate Medical Service* (1958); Katherine M. Jones, *Ladies of Richmond: Confederate Capital* (1962); Jacob R. Marcus, *American Jewish Women: 1654-1980* (1981); *Notable American Women* (1971), III: 44-45; Margaret E. Parsons, "Mothers and Matrons," *Nursing Outlook* (September-October 1983); *Savannah Morning News* (March 6, 1913); Francis B. Simkins and James W. Patton, *The Women of the Confederacy* (1936); Pember-Phillips-Myers Collection, University of North Carolina, Chapel Hill; Records of Chimborazo Hospital, National Archives, Washington, D.C.; letters and the will of Jacob Levy, American Jewish Archives, Cincinnati.

ALICE HOWELL FRIEDMAN

PFEFFERKORN, BLANCHE (January 1884, Baltimore, Maryland--June 4, 1961, Los Angeles). *Nurse-educator; author.* Daughter of Leopold Pfefferkorn, wholesale beef merchant, and Helen (Einstein) Pfefferkorn. Never married. EDUCATION: 1903, graduated from Western High School, Baltimore, Maryland; spent two months at a woman's college; 1911, graduated from Johns Hopkins Hospital Training School for Nurses,

Baltimore; 1914-1916, attended Teachers College, Columbia University, New York City, receiving her B.S. in 1916 and M.A. in 1928 (she received from Teachers College the Isabel Hampton Robb {q.v.} Fellowship for graduate study). CAREER: 1911-1912, staff nurse, Bellevue Hospital, New York City; 1912-1913, supervisor of the operating room, Harlem Hospital, New York City; 1913-1914, assistant to the superintendent of nurses, Harlem Hospital; 1916-1923, instructor and then assistant professor, University of Cincinnati (Ohio) School of Nursing and Health; 1923-1928, executive secretary, National League of Nursing Education (NLNE); 1927-1930, departmental secretary, Division of Nursing Education, Teachers College, Columbia University; 1930-1932, director of special study, Bellevue Hospital; 1932-1949, director of studies, NLNE.

CONTRIBUTIONS: Blanche Pfefferkorn, one of the distinguished graduates of Johns Hopkins nursing school, is best known for her contributions to the pioneering nursing studies, especially those produced under the auspices of the National League of Nursing Education (NLNE). She was the first author of the report of the Joint Committee on the Costs of Nursing Service and Nursing Education, which was written while she served as director of studies for the NLNE. The report, entitled *Administrative Cost Analysis for Nursing Service and Nursing Education* (1940), was based on an extensive study to examine the cost to individual hospitals of operating a nursing service without a school and with a school, and to develop methods and criteria by which a valid comparison of costs in one institution might be made with those in another. During the first phase of the study, measures were developed to quantify nursing service and education, to select cost concepts appropriate to the problem, and to develop an accounting method for cost analysis of nursing service and education as separate entities. During the second phase, the procedures developed for cost analysis were applied to specific situations. The study revealed that the cost of education was exactly that over the amount of cost of nursing service without a school, with the underlying assumption that the quality of care would be the same. The study produced important techniques for computation of nursing costs and accounting procedures for nursing time.

A second study, *An Activity Analysis of Nursing* was part of a five-year program adopted in 1926 by the Committee on the Grading of Nursing Schools. It addressed several research questions: what is good nursing? what are curricular implications of the functional aspects of nursing? how can activities be classified? and how can one compile and use nursing activity lists? The study generated three sets of data: basic lists of potential nursing conditions in the hospital and in the community, a list for classifying nursing activities, and a list of nursing activities.

The book concluded with suggestions for use of the data to determine content for teaching and to guide curriculum development.

Pfefferkorn also contributed a third important document to the nursing literature: a treatise on clinical education in nursing, published in 1932. That work was prepared to provide a guide for methodology and techniques to determine the quality and quantity of bedside care and clinical instruction for use by hospitals and schools of nursing. Included are techniques for measuring nursing, quantitatively and qualitatively, an analysis of clinical teaching in hospitals and the organization of nursing service, guidelines for assignments and rotation on services correlated with instruction, and the use of job analysis as a tool for both education and administration. In part, the book reports on the study conducted at Bellevue for which Pfefferkorn served as director.

During her tenure at the NLNE, Pfefferkorn was responsible for organization and development of the league's services and programs. She was also the principal force behind the Department of Studies, which she served as director for seventeen years. The results were pioneering efforts in nursing research and the advance of the profession as a scholarly discipline.

Her interest in nursing research apparently began in 1921, when she performed what may have been her first research study, a document with a chronology of the Johns Hopkins Hospital nursing school; her study later was used as part of the 1924 survey of the school undertaken by Carolyn E. Gray (q.v.) in response to the Goldmark Report and at the behest of the hospital's trustees. With the resignation of Euphemia Taylor (q.v.) from her position as the first executive secretary of the NLNE, in 1923, Pfefferkorn accepted the position and moved to Kew Gardens, New York. In 1932, she moved into the directorship of the Department of Studies, following completion of her master's degree and her position as director of a qualitative and quantitative investigation of nursing at Bellevue Hospital.

In 1923, she was chairperson of the program committee of the American Nurses' Association. She served on the NLNE Special Committee on Educational Problems in Wartime and on the league's postwar planning committee. In 1947, she published a study of pediatric nursing, which was completed as part of her work with the league.

After her retirement from the league on August 1, 1949, she continued to pursue her interest in writing. From August 17 to 31, 1949, she attended the Breadloaf writer's conference, in Vermont. She retired to Sierra Madre, California, but from there, she answered the call of her alma mater to write its history. For part of her work, she returned to Baltimore and lived in the nurses' residence in order to have access to important documents in the archives which were crucial for her research.

Most of the writing, however, was apparently done in California. In frail health for a number of years, she died in 1961 at the age of seventy-seven.

WRITINGS: *The Johns Hopkins Hospital School of Nursing, 1889-1949* (with Ethel Johns, 1954); *Administrative Cost Analysis for Nursing Service and Nursing Education* (1940); *An Activity Analysis of Nursing* (with Ethel Johns, 1934); *Clinical Education in Nursing* (1932, with Marian Rottman); numerous articles in professional journals.

REFERENCES: Student records and papers, Alan Mason Chesney Archives of the Johns Hopkins Medical Institutions; *American Journal of Nursing* (August 1961), p. 117; *Baltimore Evening Sun* (June 5, 1961); *Baltimore Sun* (June 14, 1961); Lyndia Flanagan, *One Strong Voice: The Story of the American Nurses' Association* (1976); Ethel Johns and Blanche Pfefferkorn, *The Johns Hopkins Hospital School of Nursing, 1889-1949* (1954); *Johns Hopkins Nurses Alumnae Magazine* (July 1954), pp. 105-106; *New York Times* (June 6, 1961); Blanche Pfefferkorn and Charles A. Rovetta, *Adminstrative Cost Analysis for Nursing Service and Nursing Education* (1940); Anna D. Wolf, "Blanche Pfefferkorn, 1911," *Johns Hopkins Nurses Alumnae Magazine* (April 1950), pp. 54-59.

JOELLEN WATSON HAWKINS

PHILLIPS, HARRIET NEWTON (December 29, 1819, Pennsylvania--August 29, 1901, Gladwyne, Pennsylvania). *Civil war nurse; missionary.* EDUCATION: 1864, enrolled in six-month course at Woman's Hospital Training School, Philadelphia; 1870, graduated from the training school and immediately was appointed head nurse at Woman's Hospital; 1878, completed the extended course at the Woman's Hospital. CAREER: 1862-1864, Civil War nurse with the western branch of the U.S. Sanitary Commission; October 2, 1862-c. October 1863, nurse, General Hospital, Jefferson Barracks, near St. Louis, Missouri; c. November 1863-c. February 1864, nurse at General Hospital, Benton Barracks, St. Louis; February 15, 1864, listed on the rolls of the Nineteenth General Hospital, Nashville, Tennessee; March 23, 1864, discharged from the Army Nurse Corps (and apparently enrolled very soon in the nursing course of Woman's Hospital, Philadelphia); 1870-1871, head nurse and instructor, Woman's Hospital Training School, Philadelphia; 1872-June 1875, missionary work among the Ojibway and Sioux Indians of northwestern Wisconsin, Odanah Station, near Ashland, Wisconsin; June 21, 1875-c. 1878, matron in San Francisco, working with Chinese immigrants and at a mission sponsored by the Presbyterian church; 1894, applied for a veteran's pension, from an address in Michigan; 1900, lived with a niece in Gladwyne, Pennsylvania, where she died.

CONTRIBUTIONS: Harriet Phillips may well be the first nurse who participated in a training program. She is credited with having received a diploma or certificate from the Woman's Hospital, Philadelphia, in 1870, after having completed a six-month course of nursing study. The hospital was chartered on March 22, 1861, and Dr. Emaline Cleveland, the first resident physician, was to be responsible for training nurses and physicians. It is believed that prior to assuming the position with the Woman's Hospital, Dr. Cleveland had conferred with Florence Nightingale while in Europe for a year of study. Therefore, it is possible that the training program at Woman's Hospital was influenced by the Nightingale model. In any case, hospital records indicate that Phillips entered training in October 1864 along with female medical students and that she had lectures in anatomy, physiology, materia medica, and chemistry, and was taught the practical arts of nursing.

Prior to her formal training, she had volunteered to serve as a nurse during the Civil War, caring for the sick and wounded in military hospitals in St. Louis and Nashville. Her name next surfaces in Philadelphia in records of the Woman's Hospital. The annual report to the board of managers for January 1864 refers to her as a novitiate preparing for nursing. The training program at Woman's Hospital seems to have been especially difficult, for the annual reports from 1863 to 1869 refer often to novitiates coming and going, many unable to withstand the rigorous course. By 1870 only four nurses had completed the course and received diplomas. In the annual report to the board of managers, January 1865, she is again referred to as the only thoroughly qualified nurse to leave the hospital and to nurse in the community. By 1870, she apparently had returned to Woman's Hospital, for once more she appears in the annual report, January 1871, as a head nurse and assistant in the training of nurses. In the monthly minutes of the hospital for October 1870, her salary was reported to be $4 per week.

Phillips' subsequent career is difficult to trace. She apparently was a missionary nurse among the Indians of Wisconsin, being mentioned in the records of the American Board of Missions, from November 1871 to November 1878. She then returned to Woman's Hospital for the extended training program of one year. Of the rest of her life, some records have been discovered, but they are incomplete. In 1883, she transferred her membership from a Presbyterian church in Philadelphia to one in Gladwyne, Pennsylvania. In 1894 she applied for a veteran's pension, giving her permanent address as Gladwyne, and in 1900 she was living as a boarder with a niece in Gladwyne.

REFERENCES: Jacob Gilbert Forman, *The Western Sanitary Commission: A Sketch* (1861), p. 107; Joan T. Large, "Harriet Newton Phillips: The First Trained Nurse in America," *Image* (October 1976), pp. 49-51; information provided by Irene Matthews, R.N., collected from various published and unpublished sources; *Norristown Daily Herald* (August 30, 1901); *Philadelphia City Directory* (1889); Victor Robinson, *White Caps* (1946); unpublished letter, Dora Ruland, executive secretary of the Woman's Hospital of Philadelphia, to Ella Best, executive secretary, American Nurses' Association, November 8, 1948; U.S. Census Report for the State of Pennsylvania, 1900; U.S. Department of the Interior, Bureau of Pensions, pension application, October 23, 1893; Roberta Mayhew West, *History of Nursing in Pennsylvania* (1926), p. 24; Woman's Hospital of Philadelphia, *Annual Report of the Board of Managers* (1870, 1871).

JOELLEN WATSON HAWKINS

POPE, AMY ELIZABETH (1868, Quebec, Canada--October 28, 1949, San Francisco). *Nurse-author.* Daughter of English parents. Never married. EDUCATION: 1894, graduated with the first class of Presbyterian Hospital School for Nurses, New York City, having also had special maternity work at Sloane Hospital; post-graduate study, St. Bartholomew's Hospital, London; studied massage, Gardner Gymnasium, New York City, and dietetics at Pratt Institute, Brooklyn, New York; enrolled in advanced courses in nursing specialties, Teachers College, Columbia University, New York City. CAREER: c. 1894-1898, public health nurse, Visiting Nurse Association of Philadelphia; 1898, army nurse, Spanish-American War; 1898-1901, served with Red Cross Auxiliary Unit in the Philippines, then 1901, at Las Animas Hospital, Havana, Cuba, and 1901-1904, in the Health Department of the Isthmian Canal Commission, Panama Canal Zone; 1904, instructor, Johns Hopkins Hospital School of Nursing, Baltimore, Maryland; 1907-c. 1909, superintendent, Government Insular Training School for Nurses, San Juan, Puerto Rico; 1904-1907 and 1909-1913, instructor, head nurse and assistant superintendent, School of Nursing, Presbyterian Hospital, New York City; house mother, Bellevue Hospital Training School, New York; 1914-retirement in 1928, instructor, St. Luke's Hospital School of Nursing, San Francisco.

CONTRIBUTIONS: Pope's greatest contribution was as an author of important nursing textbooks, one of which was translated into Chinese, Danish, Korean, and Spanish. With her colleague Anna Maxwell (q.v.), who was superintendent at Presbyterian Hospital when Pope was a student there, she wrote *Practical Nursing*, first published in 1907, a text which was so widely used that it went through many editions. She also wrote textbooks on anatomy and physiology, physics and chemistry, dietetics, materia medica, and nursing arts, as well as a quiz book for nurses and a medical dictionary.

A hard-working and restless individual, her career reflects her enthusiasm for adventure. During the Spanish-American War, she served with the army at Fortress Monroe, and later in Puerto Rico and then in the Philippines (the latter with a Red Cross Auxiliary Unit). During the 1898 yellow fever epidemic in Cuba, she served at Los Animos Hospital. When an opening in dietetics occurred at Ancon Hospital, Panama, she took it and worked under the supervision of Eugenie Hibbard (q.v.). While in Panama, Pope was appointed for service with the Health Department of the Isthmian Canal Commission. In 1907, she answered a call for a superintendent of nurses and organized the first school of nursing in Puerto Rico, the Insular Training School for Nurses, at Municipal Hospital, San Juan. The hospital opened April 2, 1908 under her direction, with a two-year course of study. In 1909, she was replaced by Pilar Cabrera. Pope clearly contributed a great deal to the organization and development of nursing in Puerto Rico. She also took positions as a private nurse and travelled with cases to Paris and Bad Nauheim, Germany.

Pope also contributed to the development of other schools of nursing. She was on the faculty at Johns Hopkins, as well as serving for an extended period at St. Luke's Hospital, San Francisco. Periodically, she served her alma mater, as a head nurse, assistant superintendent, and when the preliminary course was introduced, as an instructor. Her superintendent, Anna Maxwell, received many requests from other hospitals as to how practical nursing was taught at Johns Hopkins Hospital, and Pope was given the task of answering those letters. There were so many similar requests that it occurred to her that the solution was to write a good textbook on the subject. She approached Maxwell with the idea, and the result was their collaboration on *Practical Nursing* (1907). With the English-language edition as well as through the many translations, the book was widely used at nursing schools around the world. Pope also served as the second president of the Nurses' Alumnae Association of Presbyterian Hospital (1899). In 1926, the yearbook of the St. Luke's Hospital School of Nursing, San Francisco, was dedicated to Amy Pope, instructress in nursing. Little is known of the years after her retirement in 1928.

WRITINGS: *Practical Nursing* (1907); *Anatomy and Physiology for Nurses* (1913); *A Medical Dictionary for Nurses* (1914); *A Quiz Book of Nursing* (1915); *Physics and Chemistry for Nurses* (1916); *Essentials of Dietetics in Health and Disease* (1917); *A Practical Dietary Computer* (1917); *Manual of Nursing Procedure* (1919); *Materia Medica, Pharmacology and Therapeutics for Nurses* (1921); *A Textbook of Simple Nursing Procedure* (1921); *The Art and Principles of Nursing* (1934).

REFERENCES: *American Journal of Nursing* (February 1950), pp. 23-24; unpublished materials, Colegio de Profesionales de la Enfermeria de Puerto Rico; Minnie Goodnow, *Nursing History* (7th ed., 1943; 8th ed., 1948); Cordelia W. Kelly, *Dimensions of Professional Nursing* (2nd ed., 1968); Eleanor Lee, *History of the School of Nursing, Presbyterian Hospital, 1892-1942* (1942); Meta Rutter Pennock, *Makers of Nursing History* (1940); Mary M. Roberts, *American Nursing: History and Interpretation* (1954); St. Luke's Hospital School of Nursing archives, San Francisco.

JOELLEN WATSON HAWKINS

POWELL, LOUISE MATHILDE (March 12, 1871, Staunton, Virginia--October 6, 1943, Brownsburg, Virginia). *Nurse-educator.* Daughter of Hugh Lee Powell and Ella (Stribling) Powell. Never married. EDUCATION: 1899, received a diploma from St. Luke's Hospital Training School for Nurses, Richmond, Virginia; throughout her professional life, she returned frequently to school as a student, including post-graduate work at the Hospital for Sick Children, Mt. Wilson, Maryland, and at the Municipal Hospital for Contagious Diseases, Philadelphia, and summer sessions at the University of Virginia, Charlottesville, and Smith College, Northampton, Massachusetts; 1908-1910, enrolled in the Hospital Economics course at Teachers College, Columbia University, New York City, (during M. Adelaide Nutting's {q.v.} first years as professor of nursing, and she was a classmate there of Isabel Stewart {q.v.}, who became one of the leaders of nursing education in the United States); 1922, received a bachelor's degree in nursing education, Teachers College. CAREER: Before entering nursing school, was an elementary school teacher, Norfolk, Virginia; 1899-1904, superintendent of nurses, St. Luke's Hospital, Richmond, Virginia; 1905-1908, charge nurse of the infirmary of the Baldwin School, Bryn Mawr, Pennsylvania; 1910-1924, superintendent of nurses, University of Minnesota nursing school; 1918-1919, acting superintendent, University of Minnesota Hospital, while the medical director was on military assignment; January 1922, on leave; 1923-1924, returned and assumed her new title of director of the University of Minnesota School of Nursing; 1924-1927, dean, newly founded Western Reserve University school of nursing, resigning due to ill health; during her retirement, continued with philanthropic work, learning Braille and translating books including a biology textbook for the use of the blind.

CONTRIBUTIONS: Louise Powell is best remembered as the director during its formative years of the School of Nursing, University of Minnesota, the first baccalaureate program for nurses. An historian has said that this program changed the status of a nursing "pupil" to that of a student. Powell strengthened the curriculum, hired qualified faculty, maintained high admission standards, improved the living conditions of the students, and coordinated the clinical facilities of three hospitals into a central school for expanded clinical experiences. She worked for the full integration of the nursing students into the university community. In terms of curricular reform, she introduced sociology in 1916, public health nursing was added in 1918, and in 1919 she organized the first five-year curriculum which included the humanities as well as the sciences.

She served on various committees of professional organizations, including president of the Minnesota League of Nursing Education, vice-president and director of the National League of Nursing Education (NLNE), secretary, treasurer, and director of the Minnesota State Registered Nurses' Association, and on several committees of the American Red Cross. She was honorary president, Minnesota State Organization for Public Health Nursing, and in 1935 she was elected to honorary membership in the National League of Nursing Education.

REFERENCES: *American Journal of Nursing* (1924), p. 298 and (1943), p. 1159; Teresa Christy, *Cornerstone for Nursing Education* (1969); James Gray, *Education for Nursing* (1960); Janet James et al., *Notable American Women* (1971), pp. 89-90; Mary Marvin Wayland, "Louise M. Powell," *National League of Nursing Education Biographical Sketch* (1937).

ALICE HOWELL FRIEDMAN

R

REITER, FRANCES URSULA (June 13, 1904, Smithton, Pennsylvania--January 18, 1977, Cherry, Illinois). *Nurse-educator; researcher.* Married Harry Kreuter, December 22, 1951; two stepsons. EDUCATION: 1931, graduated from Johns Hopkins Hospital Training School for Nurses, Baltimore, Maryland; 1941, B.A. in nursing education, and 1942, M.A. in teaching biological sciences, Teachers College, Columbia University, New York City. CAREER: 1931-1934, head nurse and supervisor, Johns Hopkins Hospital, Baltimore, Maryland; 1934-1936, private duty nurse, Baltimore, Maryland, and Washington, D.C.; 1936-1938, assistant director of nursing service and nursing education, Montefiore Hospital, Pittsburgh, Pennsylvania; 1938-1939, private duty nurse, New York City; 1941-1942, taught nursing at Johns Hopkins Hospital School of Nursing, Columbia University Teachers College, and Bryn Mawr College, Bryn Mawr, Pennsylvania; 1942-1945, joint appointment with Boston University School of Nursing and Massachusetts General Hospital School of Nursing; 1946-1960, assistant professor, associate professor, then professor of nursing education, Teachers College, Columbia University; 1960-1962, director of nursing programs, Flower and Fifth Avenue Hospitals, New York City; 1960-1969, dean and professor, Graduate School of Nursing, New York Medical College (now Pace University), New York City; 1969, dean emeritus.

CONTRIBUTIONS: Frances Reiter's main contributions were to nursing education and nursing research. She was chairperson of the American Nurses' Association's (ANA) committee on education, a committee which formulated the association's first position paper on basic nursing education (December 1965). Although a response to mandates from the house of delegates at the ANA conventions of 1962 and 1964, the position paper raised a great deal of controversy within the profession, and it continues to do so. This first definitive statement of nursing education, entitled *Educational Preparation for Nurse Practitioners and Assistants to Nurses: A Position Paper*, recommended that education for all those licensed to practice nursing should take place in institutions of higher learning. It specified that the baccalaureate degree be the minimum requirement for professional nursing practice, the associate degree for technical nursing practice, and that assistants were to receive intensive pre-service programs in vocational schools. Various groups within the profession have resisted these ideas. The profession has not rallied around the position paper, as it is seen as a threat to the thousands of nurses whose education was provided by hospital schools of nursing, rather than by colleges and universities. To implement the position paper, many believe, would require legislative changes in the nurse practice acts of the various states, and extensive funding would be needed to upgrade the education of nurses already in practice.

The largest portion of Reiter's career was spent in teaching and administrative positions in collegiate schools of nursing. She was a firm advocate of the baccalaureate education of nurses, and she prepared herself for positions that offered that type of training. In her era, the doctorate was not a requirement; a master's degree in nursing education and a background of extensive clinical experience was typical of the nurse-educator of the period from 1930 to 1960. Reiter was particularly known as the one who fostered the notion of clinical specialists. She sought to prepare students for the general degree in nursing but stressed that after having completed their undergraduate nursing education, every nurse should develop a specialty, through additional clinical experience, or through a graduate program in nursing or nursing education. She sought to prepare highly knowledgeable and skillful practitioners, a rare combination at a time when the vast majority of America's nurses were graduates of hospital-based programs which required very little scientific background or study.

In addition to her contributions to nursing education, Reiter was known for her research success. She was clearly a pioneer among nurses who became researchers as well as administrators or teachers. She was a member of the executive committee of the first editorial board of *Nursing Research*, the journal which provided a forum for papers and reports based on clinical studies done by nurses. This was the profession's first journal exclusively devoted to research, and it served an important role in strengthening the scientific basis for the profession by encouraging nurses to pursue research rather than to focus their attention exclusively on patient care or on teaching. At various times, she was project director and/or consultant for research projects sponsored by the U.S. Public Health Service, the Veterans Administration, and the Montefiore Hospital Nursing Project. For the U.S. Public Health Service, she focused on

"Establishing Criteria for the Quality of Hospital Nursing Care" (1950-1954). For the Veterans Administration, she prepared "A Method of Studying the Utilization of Nursing Service Personnel in Veterans Administration Hospitals" (1954-1958). Finally, for the Montefiore Hospital Nursing Project she wrote about "Interruptions of Nursing While Giving Nursing Care" (1959-1961). She also was an associate for the Institute for Research and Service in Nursing, Columbia University Teachers College's research division. She also directed for the W.K. Kellogg Foundation a survey of advanced clinical nursing preparation, and she was the director of another Kellogg-sponsored survey of rural nursing needs in the state of Michigan.

Reiter was a member of the New York State Board of Nurse Examiners (1947-1951), a member of the editorial advisory board for G. P. Putnam's Sons (1948), a member of the advisory board to the Johns Hopkins Hospital School of Nursing (1964-1967), and a member of the medical advisory board of the National Multiple Sclerosis Society (1967-1968). She also was an associate member of the Columbia University interdisciplinary seminar on the role of the health professions (1955-1972). She was a member of a number of important committees of the ANA and the National League for Nursing (NLN). From 1951 to 1957, she was chairperson of the NLN's council of member agencies' committee on baccalaureate and higher degree programs, and from 1949 to 1952 she served as a member of the board of review of the NLN committee on the accreditation of collegiate schools of nursing.

For her contributions, Reiter received a number of important awards. In 1968, the ANA made her an honorary member. The following year, when she retired as dean of the New York Medical College's graduate school of nursing, she received from the International Red Cross the Florence Nightingale Award, from the NLN its distinguished service award, and from the New York Medical College a medal of excellence.

WRITINGS: Co-author of the American Nurses' Association's committee on education position paper, *Educational Preparation for Nurse Practitioners and Assistants to Nurses* (1965); many articles in professional journals, focusing primarily on nurse-clinicians and the improvement of nursing practice.

REFERENCES: *New York Times* (January 21, 1977), sect. D, p. 4; *Nursing Outlook* (February 1977), p. 88; manuscript papers of Frances Reiter, Nursing Archives, Mugar Memorial Library, Boston University.

ALICE HOWELL FRIEDMAN

RICHARDS, LINDA ANN JUDSON (July 27, 1841 on a farm near Potsdam, New York--April 16, 1930, Boston). *America's first trained nurse; leader in nursing education.* Daughter of Sanford Richards, a farmer, and Betsy (Sinclair) Richards. Never married. EDUCATION: Attended common schools of Lyndon and Newport, Vermont, then Barton Academy and St. Johnsbury Academy, both in Vermont; September 1, 1872-September 1, 1873, attended the nurse training program, New England Hospital for Women and Children, Boston, graduating on September 1, 1873; 1877, post-graduate study in England, France, and Scotland. CAREER: c. 1857, taught school in Newport, Vermont; 1870, ward maid, Boston City Hospital; 1872, assistant, New England Hospital, Boston; October 1, 1873-October 15, 1874, night nursing superintendent in charge of maternity wards from May-October 1874, Bellevue Hospital, New York City; November 1, 1874-April 1877, head of Boston Training School (Massachusetts General Hospital School of Nursing) and January 1875-April 1877 superintendent of nurses; January 1, 1878-August 1879 and September 1881-December 1885, organized training school at Boston City Hospital and served as superintendent (extended leave due to illness, August 1879-September 1881); January 1886-October 15, 1890, in Kyoto, Japan to set up a hospital; April-November 1891, head, Philadelphia Visiting Nurses Society; December 1891-April 1892, matron, Kirkbride Asylum, Philadelphia; April-December 1, 1892, founded training school at Philadelphia Methodist Episcopal Hospital; January 1, 1893-April 1894, reorganized and strengthened training school at New England Hospital for Women and Children, Boston; April 1894-October 1895, similar role at training school of Brooklyn Homeopathic Hospital; November 1895-November 1897, similar role at training school of Hartford Hospital; two months at Long Island Hospital, Boston Harbor; November 1897-1899, superintendent of training school, University of Pennsylvania Hospital, Philadelphia; September 1899-1904 and 1910-1911, director of nurse training school at Taunton Insane Hospital, Taunton, Massachusetts, September 1904-November 1905, superintendent and director of nurse training school, Worcester Hospital for the Insane, Worcester, Massachusetts; January 1906-September 1909, superintendent and director of nurse training school, Michigan Insane Asylum, Kalamazoo, Michigan. CONTRIBUTIONS: Linda Richards is best remembered as America's first trained nurse. Choosing the only profession open to women of her day, she began as a schoolteacher in Vermont. But this brilliant and talented woman was to give most of her life to a career as a nurse, as a founder of training schools, and as an advocate for the improvement of nursing in hospitals for the mentally ill. At the age of four, Melinda Richards, to use the name with which she had been christened, moved with her family from upstate New York to Wisconsin, where they planned to begin farming. Shortly after their arrival, however, her father died of tuberculosis, and her mother moved to Vermont, to be near her own father. They bought a small farm near Newport, Vermont, where young Linda Richards helped with the chores, attended school, and helped care for her mother, who was also suffering from tuberculosis. When she was in her teens, neighbors and family members recognized her talent for nursing, increasing her interest in becoming a nurse. After her mother's death, she lived with her grandfather and one of her sisters, and during the years that followed, she often went with old Dr. Currier on his rounds. Often she stayed with a family to nurse someone, strengthening her resolve to become a nurse. She read of Florence Nightingale's plan to begin a training school in London, but her grandfather, concerned that Linda be provided for and seeing no prospect for a husband, sent her to the academy in St. Johnsbury where, with great reluctance, she prepared to be a teacher. Even there, her best talents were not in the classroom, but in caring for her classmates, one of whom she saved from a serious infection that might have meant death had she not known what to do. She completed her year of studies and found a teaching position in Newport, where she remained from about 1860 to 1870. During some of those years, she not only taught school but also nursed the man who was her fiance through the final stages of tuberculosis.

It was in 1870, then, that she found herself in Boston, determined more than ever to become a nurse. With great trepidation and carrying her copy of Florence Nightingale's *Notes on Nursing*, she presented herself at Boston City Hospital, asking for a position as an assistant nurse. No sooner had she started work than she was struck with typhus fever, an illness which was known through history as jail fever, prison fever, and camp fever, a disease which was spread by fleas and ticks and which she most likely contracted in the hospital, known to be overcrowded and filthy. After recuperating with relatives who lived in nearby Foxborough, in 1872 she read a notice that a training school for nurses would open that autumn at New England Hospital for Women and Children. Scarcely believing her luck, she hurried to the hospital, met Dr. Susan Dimock, and, to her amazement, she was allowed to enroll as the first student. Eager to begin, she worked at the hospital during the summer of 1872, and on September 1 she officially began her training. One year later, she received her diploma, becoming the first woman to graduate from an American nursing school.

Her graduation did not pass unnoticed. Soon there were requests for her services. For her first position, she chose to go to Bellevue Hospital as the night superintendent. There, she initiated the idea of written reports on all serious cases. But the calls continued for her services, and in 1874 she responded to the invitation to become superintendent of the Nightingale training school, known as the Boston Training School for Nurses, begun the previous year. In January 1875, she became superintendent of nurses, and by the end of 1876 she finally had charge of all nursing in the hospital. She succeeded in making several changes in the difficult conditions under which the school was operating; she hired two scrubwomen to relieve the students of some of the housekeeping tasks, and she obtained a watch and a thermometer so students could measure the pulse rates and temperatures of their patients. Since relations with the medical staff were at first strained, she had to rely at first on lecturers from the medical staff of the Boston City Hospital. A new resident physician was supportive, however, and she was then able to persuade physicians at Massachusetts General Hospital to give weekly lectures to the nursing students. Some students were given the opportunity for clinical experience at the Massachusetts Eye and Ear Infirmary and the Boston Lying-in Hospital. Before she left in the spring of 1877 for post-graduate study in Europe, Richards had placed the school on a firm foundation. It had moved from McLean Street into "the Brick" adjacent to the Massachusetts General Hospital, she instituted evening classes during which she read to the pupil nurses and quizzed them, she had established uniform collars and cuffs for the students, and she had requested a sitting room for their use.

Resigning in the spring of 1877, on April 16 Richards sailed for eight months of study in Europe. She spent a few days at Florence Nightingale's summer home, and under Nightingale's guidance, she studied the training school at St. Thomas' Hospital and visited other hospitals, including King's College Hospital, London, and the Royal Infirmary, Edinburgh. She then spent a month visiting hospitals and schools in Paris, and sailed for home in October, having already accepted an offer to be matron of the Boston City Hospital, as well as superintendent of the nurse training school which was scheduled to open in 1878.

In January 1878, she set about organizing the training school, which opened in May. Due largely to her ability, the school survived the uncertainties of its early years and was established on a sound basis. Thus, when she was invited to establish the first training school for nurses in Japan, under the auspices of the American Board of Foreign Missions, she accepted. Sailing from San Francisco on December 30, 1885, she arrived in Kyoto in January 1886 and proceeded to establish a two-year program in Doshisha Hospital, a small mission hospital. In 1888, the school produced its first graduates. Again, ill health intervened, and she left Japan on October 15, 1890, travelling first to France via the Suez Canal, arriving back in the United States in March 1891.

In the early 1890s, she served a number of organizations, including the Philadelphia Visiting Nurses Society. She became matron at Kirkbride Asylum for the Insane, but was disappointed when conditions were not yet ready for a training school. She then undertook organization of the training school at Philadelphia's Methodist Episcopal Hospital, leaving in January 1893 to reorganize and strengthen the training school at the New England Hospital for Women and Children. Her tremendous talents for setting training schools on a firm foundation led to similar challenges at the Brooklyn Homeopathic Hospital, the Hartford Hospital, Long Island Hospital in Boston Harbor, and at the University of Pennsylvania Hospital in Philadelphia.

Twenty-six years after her graduation, Richards turned her career in another direction. The memories of Kirkbride Asylum continued to haunt her, and she dedicated the last twelve years of her career to improving the nursing care for the mentally ill. Her work began at Taunton Insane Hospital, where she organized a three-year course which included one year at a nearby general hospital. In 1904, the first class graduated, and Richards left to undertake similar work at Worcester State Lunatic Hospital, reorganizing the nursing department and starting a training school. At the age of sixty-five, she then moved to Kalamazoo, Michigan, where she began the training school of the Michigan Insane Asylum, remaining until the first class graduated in September 1909. When a new superintendent could not be found for Taunton, she returned there in September 1910, remaining until her retirement in March 1911, when she was given the title of superintendent emeritus.

In addition to her extensive service as a founder of early training schools, Richards was active in the early development of various professional organizations. She was a member of the American Society of Superintendents of Training Schools for Nurses when its first convention was held in January 1894, and she was elected the second president (1895), delivering a presidential address entitled "Progress in Twenty Years." In 1896 she was a member of the council, and in 1897 she served on the committee on examinations. In 1899, she was a member of the committee which approached Columbia University's Teachers College about the possibility of establishing a course for nurse-educators. She was also a member of the society's first education committee charged with the power to act on the hospital economics course to be offered at Teachers College.

When the *American Journal of Nursing* was begun, she purchased the first share of stock and for one year served as editor of its department of hospital and training school items. In 1916, already in her seventy-fifth year, she enrolled as a Red Cross nurse, and she became an ardent promoter of the bill to secure the existence of the Army Nurse Corps. She was also one of the organizers of the alumnae association of the New England Hospital for Women and Children Training School for Nurses.

Finally retired in 1911, she moved to a farm near Lowell, Massachusetts, where she lived with a cousin. Her last public appearance was at the 1923 convention of the Massachusetts League of Nurses in Swampscott, where she spoke briefly. She suffered a stroke in 1925, and for the last five years of her life she was confined to the Frances Willard Homestead, Northboro, Massachusetts. She died at New England Hospital for Women and Children in 1930, and her ashes were placed in the Columbarium at Forest Hills Cemetery, Boston. On May 16, 1930, a memorial service was held at Old South Church, Copley Square, Boston.

Over the course of her long and distinguished career, Linda Richards received numerous honors. From 1910 to 1930 she was an honorary member of the Massachusetts State Nurses' Association. In 1922, the delegates to the convention of the American Nurses' Association voted to have her likeness engraved on the corporate seal of the association. In November 1922, marking the fiftieth anniversary of the opening of the New England Hospital for Women and Children, she was presented with fifty red roses, one for each year of her service. She was honored at the Diamond Jubilee of Nursing banquet in New York City on November 16, 1948, and sixty-three cities and forty-eight states observed a Linda Richards Day in honor of her graduation seventy-five years earlier. In that year, the American Nurses' Association gave Richards Awards to an outstanding graduate in each state, a medal engraved with her likeness. In 1962, the National League for Nursing created the Linda Richards Award to honor a nurse making a pioneering contribution to the practice. In 1976, she was inducted into the American Nurses' Association Hall of Fame, as one of the original charter members.

WRITINGS: *Reminiscences of Linda Richards, America's First Trained Nurse* (1911); numerous articles in professional journals; numerous unpublished letters and reports.

REFERENCES: *American Journal of Nursing* (October 1900), pp. 12-13, (April 1902), pp. 491-494, (January 1903), pp. 245-252, (July 1909), p. 789, (June 1911), pp. 681-682, (January 1916), pp. 174-179, (August 1921), p. 805, (April 1926), pp. 323-324, and (May 1930), pp. 639-642; American Nurses' Association, *Heritage Hall/Hall of Fame* (1976); Rachel Baker, *America's First Trained Nurse: Linda Richards* (1970); *British Journal of Nursing* (December 18, 1915), p. 504; *A Century of Nursing* (1950); Lavinia L. Dock, Sarah E. Pickett, Clara D. Noyes, Fannie F. Clement, Elizabeth G. Fox, and Anna R. Van Meter, *History of American Red Cross Nursing* (1922); Mary Ellen Doona, "Nursing

Revisited: The Worcester State Hospital and Nursing," *The Massachusetts Nurse* (January 1984), p. 19; Virginia G. Drachman, *Hospital with a Heart* (1984); Wilkie Hughes, "Linda Richards," *American Journal of Nursing* (April 1941), p. 437; Agnes B. Joynes, "Linda Richards as I Knew Her," *American Journal of Nursing* (November 1920), pp. 72-77; Cordelia W. Kelly, *Dimensions of Professional Nursing* (2d ed., 1968); Helen W. Munson, "Linda Richards," *American Journal of Nursing* (September 1948), pp. 551-556; National League for Nursing, *Early Leaders of American Nursing* (1922); Linda Richards Collection, New England Hospital for Women and Children papers, Nursing Archives, Mugar Memorial Library, Boston University, Boston; *Notable American Women*, pp. 148-150; *Nursing World* (May 1930), p. 659; Sara E. Parsons, *History of the Massachusetts General Hospital Training School for Nurses* (1922); Susan Reverby, ed., *Annual Conventions of the American Society of Superintendents of Training Schools for Nurses* (1985); Meta Rutter Pennock, *Makers of Nursing History* (1940); Sylvia Perkins, *A Centennial Review: The Massachusetts General Hospital School of Nursing, 1873-1973* (1975); Linda Richards, "Progress in Twenty Years (1875-1895)," *Trained Nurse and Hospital Review* (April 1938), pp. 360-361; Mary M. Riddle, *Boston City Hospital Training School for Nurses Historical Sketch* (1928).

JOELLEN WATSON HAWKINS

RIDDLE, MARY MARGARET (June 6, 1856, on a farm near Muncy, Northumberland County, Pennsylvania--November 19, 1936, Muncy, Pennsylvania). *Leader in nursing education and in nursing organizations.* Daughter of John Riddle and Elizabeth (Bieber) Riddle. Never married. EDUCATION: Graduated from high school in Constantine, St. Joseph County, Michigan; 1889, graduated from Boston City Hospital Training School for Nurses. CAREER: Teacher in Michigan public schools; 1889-1904, assistant superintendent and night superintendent, Boston City Hospital; March 1904-December 31, 1921, superintendent, Newton Hospital, Newton Lower Falls, Massachusetts; June 17, 1918-January 1, 1919, head of Army School of Nursing, Camp Devens, Massachusetts; 1900-1904, lecturer, hospital economics course, Teachers College, Columbia University, New York City.

CONTRIBUTIONS: Mary Riddle's greatest contribution to the profession was her leadership, particularly in professional organizations but also at Boston City Hospital and Newton Hospital. Like many of her contemporaries, she began her career as a schoolteacher, deciding to attend a training school when she was about thirty years old. Following her graduation, Riddle soon became involved in nursing organizations and in the advancement of the profession. Her activities in nursing organizations were a significant part of her professional life. In February of 1896, she was elected an associate member of the newly formed American Society of Superintendents of Training Schools for Nurses. At the convention in February 1898, she delivered a paper, "How to Attain Greater Uniformity in Ward Work." She served on the council of the organization and on the committee on relations of nurses to municipal boards. In 1910, she was elected president of the society, which was then called the National League of Nursing Education.

Riddle was also a leader in the Massachusetts State Nurses Association, serving as its president from 1903 to 1910. She was active and instrumental in the development and eventual passage of the state law for registration and licensure of nurses. Indeed, her contribution was recognized when on November 15, 1910, she was issued Massachusetts registered nurse license number 1. From 1910 to 1926, she served as the first chairperson of the Massachusetts Board of Registration in Nursing. Later in her career, she was historian of the state nurses' association, and at its twenty-fifth anniversary (October 23, 1928), she presented a retrospective, "Looking Back."

She was also active in national organizations, serving as president of the Associated Alumnae of the United States and Canada from 1902 to 1905. That organization became the American Nurses' Association. From 1903 to 1932, she was treasurer of the board of directors of the *American Journal of Nursing* and was on the editorial staff for a number of years from 1912 to 1919 as editor of the department of hospital and training school administration. She was treasurer of the Isabel Hampton Robb (q.v.) Fund from May 1911 to January 1932 and treasurer of the McIsaac Loan Fund for Nurses for many years until 1932. Her editorial work was not confined to the *American Journal of Nursing*. Beginning in February 1914, she served as an editor for the department of nursing of the *Modern Hospital*. For many years, she served as president of the alumnae association of the Boston City Hospital nursing school.

In addition to her service to the profession through her organizational activities, she served the Boston City Hospital for fifteen years in various capacities: as assistant to the superintendent, Lucy Drown (q.v.), as night superintendent and superintendent of the convalescent home, and as assistant superintendent of nurses and matron of the south department. In 1904, she became superintendent of the Newton Hospital, as well as superintendent of nurses, and director of the training school. During the seventeen years she served the Newton Hospital, she exhibited not only qualities of leadership but a forward-looking approach to nursing practice. Being aware of the need for nurses to have greater knowledge of the newly developing science of psychology, as well as an appreciation of the ethical questions facing nurses on a day-to-day basis, she instituted a short course in psychology and lectures in ethics, as important aspects of the nursing curriculum. As early as 1906, her students gained experience in public health nursing through affiliation with the Newton District Nursing Association, and from 1918 to 1926, selected students could enroll in a four-month course in public health nursing co-sponsored by the Henry Street Settlement (New York City) and Teachers College of Columbia University. In 1918, the hospital was designated as an educational institution; stipends for students were discontinued, and the focus was shifted to education for the students rather than service to the hospital. Riddle instituted the eight-hour day and encouraged both rest and recreation for the students.

World War I posed special challenges for nurses, and Riddle was no exception. She organized fifty-five nurses for the first Harvard Nursing Unit, which was sent overseas in 1915. Granted a short leave of absence in 1918, she took charge of the nurses at Camp Devens, remaining long enough to help organize an induction service for the Army Nurse Corps. In 1918, Newton Hospital Training School admitted six students from the Vassar Training Camp, Poughkeepsie, New York, graduating them in 1920.

In 1922, when she retired at the age of sixty-five, she returned to Muncy, Pennsylvania, to live with her sister. She was far from inactive, however. Until 1936, she continued to attend the annual commencement exercises of the Newton Hospital, and colleagues from Boston periodically visited her in Pennsylvania. She continued to write, and in 1928, as historian for her own school and president of its alumnae association, she produced an historical sketch which was published as a book. Her contributions to professional organizations continued into the 1930s, including her service as treasurer of several funds.

Riddle suffered from an arteriosclerotic condition in her last few months that rendered her blind in one eye and confined to bed. She died in Muncy, Pennsylvania, where she was buried on November 21, 1936. On May 12, 1937, a memorial service was held in her honor at Trinity Church, in Boston's Copley Square.

Through her career, her service to the profession and to humanity was recognized in various ways. On November 20, 1918, she was commended by the governor of Massachusetts for her service as a member of the Massachusetts Divison of the Woman's Committee of the Council of National Defense. On October 10, 1919, in a letter from King George to those associated with the Harvard University Hospital Unit (World War I), she was recognized for her service in organizing the nurses' unit. Beginning in 1922 and continuing into the 1980s, selected students in each graduating class at the Newton Hospital School of

Nursing have been recognized as Mary M. Riddle Scholars, and from 1922 to 1936 she was at commencement to present the awards. In 1931, she received honorary membership in the Massachusetts State Nurses' Association.

WRITINGS: *Boston City Hospital Training School for Nurses: Historical Sketch* (1928); many articles in professional journals, as well as editorials in the *American Journal of Nursing* and the *Modern Hospital*; numerous unpublished diaries and letters.

REFERENCES: *American Journal of Nursing* (February 1914), pp. 333-334, (June 1921), p. 619, (January 1937), pp. 112-113, (June 1937), p. 677; *British Journal of Nursing* (January 31, 1914), p. 83; Lavinia L. Dock, Sarah E. Pickett, Clara D. Noyes, Fannie F. Clement, Elizabeth G. Fox, and Anna R. Van Meter, *History of American Red Cross Nursing* (1922); Mary Ellen Doona, "Nursing Revisited: Mary M. Riddle," *The Massachusetts Nurse* (October 1983), pp. 4, 14; Kathleen M. Downes, *A Tradition of Excellence: A Centennial Review of the Newton-Wellesley Hospital School of Nursing, 1886-1986* (1986); Lyndia Flanagan, *One Strong Voice: The Story of the American Nurses' Association* (1976); National League of Nursing Education, *Twelve Nursing Leaders* (1922); American Journal of Nursing and Boston City Hospital Collections, Nursing Archives, Mugar Memorial Library, Boston University; Susan Reverby, ed., *Annual Conventions of the American Society of Superintendents of Training Schools for Nurses* (1985); Mary Riddle, *Boston City Hospital Training School for Nurses: Historical Sketch* (1928); *Trained Nurse and Hospital Review* (June 1937), p. 617; unpublished papers, letters, and other documents of Riddle and correspondence with Elizabeth W. Hartman, Riddle's niece, Muncy, Pennsylvania, August 26 and September 16, 1986.

JOELLEN WATSON HAWKINS

RINEHART, MARY ELLA {ROBERTS} (August 12, 1876, Allegheny, Pennsylvania--September 22, 1958, New York City). *Nurse; author.* Daughter of Thomas Beveridge Roberts, sewing machine salesman and inventor, and Cornelia (Gilleland) Roberts, homemaker and boarding house proprietor. Married Stanley Marshall Rinehart, surgeon, April 21, 1896; three children. EDUCATION: June 1893, graduated from Allegheny (Pennsylvania) High School; August 18, 1893-1896, attended Pittsburgh Training School for Nurses, Homeopathic Medical and Surgical Hospital and Dispensary. CAREER: 1903, began to write to help the family's finances, and in her first year sold forty-five stories and novelettes; 1908, published her first book, *The Circular Staircase*; June

1918, accepted as a nurse by the American Red Cross, toured camps in France in November 1918 for the Red Cross; during World War II, served the Red Cross War Fund, Authors' Division, and the Advisory Committee of the Writers War Board.

CONTRIBUTIONS: Mary Rinehart was the most prolific and the most famous nurse-author of all times. As a nursing student, she met a young surgeon, Stanley Marshall Rinehart, and they married shortly after completing her program. They had three sons between 1897 and 1902. In 1903, a stock market panic wiped out their investments, and she turned to writing, publishing her first piece in 1904. In that year, she sold forty-five stories and novelettes, earning $1,842.50. She produced nearly five dozen more from that year to 1908, when her first book, *The Circular Staircase*, was published.

During her long career, she produced more than sixty books, hundreds of articles, stories, and poems, serialized novellas, and plays, and several of her works were made into movies as well as radio and television programs. Her sons became her publishers when in 1929 they founded Farrar and Rinehart. She wrote more best-selling novels over a longer period of time than virtually any other American author; between 1895 and 1944, she headed the list of best-selling American novelists. At the age of seventy-five, it was estimated that her books had sold more than 10 million copies in regular editions and in thirteen translations.

In her works, Rinehart almost always portrayed nurses as bright, caring, and above reproach in their conduct. The heroine of some of her early short stories and two of her novels was Hilda Adams (alias Miss Pinkerton), a nurse-detective who was characterized as intelligent, ingenious, and courageous.

During World War I, Rinehart sailed to London (January 1915) to prepare a series of articles for the *Saturday Evening Post*. She reported on the armistice and she continued to write articles on events such as the 1921 disarmament conference and the 1937 coronation of England's King George VI. After World War I, she and her husband moved to Washington, D.C., remaining there until 1935. On October 2, 1932, her husband died, and in 1935 she took an apartment in New York City, which was to be her home for the rest of her life.

She tried to spend summers in Wyoming, but when that became too much for her physical strength, she bought a home in Bar Harbor, Maine. Trips through the West introduced her to the plight of native Americans, and she raised funds for the Blackfeet Indians. She was a late convert to the cause of woman's suffrage, and she wrote several articles on the "new woman." In 1936 she underwent a radical mastectomy for breast cancer, and hoping that her experience would help other women, in 1947 she made public her experience in a *Ladies Home Journal* interview entitled "I Had Cancer."

Through her writing, she sometimes earned more than $100,000 a year, and she enjoyed the luxuries of travel, many homes, the best clothing, and jewelry. Although she was famous and hobnobbed with the upper classes, her life was touched by tragedy, through the suicide of her father on October 23, 1895, the death of her mother, periods of ill health including major surgery for cancer, the death of her husband, and a quarter of a century of widowhood. She was news in whatever she did and made headlines often, notably when her cook tried to kill her in 1947 and in October of that same year when her Bar Harbor home was destroyed in a fire which devastated the town.

The many experiences of her life are interwoven into her stories and her novels, and her work reflects her nursing background and her husband's profession. In 1923, she was awarded an honorary doctor of letters degree from George Washington University. In 1950 she was featured in articles in the *New York Times Book Review*. In 1954, she was honored with a special award by the Mystery Writers of America. A second heart attack in 1958 left her able to do little, and on September 22 of that year she died.

WRITINGS: More than sixty books, including *K* (1915), *Long Live the King* (1917), *The Amazing Interlude* (1918), *The Breaking Point* (1921), *Miss Pinkerton* (1932), and *The Doctor* (1936); several plays, including *Seven Days* (1909) and *The Bat* (1920); some of her writings were made into motion pictures, including *The Doctor and the Woman* (1918) and *Seven Days* (1925); her autobiography, *My Story* was published in 1931 and again in 1948 as *My Story: A New Edition and Seventeen New Years*; a third autobiographical piece was written, but never published.

REFERENCES: *American Authors and Books, 1640-Present*, p. 618; Jan Cohn, *Improbable Fiction: The Life of Mary Roberts Rinehart* (1980); Julie E. Miale, "Interview with Mary Roberts Rinehart, R.N.," *Nursing World* (October 1958), pp. 18-20; *National Cyclopedia of American Biography*, C: 486-487; *New York Times* (September 23, 1958); *Notable American Women*, pp. 577-578; *Nursing World* (October 1958), pp. 18-20; Gretta Palmer, "Face Your Danger in Time," *Ladies Home Journal* (July 1947), pp. 143-148, 150-153; *Mary Roberts Rinehart: A Sketch of the Woman and Her Work, with an Appreciation by Robert H. Davis* (c. 1925); Mary Roberts Rinehart, *My Story: A New Edition and Seventeen New Years* (1948), and "Writing Is Work," *Saturday Evening Post* (March 11, 1939), pp. 10ff; *Twentieth Century Authors*, pp. 1177-1178; *Twentieth Century Authors, First Supplement*, pp. 832ff.

JOELLEN WATSON HAWKINS

ROBB, ISABEL ADAMS {HAMPTON} (1860, Welland, Ontario, Canada--April 15, 1910, Cleveland, Ohio). *Nurse-educator; administrator.* Daughter of Samuel James Hampton, proprietor of a tailor shop, and Sarah Mary (Lay) Hampton, homemaker. Married Hunter Robb, obstetrician and gynecologist, July 11, 1894 (carrying a floral bouquet that was the gift of Florence Nightingale); two sons. EDUCATION: Attended preparatory school in Welland; received teaching certificate from the Collegiate Institute of St. Catharine's, Ontario, Canada; 1881-1883, attended Bellevue Hospital Training School for Nurses, New York City, graduating in 1883. CAREER: Taught for four years in Merritton, Ontario; 1883-1885, nurse, St. Paul's Hospital, Rome, Italy; 1886-1889, superintendent of nurses, Illinois Training School for Nurses, associated with the Cook County Hospital, Chicago; 1889-1894, superintendent of nurses, Johns Hopkins Hospital, Baltimore, Maryland; resigned to move to Cleveland with her husband, who became professor of gynecology at Western Reserve University.

CONTRIBUTIONS: During her three years at the Illinois Training School, Isabel Hampton Robb began a campaign to raise the educational standards of nursing schools by introducing a systematic course of study. While at Illinois, she advocated the novel idea of affiliating institutions so nursing students might have experience in areas not available at their home hospitals. She arranged for the Illinois students to care for patients at a private hospital, so they would gain experience in nursing patients other than those who were indigent and at Cook County Hospital.

As the founding superintendent of nurses and principal of the Johns Hopkins School of Nursing, she implemented as many of Florence Nightingale's ideas as possible. She introduced a systematic program that was the first graded course for nurses in America. She worked to develop a three-year course of study and an eight-hour day for nurses. Lavinia Dock (q.v.), a student at Hopkins during Robb's tenure, described her as beautiful and majestic as a Greek statue. She became known by her black silk uniform with white collars and cuffs, and by a white cap which she had designed herself. While at Hopkins, she arranged an affiliation with the Mount Wilson Sanatorium for Infants, since Hopkins could not provide such an experience at that time.

At the end of her busy days at Johns Hopkins, she spent time at her desk writing her first book, *Nursing, Its Principles and Practice*, which became a well-known textbook at nursing schools around the country. In 1893 she served as chairperson of the nursing subsection of the International Congress of Charities, Correction, and Philanthropy, which was held in Chicago during the World's Fair. It was thus that the Society of Superintendents of Training Schools for Nurses of the United States and Canada was born, becoming the National League of Nursing

Education in 1912. After her marriage and move to Cleveland in 1894, she became the chairperson of the Committee on Nursing of the Board of Lady Managers of the Lakeside Hospital, and she was active in the organization of the Training School for Nurses at the Cleveland City Hospital. In 1897 she was one of the founders of the Nurses' Associated Alumnae of the United States and Canada, which in 1911 became the American Nurses' Association. She served as its first president, from 1897 to 1901. In 1899 she collaborated with Dean Russell to establish the course in hospital economics at Columbia University, where she presented a few lectures each year until her premature death. The purpose of the course was to prepare nurses for superintendent positions in nursing. In 1900 she was a founder of the *American Journal of Nursing.* In 1909, she was a delegate to the Congress of the International Council of Nurses, which met in London, and she served as chairperson of its committee to establish international educational standards.

During her entire career, she stressed the importance of intellectual and skill development, a code of ethics for the profession, and high standards and uniformity in education. She argued for the necessity of nurse registration legislation, and to that end travelled extensively in Ohio to speak in favor of that state's proposed Nurse Practice Act, which was finally enacted in 1915, five years after her death. She died while stepping out of the way of an automobile and into the path of a moving trolley car.

WRITINGS; *Nursing, Its Principles and Practice* (1893); *Nursing Ethics* (1900); *Educational Standards for Nurses* (1907); numerous articles in the *American Journal of Nursing.*

REFERENCES: *American Journal of Nursing* (May 1910), pp. 531-532, (June 1910), pp. 625-629, and (July 1910), p. 741; *British Journal of Nursing* (April 23, 1910), p. 330 and (May 7, 1910), p. 378; Teresa E. Christy, "Nurses in American History: The Fateful Decade, 1890-1900," *American Journal of Nursing* (July 1975), pp. 1163-1165; Edith A. Draper, "Isabel Hampton Robb," *American Journal of Nursing* (January 1902), pp. 243-245; J. W. James, "Isabel Hampton and the Professionalization of Nursing in the 1890s," in Morris Vogel and Charles Rosenberg, *Therapeutic Revolution* (1979); Selma Moody, "Isabel Hampton Robb," *American Journal of Nursing* (October 1938), pp. 1131-1139; *National League of Nursing Education Calendar* (1922); *Notable American Women*, III: 170-172; Nancy Noel, *Notes on Isabel Hampton Robb* (n.d.); Meta Rutter Pennock, *Makers of Nursing History* (1928); James H. Rodabaugh and Mary Jane Rodabaugh, *Nursing in Ohio: A History* (1951).

LORETTA P. HIGGINS

ROBERTS, MARY MAY (January 31, 1877, Duncan City, Michigan, which later was part of Cheboygan--January 11, 1959, New York City). *Nurse-editor.* Daughter of Henry W. Roberts, sawmill worker, and Elizabeth Scott (Elliot) Roberts. Never married. EDUCATION: Attended company school in Michigan (sawmill company); 1885, graduated from high school, Cheboygan, Michigan, and was valedictorian; 1899, graduated from Jewish Hospital Training School for Nurses, Cincinnati, Ohio; 1919-1921, attended Teachers College, Columbia University, New York City, receiving a B.S. and diploma in nursing school administration in 1921. CAREER: 1899, member of the nursing staff, Baroness Erlanger Hospital, Chattanooga, Tennessee; 1900-1903, superintendent of nurses, Savannah Hospital, Georgia; 1904-1906, assistant superintendent and acting superintendent, Jewish Hospital, Cincinnati; 1906, private duty nursing, Evanston, Illinois; 1906-1908, acting supervisor, obstetric department, Evanston Hospital; 1908-1917, superintendent, Christian R. Holmes Hospital, Cincinnati; 1917-1918, director, American Red Cross Lake Division, directing recruitment of nurses from the area; July 22-October 3, 1918, reserve nurse, Camp Sherman; October 4, 1918-September 8, 1919, member, Army Nurse Corps, serving as director of the Army School of Nursing, Camp Sherman; 1921-1949, editor, *American Journal of Nursing.*

CONTRIBUTIONS: Throughout her long and productive life, Mary Roberts was a leader in many dimensions of the profession. She is best remembered for her many years as editor of the *American Journal of Nursing*; in fact, during her editorship, she was the *Journal.* At the urging of the board of directors, in 1920 she accepted the position as co-editor with Katharine DeWitt (q.v.), on the condition that she be allowed to complete her degree at Teachers College. In order to be better prepared for her future work on the editorial staff of the *Journal*, she enrolled in some journalism classes while she completed requirements for her bachelor's degree. In 1921, she became co-editor with DeWitt, assuming the editorship in 1923, when her colleague became managing editor. In 1948, Roberts' title was changed to editor-in-chief.

During her twenty-eight years with the *Journal*, Roberts became known for her aggressive editorial policy. She campaigned tirelessly for elevation of professional standards, while developing the clinical side of the journal so it would be an up-to-date source of information on new developments in nursing practice. Using her editorial column to speak out on behalf of the profession, she wrote on virtually every aspect of nursing, including nursing research, and the importance of public relations for the nursing profession. She was characterized by one nurse who worked on the editorial staff as a hard taskmaster who expected devotion to the tasks at hand, but whose wit and sense of humor would often save the day. Roberts knew how to stimulate others and get them to produce their best. She saw the journal through hard times, including the Depression and a second world war. During her tenure as editor, circulation grew from around 18,000 to over 100,000.

Roberts also expressed her devotion to the profession through her work in nursing organizations. Before joining the staff of the *Journal*, she was president of the Ohio State Association of Graduate Nurses (1915-1917) and a member of the Ohio State Board of Nurse Examiners. During her presidency, the state headquarters was established in Columbus, and she worked hard for passage of the Ohio nurse practice act. Governor James M. Cox appointed her to a committee on health, hospitals, and nursing. She served as a nursing consultant for the Committee on Grading of Nursing Schools from 1928 to 1934 and from 1929 to 1933 she was a member of the Committee on the Costs of Medical Care. For her alma mater, Teachers College division of nursing education, she served as a member of the committee on the function of nursing and was an alumnae representative on the board of trustees (1930-1932).

For the American Red Cross, she held not only salaried positions but also served on the national committee on nursing service between 1923 and 1944. She had enrolled as a Red Cross nurse in 1914 and was a member of the original nursing advisory committee which was appointed in 1938. In the New York chapter, she was a member of the board of directors and served on a variety of committees. During World War II, she was a member of the Nursing Council on National Defense and of the public information committee of the National Nursing Council for War Service. From July 1943 to October 1945, she was consultant to the procurement and assignment service of the War Manpower Commission.

The New York Academy of Medicine committee on medicine in the changing order counted her among its members between 1944 and 1947. From 1932 to 1942, she was on the advisory committee for what is now Cornell University-New York Hospital School of Nursing. She was a life member of the American Hospital Association. The National League of Nursing Education (NLNE) also benefitted from her expertise. In 1932, she helped work out the plan to make NLNE the educational department of the American Nurses' Association. She chaired the NLNE committee on early nursing source materials. From 1921 to 1923, she was on the board of directors of the league, and for two years she was president of the New York City League of Nursing Education.

Nor was the American Nurses' Association (ANA) bereft of her contributions. Between 1934 and 1948, she ran the nursing information bureau of the ANA. From 1934 to 1945, she was chairperson of the ANA committee on the Florence Nightingale International Foundation.

For two years she served as vice-president of the International Council of Nurses (ICN). She was also chairperson of its publications committee and a member of the ethics committee, chairing it in 1929. During 1931 and 1932, she travelled throughout Europe visiting nursing centers under sponsorship of the Rockefeller Foundation. She also attended many of the ICN congresses.

When Roberts retired, she was made editor emeritus, a title she more than lived up to. During her ten years as emeritus, she wrote countless editorials, articles, book reviews, and personal biographies for the *Journal* and for *Nursing Outlook*, along with several books. Her extensive involvement in professional organizations and activities makes it clear that she was rarely without something important to do for the profession. She was at her desk, preparing an editorial for the *Journal*, when she suffered a stroke. She died two days later at Columbia Presbyterian Medical Center in New York City.

She received many awards over the course of her career. In 1933, she received the bronze medal of the Ministry of Social Welfare, France. In 1949, the year she retired as editor of the *American Journal of Nursing*, she received numerous awards. On May 2, she was given the M. Adelaide Nutting Award for Leadership in Nursing. Less than two weeks later, on May 10, she received the Army Certificate of Appreciation. On May 11, a tea was held by the nursing services of the federal government, and a dinner with Congressman Frances Payne Bolton (Ohio) present was held in Washington, D.C., both in her honor. On May 20, she was "Woman of the Day" on the Eleanor and Anna Roosevelt radio program, broadcast over WJZ, New York City. On May 26, the *American Journal of Nursing* paid tribute to her with a tea in her honor. On June 27, the ANA held a banquet in her honor, and the following day the International Red Cross awarded her the Florence Nightingale Medal. The board of the ANA passed a resolution in her honor on August 5, 1949. On September 25, she was made an honorary fellow of the American College of Hospital Administrators. Two days later, on September 27, the American Hospital Association passed a resolution honoring her contributions to the profession. On October 19, the New York State Nurses' Association established the Mary M. Roberts Award, which is presented to a member who has contributed to the welfare of the profession through writing. In 1950, the *American Journal of Nursing* established the Mary M. Roberts Fellowship in Journalism. In 1956, the Skidmore College department of nursing gave her a citation for her leadership in the profession. Finally, in 1982, Roberts was elected to the ANA Nursing Hall of Fame.

WRITINGS: Countless articles, editorials, book reviews, and biographical sketches for professional journals; books include *American Nursing:*

History and Interpretation (1954); *The Army Nurse Corps--Yesterday and Today* (1957).

REFERENCES: *The American Journal of Nursing and Its Company: A Chronicle, 1900-1975* (1975); *American Journal of Nursing* (May 1949), pp. 261-271, and (October 1950), pp. 583-584; Daisy Caroline Bridges, *History of the International Council of Nurses, 1899-1964* (1967); Katharine DeWitt, "Mary M. Roberts," *National League of Nursing Education Biographical Sketches, 1937-40* (n.d.); Lavinia L. Dock, Sarah E. Pickett, Clara D. Noyes, Fannie F. Clement, Elizabeth G. Fox, and Anna R. Van Meter, *History of American Red Cross Nursing* (1922); *International Nursing Review* (April 1959), p. 16; Cordelia W. Kelly, *Dimensions of Professional Nursing* (2d ed., 1968); Portia B. Kernodle, *The Red Cross Nurse in Action, 1882-1948* (1949); Edith Patton Lewis, "Mary M. Roberts, Spokesman for Nursing," *American Journal of Nursing* (March 1959), pp. 336-343; M. Adelaide Nutting Historical Nursing Collection, Teachers College, Columbia University (unpublished documents); Mary Roberts Papers and the American Journal of Nursing Collection, Nursing Archives, Mugar Memorial Library, Boston University; *Notable American Women: The Modern Era*, pp. 581-583; *Nursing Outlook* (February 1959), pp. 72-74; *Nursing Research* (Winter 1959), p. 3; *Nursing World* (March 1959), p. 8; James H. Rodabaugh and Mary Jane Rodabaugh, *Nursing in Ohio* (1951).

JOELLEN WATSON HAWKINS

ROBINSON, ALICE MERRITT (December 4, 1920, Islip, New York--March 18, 1983, New York City). *Nurse-author; editor.* Daughter of William Beverly Robinson and Le Van (Cowell) Robinson. Never married. EDUCATION: 1944, graduated from Duke University School of Nursing, Durham, North Carolina; 1948, B.S., Catholic University of America, Washington, D.C.; 1950, M.S., Boston University. CAREER: 1944-1946, member, U.S. Army Nurse Corps; 1946-1948, psychiatric coordinator, George Washington Hospital, Washington, D.C.; 1948-1949, psychiatric nurse supervisor, Veterans Administration Hospital, North Little Rock, Arkansas; 1949-1950, director of nursing service and education, Menninger Foundation, Topeka, Kansas; 1950-1955, director of nursing and nursing education, Boston State Hospital, Dorchester, Massachusetts; 1956-1963, director of nursing education, Vermont State Hospital, Waterbury, Vermont; 1963-1967 editor, and 1967-1970, editor-in-chief, *Nursing Outlook*; 1971-1975, senior nursing editor, *RN Magazine*; 1975-1983, director, Specialized Consultants in Nursing, New York City.

CONTRIBUTIONS: Alice Robinson was a spokesperson for the profession through her editorial work, as well as through her writing. Her psychiatric background perhaps gave her special insight into the profession, for as an editor she observed and commented with an especially analytical manner on its maturation. She was a prolific writer, her work ranging from editorials and articles to textbooks and clinical guides, as well as books about nursing as a career (written for young people) and one novel. Her years in education and administration also gave her the dual perspective that was reflected in her writing. As an administrator in psychiatric institutions, employing a large number of attendants, she wrote guides for those individuals, addressing their role in patient care.

In 1975, she founded a company, Specialized Consultants in Nursing, with headquarters at Sayville, Long Island, and she served as its director until her death from a heart attack in 1983. This company provided educational programs in nursing administration, psychiatric nursing, clinical writing, and communication skills and human relations. She continued to write and lecture, in addition to serving as a nursing consultant.

Robinson was also active in professional organizations. While living in Vermont, she was president of the Vermont League for Nursing from 1960 to 1963. From 1958 to 1962, she was chairperson of the National Conference of Group Psychiatric Nursing. In 1975, she served on the National Task Force on Nursing in Hypertension. She was a director of Nurse's House, Inc., a consultant to the Veterans Administration, and a member of the American Heart Association and the Council on Cardiovascular Nursing.

WRITINGS: *The Psychiatric Aide: His Part in Patient Care* (1954); 2d edition published as *The Psychiatric Aide: A Textbook of Patient Care* (1959) which she also illustrated; 4th edition published as *Working with the Mentally Ill* (1971); *The Unbelonging* (a novel, 1958); *Your Future in Nursing Careers* (1972, 1978); *Clinical Writing for Health Professionals* (1981); numerous editorials and articles in professional journals.

REFERENCES: *American Journal of Nursing* (January 1967), p. 47 and (May 1983), p. 821; *Contemporary Authors*, CVIII (1983), p. 401 and CIX (1983), p. 404; *Nursing Outlook* (May-June 1983), p. 145; Alice Robinson and Mary Reres, *Your Future in Nursing Careers* (1972).

JOELLEN WATSON HAWKINS

ROGERS, LINA. See **STRUTHERS, LINA LAVANCHE (ROGERS)**.

ROPES, HANNAH ANDERSON {CHANDLER} (June 13, 1809, New Gloucester, Maine--January 20, 1863, Washington, D.C.). *Civil War nurse.* Daughter of Peleg Chandler, attorney, and Esther (Parsons) Chandler. February 1834, married William Henry Ropes, a graduate of Waterville College and a Bangor, Maine, educator; three surviving children. EDUCATION: Probably attended local elementary schools in Maine. CAREER: 1834-1835, wife and mother; after her husband left her (sometime between 1847 and 1855), supported herself as a private duty nurse; September 1855, went to homestead and support the free-soil cause in Lawrence, Kansas; fearing attack by the pro-slave Southerners in Kansas, returned east in April 1856, settling in Massachusetts; July 1862-January 1863, matron of the Union Hotel Hospital, Georgetown, Washington, D.C.

CONTRIBUTIONS: During the Civil War, Hannah Ropes offered her services to the Union army. In 1860, she had read Florence Nightingale's *Notes on Nursing*, which seemed to crystallize her thoughts concerning her possible contributions to the Union war effort when the war began in April 1861. In the few months which she served as matron of the Union Hotel Hospital, she fought dishonesty, poor care, and general disregard for and mistreatment of the wounded. On November 1, 1862, she went to the office of Surgeon-General William A. Hammond to complain about the mistreatment of the men. When she was unable to see Hammond, she went to Secretary of War Edwin M. Stanton. As a result of her perseverance, cruel treatment of wounded soldiers decreased. Her complaints about Dr. Clark, head surgeon of the hospital, resulted in his being imprisoned, released only at her behest. She served as matron at the same time when Louisa May Alcott (q.v.) served as a nurse in the hospital, and they often worked together. Ropes' diary records episodes of her work with Alcott and of the latter's illness.

Perhaps the most important contribution Ropes made was the letters and diaries she kept during her short time as matron, for they record a first-person account of the life of volunteer nurses in the hospital and the struggles to improve hospital care. She became ill late in December 1862, and she died of typhoid pneumonia on January 20, 1863.

WRITINGS: *Six Months in Kansas: By a Lady* (1856); *Cranston House: A Novel* (1859); numerous letters and diaries.

REFERENCES: Louisa May Alcott, *Hospital Sketches* (1863); John R. Brumgardt, ed., *Civil War Nurse: The Diary and Letters of Hannah Ropes* (1980).

JOELLEN WATSON HAWKINS

S

SANBORN, KATHARINE ANNE ALEXIS (October 14, 1859, Sharon, Vermont--February 23, 1941, New York City). *Leader in nursing education.* Daughter of Ebenezer Cummings Sanborn, mechanical engineer, and Clara (or Clarissa) Gould (Stevens) Sanborn. Never married. EDUCATION: Attended Villa Anna Academy, Lachine, Quebec, and Convent of Our Lady of Mercy, Newburg, New York; decided to become a nurse because of her admiration of her aunt, Kate Stevens, a professional nurse; 1890, graduated from New York Hospital Training School for Nurses; post-graduate courses in education and in hospital and training school administration, Teachers College, Columbia University, New York City. CAREER: Taught music in Jersey City and New York City for five years, then served as a companion to her sister in Nyack, New York, until enrolling in New York Hospital Training School; 1890-1891, private duty nursing; April 1, 1891-July 1, 1892, matron at county branch of the New York Skin and Cancer Hospital, New York City; July 15, 1892-September 1, 1934, superintendent, St. Vincent's Hospital, New York City.

CONTRIBUTIONS: Katharine Sanborn was one of the pioneers in nursing education. She was the first superintendent and founder of the training school at St. Vincent's Hospital (1892). At the recommendation of Irene Sutliffe (q.v.), Sanborn was invited to organize and found the training school. The hospital was operated under the Sisters of Charity but would enroll Protestants as probationers. In the early years, the teaching staff consisted of Sanborn, the hospital's physicians, and the sisters who provided nursing care to the patients. After one year, she recognized the need for nurses to have more education, and she arranged affiliations with St. Mary's Maternity Hospital, Brooklyn, and later with Lying-in Hospital, New York City. Under her leadership, the school grew rapidly and was considered one of the best in the state.

Sanborn was known as an efficient teacher, an inspiration to those who worked with her, and one who always maintained the ideals of the pioneers of nursing history. More than these attributes was her deep personal interest in every student who attended the school. She was progressive in her vision for the profession, for by 1898, students were given two weeks of annual vacation a year, duty hours were nine and a half for the day shift and twelve hours for the night shift, with each having fifteen off-duty hours per week. By 1895, the school had become so well known for its excellent training that there were 350 applications for places for only fifteen probationers. The two-year course was extended to three years in 1903. In 1905, the Regents of the University of the State of New York granted a registration certificate, making it an officially recognized school of nursing.

When the American Society of Superintendents of Training Schools for Nurses was organized and held its first convention in the Academy of Medicine, New York City (January 1894), Sanborn enrolled as a member. At the 1899 annual meeting, she gave an address on the care of patients with infectious diseases. She was also a member of the Associated Alumnae from its inception, and was recognized by the state department of education as a leader in the profession. In 1902, she was elected first vice-president of the Alumnae Association of New York Hospital Training School.

During the Spanish-American War (1898), Sanborn spent some time at Camp Black, Long Island, caring for recruits who had contracted typhoid fever. She supervised the removal of patients when the camp was disbanded and arranged their transfer to area hospitals, including St. Vincent's. The graduates of St. Vincent's also cared for survivors of the sinking of the *Titanic*.

Sanborn retired in 1934 and died in 1941, just a little too soon to have celebrated the golden anniversary of the school she founded. At the time of her retirement, 1,063 students had graduated from the school. She spent her retirement in the nurses' residence, keeping active her interest in the profession and in her nurses. Over the course of her career, she received a number of honors in recognition of her contributions to the profession. In 1923, she was given honorary membership in the Alumnae Association of St. Vincent's Hospital Training School. On November 22, 1928, the Alumnae Association held a reception in honor of Sanborn's thirty-sixth anniversary as director of the school of nursing. The following year, the Alumnae Association established in her honor the Katharine A. Sanborn scholarship, granted annually to a graduate who intended to pursue post-graduate training.

WRITINGS: Numerous unpublished records of the Training School, St. Vincent's Hospital, and numerous letters.

REFERENCES: *American Journal of Nursing* (January 1929), pp. 106-107, (November 1934), p. 1065, and (April 1941), p. 509; Jane Hodson, *How to Become a Trained Nurse* (1898); *New York Times* (February 25, 1941); *Trained Nurse and Hospital Review* (April 1941), p. 284; V. C. Sanborn, *Genealogy of the Family of Samborne or Sanborn in England and America, 1194-1898* (1899); Archives of the St. Vincent's Hospital School of Nursing.

JOELLEN WATSON HAWKINS

SANGER, MARGARET LOUISE (September 14, 1879, Corning, New York--September 6, 1966, Tucson, Arizona). *Leader in birth control movement.* Daughter of Michael Hennessy Higgins, sculptor of tombstone angels, owner of a stone monument shop, military hero, and member of the Knights of Labor, and Anne (Purcell) Higgins, homemaker. Married William Sanger, artist and architect, August 18, 1902 (divorced 1920); three children. Married J. Noah Slee, oil tycoon, September 18, 1922 (died June 1943). EDUCATION: Attended public schools of Corning, New York, to the eighth grade; 1896-1899, attended Claverack College, a coeducational Methodist preparatory school in the Catskills of New York; 1900-1902, attended two-year nursing school course at White Plains Hospital, White Plains, New York.; 1902, post-graduate course at Manhattan Eye and Ear; 1914, study in England with Havelock Ellis, and self study on population problems, at the British Museum, London. CAREER: Taught first grade at Little Falls, New Jersey, returning home to care for her dying mother and younger siblings; left the post-graduate course to marry, spent her pregnancy in a sanitorium, and from 1902-1908, devoted time to convalescence and to having and raising children in Hastings-on-Hudson, New York; 1910, returned to New York City, where she worked for Local 5 of the Socialist party, and for the Visiting Nurses Association of the Lower East Side, specializing in obstetrical cases; 1912-death, devoted her life to promoting birth control; October 1916, opened the Brownsville Clinic, Brooklyn, New York, to provide birth control information and education; 1916-1934, worked to establish birth control clinics, published articles and pamphlets on birth control, in defiance of the Comstock Act, worked to change legislation against birth control in the 1920s and 1930s, attended national and international confrerences on birth control, lectured across the world, smuggling diaphragms into the United States until they were manufactured here in 1925, and more than once was jailed for her activities; 1934, moved with her husband to Tucson, Arizona, where she continued her work.

CONTRIBUTIONS: Margaret Sanger was a pioneer in the birth control movement. Her work began as the result of her own mother's health problems and subsequent death from tuberculosis in 1896, after having had eleven children. In addition, she was influenced by her observations of women on the Lower East Side of New York, many of whom died during childbirth or from illegal abortions. Her work on behalf of the socialist movement led her to meet and be influenced by Emma Goldman (q.v.) and Bill Haywood. In the winter of 1912, she organized the evacuation to New York City of 250 children from Lawrence, Massachusetts, the scene of a textile workers' strike, providing care for them and in the process enabling the workers to continue the strike without fearing their children would starve.

On November 17, 1912, Sanger began a series of articles describing puberty and the functions of a woman's body, published in *The Call*, a socialist newspaper. These became the basis for *What Every Girl Should Know*, published first in 1915 as a pamphlet. In October 1913, she travelled to France to discover the secret of birth control, and upon her return to the United States she began publication of her own magazine, *The Woman Rebel* (March 1914). In the same year she prepared the pamphlet *Family Limitation* and organized the National Birth Control League. Because the Comstock Laws considered birth control information as obscenity, in October 1914 she was forced to flee to England to avoid prosecution for violation of those laws.

In England, she met C. V. Drysdale, head of the English birth control movement, and studied with Havelock Ellis, the pioneering sociologist. In January-February 1915, she visited Holland where a Dr. Rutger tutored her in the fitting of pessaries (diaphragms), and where she studied the clinic system. In 1915, she returned to the United States to stand trial on charges which were eventually dropped by the government. Buoyed by her legal victory, she gave lectures across the country. In October 1916, she began America's first birth control clinic, the Brownsville Clinic, in Brooklyn, New York, with her sister Ethel, who also was a nurse. At the end of the first day of the clinic's operation, she was arrested, charged with violating the state's laws against disseminating birth control information, tried, found guilty, and sentenced to thirty days in prison. After her release in 1917, she continued to write and lecture, and in 1920 she published *Woman and the New Race.*

In 1921, she devoted her energies to planning the first National Birth Control Conference, and launching the American Birth Control League (which in 1942 became Planned Parenthood Federation of America). After attending the fifth International Neo-Malthusian and Birth Control Conference, in London (1922), she substantially expanded her operations, engaging Dr. Dorothy Becker to run a Clinical Research

Bureau, commissioning Dr. Hannah Stone to establish a clinic, and hiring Dr. James F. Cooper to lecture to physicians about birth control. Until 1925, when she convinced two of her supporters to found the Holland-Rantos Company to produce diaphragms, she had to smuggle them into the country, with her husband, Noah Slee, importing them through his Canadian factory. In 1926, she travelled to London, Paris, and Geneva to prepare for the 1927 International meeting, out of which came the Population Union. In 1928 she resigned the presidency of the league but continued to edit the *Review* until 1929, when she withdrew from both the league and the paper. In April 1929, the Clinical Research Bureau was raided by the police, indicating that the fight to promote birth control was not yet over. By 1938, largely due to the work and influence of Margaret Sanger, over 300 birth control clinics were in operation in the United States. In 1936, the Comstock Acts' classification of birth control as obscenity was finally revised, and in January 1937 she won a great victory, opening up the mails for the transmission of materials and literature on birth control to qualified persons.

Another victory occurred in June 1937, when the American Medical Association adopted a resolution that contraception was a legitimate medical service. In 1939, the American Birth Control League and the Voluntary Parenthood League were merged, and Sanger was made honorary president. In 1952, she travelled to India for a conference where the International Planned Parenthood Federation was organized; the following year she was elected president of that organization. In 1952, she was instrumental in persuading Katherine McCormick, widow of the founder of International Harvester, to fund the research that Dr. Gregory Pincus was conducting that would produce the birth control pill. In 1965, as a result of the decision in the case of *Griswold v. Connecticut*, that state struck from its books the anti-birth control law; two years later (and one year after Sanger's death), the last law prohibiting the distribution of birth control devices and information was repealed, in Massachusetts. Her last years were spent in decline with angina, and she was heavily dependent upon demerol and wine, finally dying in Arizona in 1966.

Over the years, Sanger received numerous honors for her work, including the Medal of Achievement from the American Women's Association (1931), the Town Hall Club annual medal (1937), an honorary L.L.D. degree from Smith College (1949), a world luncheon in New York City hosted by Sir Julian Huxley as a tribute to her work (1961), and a Gold Medal from the emperor of Japan (1962). Planned Parenthood Federation of America presented her with the Albert and Mary Lasker Foundation Award (1950) and created in her honor the Margaret Sanger Medallion (1966), which is awarded to persons who have made distinguished contributions on the community level. In 1966, Sanger

received an honorary L.L.D. degree from the University of Arizona. In 1976, she was elected to the American Nurses' Association Hall of Fame.
WRITINGS: *The Case for Birth Control* (1917); *What Every Mother Should Know* (1917); *Woman and the New Race* (1920); *What Every Girl Should Know* (1920); *Pivot of Civilization* (1922); *Married Happiness* (1926); *Motherhood in Bondage* (1928); *The Practice of Contraception, an Introductory Symposium and Survey* (with Hannah M. Stone, 1930); *My Fight for Birth Control* (1931); *Margaret Sanger, An Autobiography* (1938); *Hear Me for My Cause: Selected Letters of Margaret Sanger* (1967); diaries, letters, and other papers are at the Sophia Smith Collection, Smith College, Northampton, Massachusetts.
REFERENCES: Joan Dash, *A Life of One's Own* (1973); Emily Taft Douglas, *Margaret Sanger: Pioneer of the Future* (1970); Linda Gordon, *Woman's Body, Woman's Right* (1977); Madeline Gray, *Margaret Sanger* (1979); Lawrence Lader, *The Margaret Sanger Story* (1955); Joan Marlow, *The Great Women* (1979); *National Cyclopedia of American Biography*, 52:325-326; *Notable American Women: The Modern Period*, pp. 623-627; Margaret Sanger, *Margaret Sanger, An Autobiography* (1938) and *My Fight for Birth Control* (1931).

JOELLEN WATSON HAWKINS

SARGENT, EMILIE GLEASON (April 26, 1894, St. Paul, Minnesota--April 17, 1977, Detroit, Michigan). *Public health nurse.* Daughter of Henry Curtis Sargent and Evelyn Flora Sargent. Never married. EDUCATION: 1911-1912, attended Tift College, Forsyth, Georgia; 1916, B.A., University of Michigan, Ann Arbor; 1918, completed course, Vassar Training Camp for Nurses, Poughkeepsie, New York; 1920, graduated from Mt. Sinai Hospital School of Nursing, New York City; 1938, M.P.H., University of Michigan. CAREER: 1916-1918, high-school teacher, Ypsilanti, Michigan; 1920, staff nurse, Detroit Visiting Nurse Association; 1924-1964, executive director, Visiting Nurse Association of Detroit.
CONTRIBUTIONS: Emilie Sargent was nationally known for her contributions to public health nursing, especially for her role in improving and diversifying the services provided by the Visiting Nurse Association (VNA) of Detroit, which she directed for forty years. Other nursing associations across the country followed her lead in introducing physical and occupational therapy, nutritional services, providing mental health screening and care and services in industrial health, and in employing practical nurses and home aides to the field of visiting nursing. Sargent was the first to develop a program of supervised field experience for students of public health nursing, which was done through a

cooperative agreement with the Wayne State University public health nursing program. With the VNA of Detroit, she required staff members not only to have graduated from a recognized nursing school, but also to have graduated from high school. (There were quite a few nurses at that time without the high-school equivalency certificate). She upgraded those on her staff by making it possible for them to graduate from high school through evening classes.

Sargent was one of the first public health nursing administrators to recognize the need to improve conditions for the aged and the chronically ill. She did this long before those needs were generally recognized as major problems facing American society. As a solution to these needs, she was the moving force behind the Home Care Demonstration Project for Detroit, which was funded by the McGregor Fund in 1955. The goal was to provide more home care for the aged and chronically ill. She was a leader in the movement to coordinate hospital and home-care. She wrote, published, and spoke frequently on this subject, and she was responsible for developing the pilot program which demonstrated the feasibility of a home-care program for patients who had recently been discharged from a stay in the hospital. She conceived of the need for planning services for the aged many years before Congress enacted legislation which established the Medicare program. She was one of the first to recognize the growing need for home-care services for elderly patients who were being discharged from hospitals before their families could properly provide for their needs, and before they could care for themselves. She published in nursing journals accounts of this project, which undoubtedly served to encourage thought and action by others with similar concerns.

Sargent was active in numerous nursing and public health organizations. She served as president of the National Organization for Public Health Nursing (1950-1952), president of the Michigan Public Health Association (1943), vice-president of the American Public Health Association (1948), president of the Michigan State Nurses' Association (1934-1936), and a member of the board of the American Journal of Nursing Company (1952-1955) and the National League for Nursing (1954-1955). She was active in community service agencies, including the United Community Service of Detroit and the National Foundation for Infantile Paralysis, and she served as a member of the advisory committee to the Harper Hospital School of Nursing (Detroit) and as chairperson of region 10 of the Michigan White House Conference on Aging. She was a fellow of the American Public Health Association, served as a member of its committee on chronic disease and rehabilitation, and was a member of the U.S. Public Health Service's national advisory committee on chronic disease and health of the aged. She was also a member of the national committee on aging of the National Social Welfare Assembly.

Over the course of her long career, she received a number of awards in recognition of her distinguished service to humanity and to the profession. In 1935 she was granted life membership in the National Organization for Public Health Nursing. In 1946 she received an honorary doctor of science in nursing degree from Wayne State University (Detroit). In 1960, the American Nurses' Association gave her the Pearl McIver Award, and she received an outstanding achievement award from the University of Michigan. In 1962 she was given honorary membership in the Michigan Public Health Association. In 1964, the year of her retirement, the University of Michigan School of Public Health created the Emilie Gleason Sargent Prize.

WRITINGS: Articles in many journals, including *Public Health Nursing* and the *American Journal of Nursing*.

REFERENCES: Gladys B. Clappison, *Vassar's Rainbow Division* (1964), pp. 259-261; *Nursing Outlook* (1977), p. 303; Emilie Sargent papers, Nursing Archives, Mugar Memorial Library, Boston University.

ALICE HOWELL FRIEDMAN

SCHUTT, BARBARA GORDON (March 25, 1917, Ithaca, New York--December 26, 1986, Montville, Connecticut). *Editor.* Daughter of a journalist father and housewife mother. Never married. EDUCATION: 1939, graduated from Jefferson Medical College Hospital School of Nursing, Philadelphia; 1942, B.A., Bethany College, Bethany, West Virginia; 1949, M.S. in nursing education, University of Pennsylvania, Philadelphia. CAREER: Staff nurse and instructor, Jefferson Medical College Hospital; 1939-1944, camp nurse and assistant counselor, assistant, Bethany College student health service; 1944-1946, U.S. Army Nurse Corps; 1946-1957, assistant executive secretary, Pennsylvania State Nurses' Association; July 1957-November 1958, executive secretary, Pennsylvania State Nurses' Association; December 1, 1958-1971, editor, *American Journal of Nursing*; 1974-1979, director, division of nursing, Mohegan Community College, Norwich, Connecticut, retiring in 1979.

CONTRIBUTIONS: Barbara Schutt's greatest contribution to nursing was through her service as editor of the *American Journal of Nursing* from 1958 to 1971, when she became known for her perceptive and forceful editorials. During the years of her editorship, nursing was struggling with critical issues; Schutt was particularly noted for her advocacy of nurses' rights to organize for collective bargaining and for her belief in nurses' rights and responsibilities for control of their own practice. Her editorials often focused on issues crucial to the development of nursing as a profession.

Her organizational work began seven years after her graduation and immediately after her discharge from the Army Nurse Corps during World War II. In 1946 she accepted the offer to serve as assistant executive secretary of the Pennsylvania State Nurses' Association (PSNA), becoming the executive secretary in 1957. One of her accomplishments was to help establish the association's economic and general welfare program. She also served as editor of *Pennsylvania Nurse*, the official organ of the PSNA. One can surmise that members of the board of the American Nurses' Association (ANA) recognized her excellent work as editor of *Pennsylvania Nurse* and were familiar with her as a result of her extensive work for the national association as well as the PSNA. From 1952 to 1958, she served as chairperson of the ANA committee on economic and general welfare, was a member of the ANA special groups section committee on functions, standards, and qualifications for practice for executive secretaries, and was a member of the American Journal of Nursing Company board of directors. After retirement from the *Journal*, she served as chairperson of the ANA nominations committee (1972-1974) and as president of the Connecticut Nurses' Association (1977-1979). She was, in the words of a colleague, an eloquent and influential voice at many ANA conventions, always committed to organized nursing.

Although her retirement from the *Journal* ended a long commute to New York from her pre-Revolutionary home in Connecticut, Schutt never retired from nursing. She directed the division of nursing at Mohegan Community College, and when she left that position in 1979, she received the presidential citation for her five years of service. She served in various capacities for Eastern Connecticut's Health Systems Agency and Southeastern Connecticut's Commission on Aging and participated in Senator Lowell Weicker's Senior Intern Program in Washington, D.C. She was a volunteer at Mystic Seaport, with the Literacy program, and also volunteered at the Woman's Center of Southeastern Connecticut.

She received several honors in recognition of her service to the profession. In 1973, she was made a charter member of the American Academy of Nursing. That same year, she received an honorary doctor of science degree from Bethany College. She received the honorary recognition award from both the ANA and the Connecticut Nurses' Association. The Connecticut Nurses' Association established a nursing scholarship named in her honor. She also received other honors from the Connecticut and Pennsylvania Nurses' Associations.

WRITINGS: Countless editorials and articles in professional journals.

REFERENCES: *American Journal of Nursing* (August 1985), p. 1114, (January 1959), p. 22, and (February 1987), p. 249; *The American Journal of Nursing and Its Company: A Chronicle 1900-1975* (1975); *Canadian Nurse* (July 1959), p. 637; unpublished material provided by Edith P. Lewis, 1987.

JOELLEN WATSON HAWKINS

SCOTT, ALMA {HAM} (January 31, 1885, Frankfort, Indiana--July 7, 1972, Rossville, Indiana). *Nurse-administrator.* Daughter of Charles W. Ham and Corabelle (Blake) Ham. Married (and divorced) Dr. Scott; no children. EDUCATION: Graduated from high school in San Bernardino, California; 1907, graduated from Presbyterian Hospital School of Nursing, Chicago; 1921-1922, post-graduate study at Teachers College, Columbia University, New York City. CAREER: 1907-1917, private duty nursing in Chicago; 1918-1919, army nurse, Base Hospital Number 13, Limoges, France, and Evacuation Hospital Number 7, Coulonmiers, France; 1919, night supervisor, Robert W. Long Hospital, Indianapolis, Indiana; 1924-1929, educational director, Indiana State Board of Examination and Registration for Nurses, and executive secretary, Indiana State Nurses' Association; 1929-1935, field secretary, American Nurses' Association, New York City; 1935-1946, executive secretary, American Nurses' Association.

CONTRIBUTIONS: Alma Scott was for twelve years the executive secretary of the American Nurses' Association (ANA), and prior to that time she was acting director for one year. During those thirteen years (1934-1946), membership in the ANA passed the 157,000 mark. She brought to the position knowledge of the various aspects of administering the ANA, having previously served as field secretary, assistant director, associate director, and acting director prior to being appointed executive secretary. One of her major responsibilities was to make plans for the association's annual conventions and to ascertain that those plans were being implemented accurately. She also handled questions and complaints, both from the membership and from the officers of the ANA. It was said that administration of the ANA during that time gave "full scope" to her "organizational genius."

Scott was instrumental in establishing the ANA professional counseling and placement service, which would serve to help unemployed nurses find appropriate positions, and to assist nurses who wanted to relocate to other parts of the country or to leave their positions. While she was executive secretary, the Great Depression was wreaking havoc with the nation's economy, and the ANA had to focus attention on the economic conditions of the American nurse. Of particular concern to nurses was the important question of whether hospitals would reduce salaries of nurses, or even fire nurses and replace them with non-professionals who were available at lower wages. At the twenty-ninth convention of the ANA, Scott explained to her audience that "from a professional standpoint, the ANA had definite responsibility toward each community in the United States which is either adequately or inadequately supplied with nursing." Not only did she see that professional guidance was available for members of the ANA when it came to placement, but she insisted that schools of nursing examine their programs with a view toward training nurses in specialties which were in short supply in specific geographical areas of the country. In the midst of the Depression, Scott recommended to the ANA board of directors that a study of the economic status of nurses was desperately needed; the result was a study of twenty-three states which began a long practice of studying personnel needs and conditions within the profession.

When World War II began and there was a desperate need for military nurses, Scott represented the ANA when it was proposed to draft nurses into the military. Although the legislation was not enacted into law, the issue flooded the ANA headquarters with comments and questions from both members and from the general public. As executive secretary, Scott was responsible for the public relations of the association, and she represented the American nurse quite well in the process.

Prior to becoming executive secretary, she served as field secretary, which gave her considerable insight into the problems of nursing on the national scene. She was meticulous in her evaluation of the various schools and the way they prepared students to become professional nurses. Before she visited a school, she provided an outline explaining how she would conduct the visitation, and in the process she made it easier for the administrators and instructors to cooperate by having everything available which would be necessary at the time of the visit. Her practice was to devote several days to each school, meeting with administrators, instructors, and students, visiting the facilities, and examining the records of the school and hospital. She was known for her tact in recommending that certain schools phase out their nursing programs, especially in the case of small hospitals whose nursing schools were intended to provide a source of inexpensive labor rather than to provide high-quality education. In such cases, Scott carefully and correctly explained how a staff consisting of graduate nurses would be no more costly and how it would satisfy both physician and patient.

At the same time, she joined others in seeking to recruit the best-qualified applicants to the various nursing schools. She published a pamphlet on nursing which was addressed to high-school girls; this was quite revolutionary at a time when young women learned about opportunities in the profession and about specific nursing schools by word of mouth, and when it was impossible for them to evaluate the information or to determine whether one school was better able than another to provide high-quality training.

In addition to her work on the national scene, Scott was president of the Indiana League of Nursing Education. Her major work, however, was clearly with the ANA. She chaired a number of committees of that association and served in several positions with the International Council of Nurses (ICN). She was chairperson of the special study committee on the constitution and by-laws of the ICN, as well as the committee which dealt with the relationship between the ICN and the Florence Nightingale International Foundation. She presented the findings of both committees, along with recommendations, at the International Congress which was held in Atlantic City in 1947.

WRITINGS: Numerous articles in professional journals.

REFERENCES: *American Journal of Nursing* (1929), p. 734, (1946), p. 200, and (1950), p. 789; Ethel P. Clarke, "Alma Ham Scott," *American Journal of Nursing* (1936), p. 149; Lyndia Flanagan, *One Strong Voice: The Story of the American Nurses' Association* (1976); information from volunteer-genealogist, Frankfort, Indiana, Public Library.

ALICE HOWELL FRIEDMAN

SELLEW, GLADYS (July 29, 1887, Cincinnati, Ohio--July 6, 1977, Oberlin, Ohio). *Pediatric nursing leader; author.* Daughter of Ralph Sellew and Rachel Ella (Moore) Sellew. Never married. EDUCATION: Probably attended local schools and graduated from high school in Cincinnati; 1918, A.B. in economics, 1920, B.S. in nursing, 1921, M.A. in economics, all from the University of Cincinnati; studied child development and family life for three months at Merrill-Palmer School, Detroit, Michigan; 1938, Ph.D. in sociology, Catholic University of America, Washington, D.C.; c. 1938-1944, attended summer classes at Columbia University, New York City, and the University of Chicago. CAREER: 1907-1917, volunteer social work in the tenement districts of Cincinnati; 1920, head nurse, children's ward, Cincinnati General Hospital; 1921-1925, instructor, school of nursing and health, University of Cincinnati, and supervisor of all children's departments of the hospital; 1925-1928, assistant professor of nursing education, Western Reserve University, Cleveland, Ohio, and director of the nursing service, Babies and Children's Hospital, Cleveland; 1928-1930, assistant director in charge of pediatric and communicable disease nursing service, Cook County

Hospital, Chicago; 1928-1929, assistant to the dean, Illinois Training School for Nurses and 1929-1930, assistant to the dean, Cook County School of Nursing, which succeeded the Illinois Training School; 1930-1932, assistant dean, Cook County School of Nursing, and assistant director, nursing service, Cook County Hospital (during these years, also taught at Tulane University and the University of Wisconsin); 1932-1935, served at St. Vincent's, a 250-bed asylum and home for unmarried mothers in the heart of Chicago's tenement district; winter of 1934-1935, taught four days a week in the University of Indiana extension program, while working the remaining time at St. Vincent's; 1932-1935, also taught nursing at DePaul University, Chicago; 1933-1943, assistant professor of sociology and nursing, Catholic University of America, Washington, D.C.; 1943-1944, director, Kansas City General Hospital, Kansas City, Missouri; 1944-1946, director of the department of nursing, St. Catherine College, St. Paul, Minnesota; 1946-1949, associate professor and, 1949-1956, professor and chairperson of sociology and social work, Rosary College, River Forest, Illinois; 1948-1956, visiting professor, and 1956-1958, professor of pediatric nursing, University of Maryland, College Park, Maryland; 1958-1977, retired to Oberlin, Ohio, and devoted her time to a private, nonprofit program to assist families to purchase their own homes and to the more than one hundred Oberlin College students she housed in her home.

CONTRIBUTIONS: Devotion to serving others was the hallmark of Gladys Sellew's long and distinguished life. In 1900, at the age of thirteen she was introduced to the tenements of Cincinnati, an experience which made a considerable impression, for from 1907 to 1917, she was a volunteer social worker through various agencies, including the University Settlement of the University of Cincinnati, the Cincinnati Union Bethel (a settlement house endowed by the Taft family of Cincinnati), the neighborhood activities of Christ Church and the Cathedral (both Episcopal churches, the Italian Mission, and the Hospital Social Service Department of the Cincinnati General Hospital (a University of Cincinnati affiliate). For three years, she also held a salaried position teaching sewing in the first vacation schools organized in Cincinnati. Her activities in social service with the Hospital Social Service Department included membership on the board of directors and as secretary, as well as follow-up work with children and unmarried mothers, and assisting in the organization of the occupational therapy department.

After graduation from nursing school in 1920, she continued her work in the ghettoes, first in Cincinnati, then in Cleveland and Chicago. While working at the Babies and Children's Hospital of Cleveland, she conducted a study of time required for nursing care in a pediatric ward, later published in 1932 in her book, *Ward Administration.* Her work at

Chicago's Cook County Hospital enabled her to continue working in the ghettoes; the hospital was not only the largest active hospital in the country, with 2,500 beds, but it is also located in the heart of what were then the tenement districts of Chicago. Her dual interests in nursing and the ghettoes led her to the Catholic University of America, Washington, D.C., where she earned a Ph.D. in sociology and held dual appointments in nursing and sociology. Her thesis on black families was the first one in nursing to be based on original investigation and participant observation. From the ghettoes of Washington, her academic appointments and continuing concern for the poor led her to Kansas City, St. Paul, Forest Park, Illinois, and Maryland.

Her publications were important in the development of nursing as a mature profession, especially in bringing to nursing the work of sociologists, and in promoting the use of sociology in nursing. Two of her books were especially important in this respect: *Sociology and Social Problems in Nursing Service* (fifth edition, 1962) and *Sociology and Its Use in Nursing* (1962, in its fourth edition in 1977).

Although she devoted her life to helping the poor, she was active in the nursing profession. She served on the board of the National League of Nursing Education, and recruited and educated cadet nurses during World War II. She gave an address at the American Nurses' Association convention in Detroit in 1924 and wrote articles on recruitment of students and on nursing as a profession for women. She also gave talks on nursing to lay groups. In 1956 she was honored by her inclusion in the well-known biographical directory, *American Men of Science*, and in 1970 was named Senior Citizen of the Year by the Oberlin City Health Commission and was named Man of the Year by the *Oberlin News Tribune*. In 1971, she was awarded the First Annual Community Service Award by Oberlin College and received a commendatory letter from President Richard M. Nixon, as well as recognition by the Ohio Planning Conference.

In 1929, she purchased for her mother a home in Oberlin, Ohio, beginning her long association with that community. Her mother, until her death in 1932, housed college students, and when Gladys retired in 1958, she resumed her mother's practice, asking the dean of men to send her some likely candidates. Over the next twenty years, she provided rent-free housing for over one hundred students, sharing her house from cellar to attic with seven or eight men a year. Sellew House, as it came to be known, was often used by students in the Oberlin Conservatory for their senior recitals.

Using her savings, she began a nonprofit, private program to finance the purchase of homes by families ineligible for any other kind of assistance. Several of the fifteen homes she built are located on Gladys

Court, named in her honor. For eleven years, she was active in the Oberlin Health Commission. A scholarship fund that she endowed, named by the college in her honor, and the homes she financed and built, are evidence of her continuing work. For the last two years of her life, she was in the Welcome Nursing Home in Oberlin, where she died at the age of eighty-nine.

WRITINGS: *Pediatric Nursing* (1926) that went into several editions and was translated into Japanese and Chinese; *Ward Administration* (1932), the first book in any language to use a time study in nursing; *Sociology and Its Use in Nursing* (1962, 4th ed., 1977); *A History of Nursing* (1946, 1951), with a Japanese edition in 1946; *Sociology and Social Problems in Nursing Service* (5th ed., 1962); *Ward Administration and Clinical Teaching* (1949); numerous articles in professional journals.

REFERENCES: *American Men of Science: The Social and Behavioral Sciences* (10th ed., 1962), p. 972; "Biographical Note on Distinguished Community Service Award Recipient," p. 21 in Oberlin College, *1971 Commencement Program*; "Biographical Notes on Miss Sellew," typed notes in the Catholic University of America Department of Archives and Manuscripts, Washington, D.C.; Geoffrey Blodgett, *Oberlin Architecture College and Town: A Guide to Its Social History* (1985), pp. 163-164; *The Catherine Wheel*, February 3, March 9, March 30, April 3, April 19, September 27, November 9, and November 24, 1944, February 1, May 24, and September 27, 1945, February 23 and September 26, 1946, and May 7, 1947; certificate of death, Ohio Department of Health; Cook County Hospital Archives, letter from Terrence S. Norwood dated July 8, 1986, detailing Sellew's positions; "Distinguished Community Service Award Citation," May 23, 1971, Oberlin College Archives; *Elyria Chronicle-Telegram* (July 7, 1977); "Gladys Sellew, 1887-1977: A Life of Service," Oberlin publication (1977); Annie Warburton Goodrich, *The Social and Ethical Significance of Nursing* (1932); Peggy Kahn, "Sellew Sponsors Option to Federal Housing," *Oberlin Review* (September 21, 1971); Laura Logan, "Gladys Sellew, A.B., B.S., A.M., R.N.," *American Journal of Nursing* (May 1929), pp. 565-566; *Oberlin Review* (September 21, 1971); *Oberlin Alumni Magazine* (September-October 1977), p. 28; Meta Rutter Pennock, ed., *Makers of Nursing History* (1928), pp. 96-97; Grace Fay Schryver, *History of the Illinois Training School for Nurses, 1880-1929* (1930).

JOELLEN WATSON HAWKINS

SHAW, CLARA {WEEKS} (February 28, 1857, Sanborton, New Hampshire--January 14, 1940, Mountainville, New York). Daughter of

Dr. Alpheus Weeks and Anna (Coe) Weeks, a teacher. Her father died when Clara was five years old, and her mother moved to Kingston, Rhode Island, where she directed a boarding school. *Nurse-educator; author.* September 28, 1888, married Cyrus W. Shaw, retired from nursing, and moved to Cornwall, New York, and later to Mountainville, New York; two children, including Elizabeth Comfort Shaw, who graduated from Methodist Episcopal Hospital School of Nursing, Brooklyn, New York and who for many years ran a nursing home in Mountainville, New York. EDUCATION: Graduated from East Greenwich (Rhode Island) Seminary; January 22, 1875, graduated from Rhode Island State Normal School, Providence, Rhode Island; c. 1878-1880, attended the New York Hospital Training School for Nurses, New York City, graduating in 1880. CAREER: c. 1877-1878, taught in a Newport, Rhode Island, school; 1880-1884, private duty and institutional nursing; 1884-1887, superintendent, Ladies Hospital Training School for Nurses (New Jersey's first nursing school; it became Paterson General Hospital and then Wayne General Hospital, Paterson, New Jersey); retired from nursing upon her marriage in 1888.

CONTRIBUTIONS: Clara Weeks Shaw's greatest contribution was the first textbook for nurses written by a nurse in the United States. *A Text-book of Nursing for the Use of Training Schools, Families, and Private Students* was published in 1885 by D. Appleton and Company, New York City. Prior to that time, the only texts in which nurses had any part as authors were two manuals of nursing published by Bellevue and the Connecticut Training School, written by physicians and nurses. Those manuals were also designed to be used by trained graduate nurses and not as texts for students. In the first chapter, she addressed the need for training of nurses and differentiated between trained and untrained nurses. The book had a number of black and white illustrations, questions for students to use for each chapter, a glossary, and an index. The book was very successful, with fifty-eight printings and sales of over 100,000 copies. The second edition in 1892 contained a new chapter, "Gynecology," as well as chapters on surgical nursing and nursing of infants, reflecting changes in nursing practice and responsibility. The book, typical of the times in which it was written, emphasized obedience to the physician and deference to his orders. In the preface, Shaw stated that she did not consider the book to be original work, since she had compiled materials from many sources and added practical points based on her experience as a nurse and educator.

The book became a standard text for many of the early schools of nursing. It is mentioned as one of the texts in use at the Johns Hopkins Hospital Training School during its first year of existence (1889). On May 10, 1932, Clara Weeks Shaw was the guest of honor at a banquet celebrating the golden anniversary of Paterson General Hospital School of Nursing.

WRITINGS: *A Text-book of Nursing* (1885, 1892, 1902).

REFERENCES: *American Journal of Nursing* (March 1940), p. 356; Archives of Rhode Island College, James P. Adams Library, Providence; Bicknell, *History of the Rhode Island Normal School* (1911); unpublished biographical material (xerox copy of obituary, pages from her family Bible, etc.) from the collections of the Cornwall Public Library, Cornwall-on-Hudson, New York; *The Cornwall Local* (January 18, 1940); Minnie Goodnow, *Nursing History* (7th ed., 1943); Ethel Johns and Blanche Pfefferkorn, *The Johns Hopkins Hospital School of Nursing 1889-1949* (1954); Helene J. Jordan, *Cornell University-New York Hospital School of Nursing* (1952); Cordelia W. Kelly, *Dimensions of Professional Nursing* (2d ed., 1968); Doris Troth Lippman, "Early Nursing Textbooks," *Journal of Nursing History* (April 1986), pp. 52-61; Jane E. Mottus, *New York Nightingales: The Emergence of the Nursing Profession at Bellevue and New York Hospital, 1850-1920* (1980); Paterson General Hospital, *Centennial Publication* (1971); Shaw family Bible, Cornwall-on-Hudson, New York; Clara S. Weeks, *A Text-book of Nursing for the Use of Training Schools, Families, and Private Students* (1885).

JOELLEN WATSON HAWKINS

SIMPSON, CORA E.. *Missionary nurse; educator.* EDUCATION: Attended Methodist Hospital School of Nursing, Omaha, Nebraska; studied theology, Bible, and social service; four-year course in the Chinese language; course in public health nursing, Simmons College, Boston. CAREER: 1907-1944, missionary nurse, teaching at Florence Nightingale School of Nursing, Magaw Memorial Hospital, Foochow, China.

CONTRIBUTIONS: Cora Simpson played a major role in the development of the China Nurses' Association (CNA), an organization of the missionary nurses who devoted their lives to assisting the Chinese people. In 1907, she suggested that the missionary nurses of China unite and establish such an organization, and two years later, the CNA was founded with seventeen charter members. In 1910, she was invited to be the first nurse delegate to the Medical Conference in China, and at that meeting support of the medical community was attained for registration of nurses and for a nursing organization. By 1912, the CNA had drawn up a curriculum for nursing schools, and by 1914 examinations were being given for admission to those schools. These accomplishments were remarkable, for they not only occurred in a relatively short period of time but they changed the image of nurses in China, who previously had been considered to be doing the work of coolies. Before most of the schools of nursing were established, a national organization had been founded and a standard curriculum was adopted, something that many more progressive countries had not yet achieved at that time. The CNA became the accrediting agency for schools of nursing, and eventually began to publish its own journal, the *Nursing Journal of China.* The word *Hu-shih* was used to describe an educated nurse. Many men were trained because in China it was not considered proper for women to care for male patients. In 1922 the organization was recognized by the International Council of Nurses (ICN), and Simpson became its executive secretary and its first paid employee.

She broadened the role of nurses from hospital based into the community, where they served in schools, ran health education campaigns, and did social work. The Magaw Memorial Hospital, Foochow, China, where she served, was used in 1919 by the Red Cross nursing committee as a cholera hospital during the epidemic of that year. Simpson's major role, however, was as executive secretary of the CNA. She was an activist who was able to establish a permanent headquarters for the CNA in Nanking. In 1928, she shared her position with a Chinese co-secretary, Mary Shih, indicating that she recognized that in order to receive acceptance by the Chinese people, and thereby to ensure that trained and educated nurses provided nursing care in the various cities, towns, and villages of China, it was necessary to have native Chinese involved in the various aspects of the work of the organization.

In 1926, Simpson wrote articles for the *American Journal of Nursing* to publicize the ICN congress which was to be held in China in 1929. Because of warfare there, however, the congress was rescheduled for Canada. Because of the unrest in China and the Japanese invasion in 1937, most of the missionary nurses were assigned to posts outside China, depriving the CNA of many of its leaders. According to Virginia Henderson's *Nursing Studies Index*, Simpson did not leave China until 1944, a time when not only was China still struggling with Japanese control, but a civil war was beginning between the Communist Chinese of Mao Tse-Tung, and the Nationalist Chinese of Chiang Kai-Shek.

WRITINGS: "On to Peking! Follow Your President to China," *American Journal of Nursing* (October 1926), p. 780; "On to Peking," *American Journal of Nursing* (November 1926), pp. 860-861; "Examinations for Nurses in China," *International Nursing Review* (May 1950), pp. 236-242; *A Joyride through China* (n.d.).

REFERENCES: Minnie Goodnow, *Nursing History* (7th ed., 1943); Deborah MacLurg Jensen, *History and Trends of Professional Nursing*

(1955); Meta Rutter Pennock, ed., *Makers of Nursing History* (1928); Cora Simpson, *A Joyride Through China* (n.d.); Isabel Stewart and Anne Austin, *A History of Nursing* (5th ed., 1962).

LORETTA P. HIGGINS

SIRCH, MARGARET ELLIOT {FRANCIS} (1867, Owen Sound, Canada--1954). *Nurse; journalist; social welfare worker.* Daughter of John G. Francis and Catherine (Chisholm) Francis. Married Charlemagne Sirch, July 18, 1899. EDUCATION: 1887, received diploma in nursing from Buffalo General Hospital, Buffalo, New York. CAREER: 1887-1889, superintendent of nurses, Buffalo General Hospital (had been acting superintendent during the last six months of her training); 1889-1894, organized two hospitals and their nursing services, one in New York and the other in Wisconsin; 1894-1899, private duty nursing, which included accompanying a patient abroad and travelling through France, Germany, and other European countries; 1910-1915, public health nurse, state of California; 1915-1937, in charge of the State Board of Charities and Corrections, California; 1937, retired upon reaching the compulsory retirement age of seventy.

CONTRIBUTIONS: Margaret Sirch was the first editor of *The Trained Nurse* (1888-1889), the first permanent nursing magazine to serve the profession in the United States (later it became *The Trained Nurse and Hospital Review* and, in midcentury, *The Nursing World*. This journal served as a channel of communication for the ninety-four nursing schools in the United States. The journal was not owned by nurses or by the profession, but a large number of nursing leaders of the day wrote for it in its early years; among them were Sophia Palmer (q.v.), Lystra Gretter (q.v.), and Anna Maxwell (q.v.).

Sirch was motivated to start the journal when she realized that nurses had no vehicle for their continuing education, and when a publisher showed interest in financing the start of the journal. She thought that a journal with articles about new medical and nursing practices would help alleviate the sense of isolation that new graduates felt. The magazine was instrumental in spreading the ideas about the need for such nursing organizations that exist today. A letter to the editor, for instance, in January 1889 outlined a proposal to band together the country's nurses into an "American Nurses Association." Mrs. Sirch solicited responses from readers, and later the same year the journal printed a proposal that each state develop local nurses' organizations. She encouraged nurses in New York State to initiate their first state organization. She also pioneered in establishing (in California) standards of sanitation and care for children in boardinghouses, for childrens' hospitals and preventoria, day nurseries, maternity hospitals, and homes for the aged.

After passing the examinations for public health nursing, Sirch had to wait a year for an appointment to the staff until the California law was passed that allowed married women to work for the state. She was considered outstanding as "founder and builder of the welfare and health departments" of the state of California. She was credited with having written many reports which helped to transform unsanitary institutions into modern hospitals.

WRITINGS: Many articles for early nursing journals, including "Fever Nursing" in the first number (August 1888) of *The Trained Nurse.*

REFERENCES: Lyndia Flanagan, *One Strong Voice* (1976); *Nursing World* (September 1954), p. 17; Meta Rutter Pennock, "Margaret Francis Sirch," in *Makers of Nursing History* (1940); Antonia Potemkina, "Meet the First Editor," *Trained Nurse and Hospital Review* (April 1938), pp. 343-351; Mary M. Roberts, *American Nursing: History and Interpretation* (1954).

ALICE HOWELL FRIEDMAN

SLY, SARAH (c. 1876, probably in Birmingham, Michigan--May 26, 1944, Birmingham, Michigan). Daughter of farmers. *Organizer.* EDUCATION: 1898, graduated from Farrand Training School, Harper Hospital, Detroit, Michigan. CAREER: Staff nurse, Pennsylvania Hospital; private duty nurse.

CONTRIBUTIONS: Because of her fragile health, after several years of nursing practice, Sarah Sly devoted her energies to work in nursing organizations. She was president of the Michigan State Nurses' Association during the campaign in that state for passage of a nurse registration law. She helped in assisting the national organization make the transition from the Nurses' Associated Alumnae of the United States to the American Nurses' Association (ANA) in 1911, and she served as president of the ANA from 1911 to 1913. She was also the interstate secretary of the ANA. For eight years, she chaired the revision committee of the ANA, which in 1916 succeeded in changing the association's organizational pattern into a system in which the various states would be unit members of the national. In 1923, she became the general secretary of the Michigan State Nurses' Association. She was also active in the International Council of Nurses, serving on its by-laws committee. For several years she served on the board of directors of the American Journal of Nursing Company, putting to use her considerable business and administrative talents to strengthen the *Journal.* Because of

ill health, she finally was forced to resign from her duties; after her retirement she lived with her sisters on a Birmingham, Michigan, fruit farm which had been in her family for a century.
REFERENCES: *American Journal of Nursing* (July 1944), p. 718; American Journal of Nursing Collection, Nursing Archives, Mugar Memorial Library, Boston University; Lyndia Flanagan, *One Strong Voice: The Story of the American Nurses' Association* (1976).

LORETTA P. HIGGINS

SMITH, MARTHA RUTH (November 14, 1894, Lebanon, New Hampshire--August 21, 1960). *Nurse-educator.* Daughter of Dr. Frank A. Smith and ? (Wanen) S. Smith. Never married. EDUCATION: 1913, graduated from Lebanon (New Hampshire) High School; 1914-1915, attended University of Wisconsin, Madison; 1919, graduated from Peter Bent Brigham Hospital School of Nursing, Boston; 1924, B.S., and 1931, M.A., Teachers College, Columbia University, New York City; 1935, completed clinical course in psychiatric nursing, Butler Hospital, Providence, Rhode Island. CAREER: 1919, head nurse, and 1920, supervisor, Peter Bent Brigham Hospital, Boston; 1920-1921, resident school nurse, Kimball Union Academy, Meriden, New Hampshire; 1921-1923, instructor, Samaritan Hospital School of Nursing, Troy, New York; 1924-1929, instructor, Massachusetts General Hospital School of Nursing, Boston; 1929-1935, instructor of nursing education, Teachers College, Columbia University; 1935-1938, instructor, Simmons College School of Nursing, Boston; 1935-1939, assistant principal, Massachusetts General Hospital School of Nursing; 1939-1946, professor of nursing education, Boston University School of Education; 1946-1963, dean, Boston University School of Nursing.
CONTRIBUTIONS: Martha Smith made significant contributions to the teaching of nursing, through innovative teaching methods and attention to curriculum design. She was motivated to improve the practice of nursing through curriculum development and experimentation with new teaching methods. Her goal was to prepare nurses who could pursue appropriate methods of nursing care by first analyzing their practice and evaluating the outcome of their practice. Using this method, students would know why they were giving a certain care, rather than acting on the basis of rigid procedures to be followed in every case. Smith was also remembered for her revolutionary approach to teaching the beginning course in nursing. She wanted students to have a broader understanding of nursing, and not to consider nursing simply as a role in the hospital. In 1935, she described her approach in a paper presented at the 1935

convention of the National League of Nursing Education, whose main theme was with curriculum advances.

She had considerable influence on developing the modern curriculum that kept the Massachusetts General Hospital School of Nursing in the forefront of nursing education among hospital schools of nursing. As supervisor of instruction, she prepared an improved plan for the correlation of theory and practice. In 1923, the Goldmark Report on the status of nursing education had recommended that schools ensure that students had an understanding of nursing theory before they were responsible for clinical practice, and Smith carried that idea to what may have been its logical conclusion: that theory and practice should be fully integrated into the nursing program from the first class to graduation. These ideas were advanced in the textbook *An Introduction to the Principles of Nursing Care*, which she co-authored with colleagues at Teachers College, and it was widely used in schools of nursing around the world. Rather than concentrating on specific procedures, the text provided the student with an overview of the elements of good nursing, the care of the individual patient, and the principles underlying the remedial procedures carried out by the nurse. In addition to her contribution to nursing theory and practice, she developed a procedure manual and a system for evaluating student practice. She provided students with a more coherent rotation through the various clinical specialties, and her curriculum ensured that students had a reasonable amount of classroom time in addition to hospital training.

Her final position, and the capstone to her career, was as professor of nursing education at Boston University (1939-1946) and as the first dean of the Boston University School of Nursing (1946-1963). Well respected among nurse-educators, she was a member of the committee which set up a plan with Boston University for graduate nurses who wished to continue their education beyond the hospital nursing school. When Boston University's division of nursing education was established in 1939, Smith became its director. Under her leadership, the nursing program flourished, and in 1946-1947 it was reorganized into a self-contained nursing school; Smith was appointed its dean, the first female academic dean in the history of the university. At the time of its establishment as a school of nursing, full-time enrollment was 170, of whom 125 were veterans of World War II taking advantage of the GI Bill to further their education.

Smith was aware of the limits of her own knowledge, and several times in her career she sought to strengthen her ability to serve as a nurse-educator. Many years after she began her teaching career, she enrolled in post-graduate courses. One took her to the Visiting Nurse Association of Boston for four months of clinical work which enabled her to learn first-hand about public health nursing. In order to strengthen her understanding of mental hygiene and psychiatric nursing, she enrolled in a clinical program offered at Butler Hospital, Providence, Rhode Island.

In addition to her role as a nurse-educator and as an influential author, she served the National League of Nursing Education, the American Nurses' Association, the American Red Cross Nursing Service, as well as many other local and national organizations in both nursing and social welfare. She also worked diligently for the Massachusetts State Mental Hygiene Association. Upon her retirement from Boston University in 1955, she was named dean emeritus, in recognition of sixteen years of devoted service to nursing education in the academic setting, and in recognition of her important role in the development of the Boston University School of Nursing.

WRITINGS: *An Introduction to the Principles of Nursing Care* (general editor, 1937).

REFERENCES: *American Journal of Nursing* (1946), p. 635, (1947), p. 420, and (1957), p. 1114; *Nursing Outlook* (1960), p. 583; Sylvia Perkins, *A Centennial Review: The Massachusetts General Hospital School of Nursing, 1873-1973*; Martha Smith Collection, Nursing Archives, Mugar Memorial Library, Boston University; *Who's Who in Massachusetts* (1946), p. 624.

ALICE HOWELL FRIEDMAN

SOULE, ELIZABETH {STERLING} (October 13, 1884, East Douglas, Massachusetts--February 19, 1972, Seattle, Washington). *Leader in nursing education.* Daughter of Edwin Sterling, a physician, and Adaline (Bates) Sterling. Married Harry W. Soule, June 11, 1912 (he died July 1, 1950). EDUCATION: 1903, graduated from Everett (Massachusetts) High School; April 25, 1907, graduated from Malden Hospital School for Nurses, Malden, Massachusetts; 1909, completed four-month course, Boston Instructive District Nursing Association; 1926, B.A. in sociology, and 1931, M.A. in sociology, University of Washington, Seattle. CAREER: 1907, staff nurse, Malden Hospital, Massachusetts; 1907-1909, private duty nurse; 1909-1912, district nurse, Everett Visiting Nurse Association; 1912-1915, public health nurse, Metropolitan Life Insurance Company, Seattle, Washington; 1915-1918, public health nurse, Washington State Tuberculosis Association and Walla Walla County Health Department; 1918-1920, supervisor of nurses, Washington State Tuberculosis Association and Washington branch of the American Red Cross; 1920, state advisory nurse, Washington State Department of Health; 1918-1920,

assistant for graduate-level course in public health nursing, University of Washington extension service; September 1920-1950, organized and directed nursing school at the University of Washington, Seattle.
CONTRIBUTIONS: Elizabeth Soule's most important contribution was as a pioneer in collegiate nursing education, developing a nursing school for the University of Washington, Seattle. After serving as an assistant teaching the course in public health nursing for graduate nurses during the summers of 1918, 1919, and 1920, she was asked by the president of the university to continue the program under a temporary appointment as an instructor (September-December 1920). In January 1921, he asked her to organize a university department of nursing, based on the various nursing courses then being offered in the college of science. By the fall of 1921, the new department had been organized, with a second quarter of nursing courses, along with a quarter of fieldwork. The public health nursing certificate program was now nine months in length.

Soule applied to the National Organization for Public Health Nursing, seeking approval of the program; approval was granted in 1923, although her own academic preparation was questioned in the report which gave the new program an A rating on every other area of evaluation. The problem was that she was teaching graduate nurses, yet she did not possess a bachelor's degree or any post-graduate degrees. She tried to resign so that a nurse with proper qualifications could assume the post. The university president responded by challenging Soule to get the necessary preparation, while continuing as the head of the University's nursing program. She accepted the challenge, enrolled in the university, and in 1926 received her B.A. in sociology, followed in 1931 by a master's degree.

Between 1923 and 1934, the university provided courses in anatomy, chemistry, nutrition, and physiology for students enrolled in hospital programs. Soule also considered and responded to the need for graduate nurses to have programs that would keep them up to date; one- and two-day institutes were offered in cooperation with the Washington State Nurses' Association and other nursing organizations in the region. The department also had five-year degree students who enrolled for three years in the university and then entered a hospital training school. As the school moved toward becoming a self-contained collegiate program in nursing, in 1926 Soule devised an experiment which was intended to develop a method for clinical teaching which would help the university's students as well as those from the hospital training school; she sent to the hospital a nursing instructor and students who were ready for hospital experience. Plans for a new and large public hospital dovetailed with Soule's thinking about the relationship between a university and a hospital that could provide the necessary clinical experience for trained nurses.

On the basis of her experiment, as well as consultation with nursing leaders like Annie Goodrich (q.v.) and Mary Roberts (q.v.), Elizabeth proposed a four-year experimental plan and secured a grant from the Rockefeller Foundation to support it for those four years and for one additional year. The grant also funded a three-month tour of European nursing schools and public health centers, providing Soule with an understanding of nursing education around the world. Harborview King County Hospital opened in March 1931 with thirty graduate nurse students enrolled to earn a bachelor's degree at the university. In July 1931, the Harborview division of the University of Washington opened with eight "basic students," who had completed four quarters of preclinical courses on campus. The university retained responsibility for the clinical nursing education of its students, and the hospital asssumed responsibility for its nursing service.

Nearly twenty more years remained of Soule's formal career, during which she not only continued to improve the University of Washington program, but she promoted collegiate education for nursing. When the University of Washington was reorganized in the 1930s, Soule's nursing department was renamed the University of Washington School of Nursing. She was instrumental in the development of teaching units in the northern and western Washington state psychiatric hospitals and in encouraging hospital schools to follow the model of the university, turning over the education to colleges and universities, and providing sites for clinical experiences.

In 1949, Soule witnessed the culmination of all her work when the University of Washington division of health sciences was created. Under this reorganization, which she had wholeheartedly supported, the schools of nursing, dentistry, and medicine would retain their independence and their own deans, but the deans would work together, serving as a planning and advisory council for the division. The new health sciences building was dedicated in October of that year.

Soule was known not only for her accomplishments in her official position, however, but also for her ability to share with students and faculty her enthusiasm and her visions for the future. She shared with faculty and former students opportunities to serve on national committees and boards and to take part in institutes at other universities.

Meeting the challenges of building what became a very large and prestigious school apparently did not consume all of her time or energy. Over the years, she played leadership roles in various professional organizations. Shortly after her move to Seattle, she helped to organize and plan activities for the Washington state branch of the National League of Nursing Education (NLNE), serving one term as its president. In 1914, she was one of ten nurses who formed the Washington State

Organization for Public Health Nursing, and she became its third president. She was on committees and on the board of the Washington State Graduate Nurses' Association, and in 1929 she was president of the northwest division of the American Nurses' Association. In 1932, she was elected to the boards of the American Nurses' Association (serving from 1932 to 1944) and the American Journal of Nursing Company.

In that same year, 1932, at the NLNE convention in San Antonio, Soule joined with representatives of twenty collegiate schools of nursing to form an organization of schools with university connections. In January 1933, a temporary association was established, and she volunteered to serve on the membership committee. Soule served as president of the Association for Collegiate Schools of Nursing in 1944.

During World War II, Soule was a member of the Nursing Council on National Defense and acted as a special consultant to the U.S. Public Health Service. She was also western representative for the American Red Cross advisory council. In Washington, she was on the board of the Seattle Visiting Nurse Service, secretary of the public health committee of the State Planning Council, on the advisory committee of the State Health Department, secretary of the Washington State Tuberculosis Association, and treasurer of the Northwest Conference on High School and College Hygiene.

Soule's father was a physician, and it has been suggested that her experience assisting him in his office and on house calls led her to nursing as a career. When her mother was very ill and attended by a nurse from Boston City Hospital Training School, Soule was an eager pupil. Still, she considered entering one of the New England colleges for women. Her father died in her final year of high school, and at that point she declared her intent to enter a training school. Hoping to dissuade her, a friend of the family offered to give her experience in a small private hospital he owned. After nearly one year of exceptional service to that hospital, the superintendent came to recognize that she was ideally suited for life as a trained nurse. At that point, he agreed to support Soule's application to the Malden Hospital School for Nurses.

After a short period of staff and private nursing, Soule was drawn to public health nursing and entered the four-month program of the Boston Instructive District Nursing Association, organized by Charlotte Macleod (q.v.), and she became the first district nurse in Everett, Massachusetts.

Her marriage to Harry Soule in 1912 resulted in the move to Washington State that was to change the entire course of her life. In Washington, she resumed the public health work begun in Everett and found that her services were in demand. Three years as a visiting nurse for the Metropolitan Life Insurance Company led to a position as the first public health nurse for the Washington State Tuberculosis Association and the Walla Walla Health Department. She gained experience in rural nursing in those positions. Her next position required her to organize and promote public health nursing, pursuading officials in small and large communities, as well as county commissioners, that they needed to support a county nurse. She then became responsible for organizing the public health nursing service for the State Department of Health. At that point she began her long service to the University of Washington, service which ended with her retirement in 1950. She was named dean emeritus and retired to a small house overlooking Lake Washington near the university. Her husband died in the year of her retirement, 1950, so instead of the around-the-world trip they had planned, she spent a year close to her brother's home in Boston. Then she returned to spend the rest of her life in the state of Washington.

Soule received a number of honors during her long and distinguished career. In 1940, she was named Alumnus Summa Laude Dignatus, the second distinguished graduate of the University of Washington to receive that designation. In 1944, she was given an honorary doctor of science degree by Montana State College. Graduates of the University of Washington School of Nursing commissioned a portrait of her in her doctoral robes, painted by the well-known artist Neale Ordayne. In 1986, she was elected to the American Nurses' Association Nursing Hall of Fame, and in 1987 the University of Washington School of Nursing established the Elizabeth Sterling Soule endowed professorship.

WRITINGS: Numerous articles for professional journals, including "Building the University School," *American Journal of Nursing* (May 1938), pp. 580-586.

REFERENCES: Kathleen M. Leahy, "Elizabeth Sterling Soule," *National League of Nursing Education Biographical Sketches, 1937-1940* (1940); Henrietta Adams Loughran, "Mrs. Soule of Washington, Part I. Her Early Career in Nursing," *Nursing Outlook* (September 1956), pp. 492-496, and "Mrs. Soule of Washington, Part II: The University of Washington School of Nursing," *Nursing Outlook* (October 1956), pp. 567-572; *The Seattle Times* (October 4, 1964); *The Washington Nurse* (Winter 1986), p. 5; unpublished materials provided by the Nursing Alumni Association, University of Washington School of Nursing, Seattle; *Who's Who of American Women* (1959), I: 1203 and (1964-1965), III.

JOELLEN WATSON HAWKINS

STERLING, ELIZABETH. See **SOULE, ELIZABETH {STERLING}**.

STEWART, ISABEL MAITLAND (January 14, 1878, Fletcher, Ontario Canada--October 5, 1963, Chatham, New Jersey). *Educator, historian; author*. Daughter of Francis Beattie Stewart, Presbyterian missionary, and Elizabeth (Farquharson) Stewart. Never married. EDUCATION: Attended and received a diploma from Manitoba Normal School; attended Winnipeg Collegiate Institution; 1900-1902, attended Winnipeg General Hospital School of Nursing, graduating in 1902; 1909-1913, attended Teachers College, Columbia University, New York City, receiving a B.S. in 1911 and an M.A. in 1913. CAREER: Taught kindergarten, first, and second grades for about four years after graduating from normal school; 1903-1905, private duty nursing and district nursing; 1905-1907, night supervisor, Winnipeg General Hospital; 1909, appointed assistant to M. Adelaide Nutting (q.v.) at Teachers College; advanced through ranks becoming professor of nursing education, and 1925-1947, director of the department (succeeding Nutting); 1947, retired.

CONTRIBUTIONS: Although distinguished in numerous areas, Isabel Stewart was indisputably a giant in the field of nursing education. Perhaps it was prophetic that with her classmates of the Winnipeg General Hospital School of Nursing's class of 1902, she made suggestions about improving the curriculum. Perhaps, too, her normal school education was to have a lifelong influence by giving her an understanding of teaching methods and educational theory, an understanding which undoubtedly was strengthened immeasurably through her studies at Columbia University's Teachers College.

She contributed to the development of nursing education both as a faculty member at Teachers College and as a member and chairperson of countless committees of various professional organizations. At Teachers College, she took many courses in the field of general education, and she transferred applicable concepts to nursing education. She established a course of study to prepare teachers of nursing. Previously, the course at Teachers College prepared only administrators of nursing service and schools of nursing.

Stewart was active in professional organizations throughout her career and was especially willing to serve on or chair the education or curriculum committees of those organizations. In 1914, she became secretary of the educational committee of the National League of Nursing Education (NLNE) until she succeeded Nutting as chair from 1920 to 1937. She also chaired the league's Committee on International Affairs. She held the posts of secretary and vice-president of the NLNE. Three important publications came out of that committee's work. In 1917, *Standard Curriculum for Schools of Nursing* was published. In 1929 it was revised as *A Curriculum for Schools of Nursing* but was deemed too rigid, so a third publication appeared, *A Curriculum Guide for Schools of*

Nursing, encouraging more autonomy for the various schools. Largely as a result of her lengthy service on that committee, her knowledge of the subject became so impressive that she was known as "Miss Curriculum."

In addition to her service on the NLNE committee, she held various positions with the International Council of Nurses, including twenty-two years as chairperson of its committee on education (1925-1947). In 1944, she was elected to the second vice-presidency of the American Council on Education.

She contributed to the recruitment of nurses during World War I, as part of a triumvirate with Elizabeth C. Burgess (q.v.) and Anne Strong (q.v.). Together they formed an advisory committee on curriculum at the Vassar Training Camp, Poughkeepsie, New York. Over 400 college graduates entered the twelve-week summer program at Vassar. Called the "Rainbow Division," they then went on to complete their education by completing two years at a school of their choosing. Forty-two percent of these women completed their nursing education, and many went on to become leaders of the nursing profession. Stewart also prepared most of the written materials used in the nurse recruitment effort during the war.

Because of her concerns about the status of nursing in the event of war, in July 1940, the Nursing Council for National Defense was organized. She chaired the first committee that was established under that group -- Educational Policies and Resources -- and she was instrumental in securing for the first time support for nursing education in federal funds earmarked for that purpose.

Stewart was a prolific author. She wrote pamphlets, books on nursing history, and numerous articles. She was able to look toward the future, writing articles such as "Preparing Nursing to Meet the Needs of a Changing Society," that appeared in the forty-second annual report of the NLNE. From 1916 to 1921 she was editor of the Department of Nursing Education of the *American Journal of Nursing*. In addition, for twenty years she edited the Macmillan Educational Monographs which were used in nursing education nationwide.

In addition to helping to make nursing history, she had a profound awareness of the need to preserve the history of her profession. She credited a trip to Great Britain in 1908 with stimulating her interest in nursing history. Other trips, including one to the Orient, increased her nursing history knowledge and her awareness of the international scope of the profession. She co-authored two nursing history texts, one with Lavinia Dock (q.v.), *A Short History of Nursing: From the Earliest Times to the Present Day*, and the other with Anne Austin, *A History of Nursing from Ancient to Modern Times: A World View*. In addition to her publications in nursing history, even into her retirement she played a major role in developing a major archive for nursing history, the M. Adelaide Nutting Historical Collection at Teachers College.

Although she devoted her life to the advancement of the nursing profession, she was concerned about the status of all women, as indicated by her support of the suffrage movement. Along with Lavinia Dock (q.v.), she marched in suffrage parades, adding her support to that important movement. Her feminist views, however, had a long history. When in high school, for example, she wrote for the school newspaper an article entitled "Votes for Women."

Stewart's contributions to her profession were legion. She shaped the course of nursing education while recording the history of her profession. She was a scholar and an activist, a researcher and a writer. During her retirement, she continued to live near Columbia University and work for the cause of nursing education. Although she was a private person, those who knew her described her as humorous, fond of telling stories, and enjoying travel and the theater. Through her life, she received recognition for her contributions to her profession. She received three honorary doctorates, along with many awards, including the M. Adelaide Nutting Award of the National League of Nursing Education (1947). In 1936 the New York League of the National Federation of Business and Profession Women named her as one of twenty-three women of achievement. In 1961, the Isabel Maitland Stewart Research Professorship in Nursing Education was established at Teachers College.

WRITINGS: *A Short History of Nursing: From the Earliest Times to the Present Day* (with Lavinia Dock, 1st ed., 1920, subsequent editions in 1929, 1931, and 1938); *A History of Nursing from Ancient to Modern Times: A World View* (with Anne Austin, 1962); *The Educational Programme of the School of Nursing* (1934); *The Education of Nurses: Historical Foundations and Modern Trends* (1943); and numerous pamphlets and articles.

REFERENCES: *American Journal of Nursing* (April 1922), p. 543 and (October 1960), pp. 1426-1430; *American Women of Nursing* (1965); *British Journal of Nursing* (April 1927), p. 79; Gladys Bonner Clappison, *Vassar's Rainbow Division, 1918* (1964); Teresa E. Christy, "Portrait of a Leader: Isabel Maitland Stewart," *Nursing Outlook* (October 1969), pp. 44-48; Grace L. Deloughery, *History and Trends of Professional Nursing* (1977); Stella Goostray, "Isabel Maitland Stewart," *American Journal of Nursing* (March 1954), pp. 302-306; Mary M. Roberts, *American Nursing: History and Interpretation* (1954); *Notable American Women*, IV: 660-662; *Nursing Outlook* (November 1963), pp. 779-780; *Pacific Coast Journal of Nursing* (January 1934), p. 21; Effie J. Taylor, "Isabel Maitland Stewart," *National League of Nursing Education Biographical Sketches 1937-1940* (n.d.), and "Isabel Maitland Stewart-Educator," *American Journal of*

Nursing (January 1936), pp. 38-44; Edna Yost, *American Women of Nursing* (1965).

LORETTA P. HIGGINS

STIMSON, JULIA CATHERINE (May 26, 1881, Worcester, Massachusetts-September 29, 1948, Poughkeepsie, New York). *Military nurse.* Daughter of Henry Albert Stimson and Alice Wheaton (Bartlett) Stimson. Never married. EDUCATION: Attended Brearley School, New York City; 1901, B.A., Vassar College, Poughkeepsie, New York; 1901-1903, graduate studies in biology, Columbia University, New York City; 1908, graduated from New York Hospital School of Nursing, New York City; 1917, M.A., Washington University, St. Louis, Missouri. CAREER: 1908-1911, superintendent of nurses, Harlem Hospital, New York City; 1911, director of hospital social service, Washington University, St. Louis, Missouri; 1911-1917, superintendent of nurses, Barnes Hospital, Washington University, St. Louis; 1918, chief nurse, American Red Cross, serving in France; 1918, director of nursing service, American Expeditionary Forces; 1919-1933, dean, Army School of Nursing; 1919-1937, superintendent, Army Nurse Corps, Washington, D.C.

CONTRIBUTIONS: During the first half of the twentieth century, Julia Stimson was one of the most prominent American nursing leaders. Her executive ability was recognized in her early work as superintendent of nurses of two large hospitals (Harlem Hospital and Barnes Hospital) and in organizing the Red Cross service after a particularly devastating flood in Ohio. Her dynamic personality was reflected in her leadership style; although she had strong beliefs and commitment to action, she was understanding of the needs of others, and she was willing to listen to recommendations and suggestions from members of her staff. As a young graduate, she recognized the plight of the underprivileged patient and their families, and she organized a social service department at each of the hospitals in which she was superintendent.

When she became chief nurse of the American Red Cross in France during World War I, she demonstrated her ability to resolve conflict and to ensure that nurses could work without interference; observers commented that she had demonstrated "sheer generalship." In 1918 she became director of nursing services for the American Expeditionary Forces, and one of her most effective contributions was her ability as a liaison officer between the Army Nurse Corps and the Red Cross. Her knowledge of both organizations and the fact that her judgment was respected made it possible for her to move nurses to the areas where they were needed regardless of the red tape involved in transfers. Her success became legendary in supervising the nursing services provided by more than 10,000 nurses overseas during the war. After the war, she was honored by the United States, Great Britain, and France for her distinguished service which undoubtedly had a major impact on reducing mortality rates in military hospitals by ensuring that nurses were available to meet the changing needs.

After the war, she succeeded Annie Goodrich (q.v.) as the dean of the Army School of Nursing. When that school closed in 1931, Stimson continued as superintendent of the Army Nurse Corps. After the Army School of Nursing closed, she devoted her energies to raising the educational and physical standards of those who entered the Army Nurse Corps. She instituted the requirement of a high school diploma, graduation from an approved nursing school, and a rigid physical examination upon enlistment and annually. She fought to improve conditions for the army nurses, and through her efforts housing at military posts was improved, opportunities were provided for post-graduate study and participation in professional organizations, and arrangements were made for retirement privileges resulting from disability or length of time in the service. All of this served to improve morale, as well as the quality of nursing service in the Army Nurse Corps.

Stimson was the first woman who was given the rank of major in the U.S. Army. When the Army Nurse Corps was granted relative rank in 1920 by an act of Congress, her position as superintendent of the corps brought her the title of major. Full commissioned rank was granted to army nurses in 1947, and in 1948, just six weeks before her death, Stimson was promoted to the rank of colonel (on the retired list).

When she retired from the Army Nurse Corps in 1937, she moved to New York City where she gave much of her time as a volunteer with the American Nurses' Association (ANA). She was elected president of the ANA, serving in that capacity from 1938 to 1944. She stressed the importance of collective action by nurses, and that through a united front their goal of improving nursing education and service could be achieved. During World War II, she was recalled to active duty for six months (1942-1943), and during that time she was active in the recruitment of nurses for the army. From 1940 to 1942, she served as chairperson of the Nursing Council of National Defense. She served on a large number of committees dealing with military nursing service, and with the American Red Cross. She was secretary-treasurer of the Isabel Hampton Robb (q.v.) Memorial Fund (1945-1947) and a board member of the National League of Nursing Education.

Over the course of her long and distinguished career, Stimson received numerous honors in recognition of her contributions. For her military service, she received the distinguished service medal, the Royal Red Cross' first class citation, the Medaille de la reconnaissance francaise and the silver Medaille d'hygiene publique (France). General John J. Pershing cited her for "exceptionally meritorious and efficient service" during World War I. In 1921, Mt. Holyoke College awarded her an honorary doctor of science degree. The medical library at Fort Sam Houston, Texas, was named for her. In 1929, she received the Florence Nightingale Medal of the International Red Cross. Finally, in 1982 she was inducted into the ANA Nursing Hall of Fame.
WRITINGS: *Nurses Handbook of Drugs and Solutions* (1910); *Finding Themselves* (1918); many articles and reports for nursing and medical journals and a large number of army medical bulletins and pamphlets.
REFERENCES: Lyndia Flanagan, *One Strong Voice: The Story of the American Nurses' Association* (1976); Portia B. Kernodle, *The Red Cross Nurse in Action, 1882-1948* (1949); *Notable American Women*, III: 378-380; Meta Rutter Pennock, ed., *Makers of Nursing History* (1940); *Public Health Nursing* (1948), p. 568; Mary M. Roberts, *American Nursing: History and Interpretation* (1954).

ALICE HOWELL FRIEDMAN

STRONG, ANNE HERVEY (January 1876, Wakefield, Massachusetts--June 17, 1925, Boston). *Public health nurse; educator.* Daughter of Rear Admiral Strong. EDUCATION: 1898, graduated from Bryn Mawr College, Bryn Mawr, Pennsylvania; 1903-1906, attended Albany Hospital Training School for Nurses, Albany, New York; summers, 1913-1914, post-graduate studies in nursing education, Teachers College, Columbia University, New York City. CAREER: 1906-1907, supervisor and instructor, Albany Hospital Training School for Nurses; 1907-1913, instructor, and 1913-1914, assistant principal, Mary C. Wheeler School, Providence, Rhode Island; 1914-1916, instructor in public health nursing, Teachers College, Columbia University; 1916-1918, instructor of public health nursing, and 1918-1925, director of the School of Public Health Nursing, Simmons College, Boston.
CONTRIBUTIONS: Although often slowed by illness, which resulted in her untimely death, Anne Hervey Strong made a significant contribution to the development of public health nursing. In 1918, she organized the School of Public Health Nursing at Simmons College, a five-year program affiliated with Massachusetts General Hospital and, in 1921, with the Children's Hospital Medical Center and Peter Bent Brigham Hospital, both

in Boston. Students who completed the course of study received a B.S. from Simmons College and a diploma from the hospital school. The course began with two years at Simmons College, followed by clinical work in medical and surgical nursing either at the Massachusetts General Hospital or the Peter Bent Brigham Hospital, with obstetrical training at the Boston Lying-in Hospital, and pediatrics at the Children's Hospital Medical Center. The fifth year consisted of upper-level courses at Simmons College and public health nursing experience.

Strong was uniquely prepared for her life long endeavor, as one of the relatively few nurses of her time who began with a college education rather than completion of a hospital training school program. Her strong science background, coupled with ten years of training school teaching and administration, provided her with the skills necessary for the successful planning and implementation of the pioneering program at Simmons College. Indeed, her teaching experience began while she was studying nursing at the Albany Hospital School of Nursing, when she taught some science classes. Her summer work at the Henry Street Settlement House, New York City, provided her with field experience in public health nursing. After her post-graduate study was completed, she became an instructor at Teachers College, where she worked closely with M. Adelaide Nutting (q.v.).

In 1916, Simmons College invited her to teach public health nursing courses in conjunction with the Instructive District Nursing Association program begun by Charlotte Macleod (q.v.), and she continued as a guest lecturer at Columbia. When the School of Public Health Nursing was established in 1918, Strong was the natural choice to head the program. Not only a fine organizer, she was also a wonderful teacher, a deeply sympathetic person, and an unprejudiced thinker. She had patience and intelligence, traits critical to a person with high idealism. It is clear that her colleagues and students were enriched by their experiences with her.

She served as assistant secretary to Josephine Goldmark on the study of nursing and nursing education which was commissioned by the Rockefeller Foundation, and which produced the 1923 report which had profound implications for the future of American nursing. From 1917 to 1922, she was chairperson of the education committee of the National Organization for Public Health Nursing. In 1918, she was an instructor and member of the planning committee for the Vassar Training Camp, Poughkeepsie, New York. From 1920 to 1923, she was on the National League for Nursing committee on education, and from 1924 to 1925 she served on its special committee on grading of schools of nursing.

Ill health plagued Strong throughout her life but never prevented her from accomplishments. A back injury after graduation from college laid her up for a number of years and necessitated hospitalization, exposing her to nursing care which she characterized as both good and bad. That experience apparently determined her to become a nurse, a goal that was not abandoned even when her training was interrupted by typhoid fever. Nor did she waver from her chosen career when in 1907 ill health forced her to put aside nursing. During the next seven years, she taught math and Latin at the Mary C. Wheeler School, while spending summers as a volunteer working with Lillian Wald (q.v.) at the Henry Street Settlement. While working at Henry Street, she returned to school, taking post-graduate courses at Teachers College, which led her to return to a career in nursing education, first at Columbia and then at Simmons College. Ill health finally led to her untimely death in 1925, while directing the Simmons program. The Nurse Instructors' Study Club she had proposed in 1923, to bring about closer cooperation between nurse-instructors at Simmons, Massachusetts General Hospital, Peter Bent Brigham Hospital, and Children's Hospital, was named in her honor. In 1984 she was inducted into the American Nurses' Association Hall of Fame.

WRITINGS: Numerous articles in professional journals, including "Teaching Problems of Public Health Instructors," *American Journal of Nursing* (July 1917), pp. 1188-1189.

REFERENCES: Josephine Goldmark, "Anne Hervey Strong," *Public Health Nurse* (October 1925), pp. 516-519; Lois Haggerty, "Nursing Revisited: Strong Public Health Nursing Leader and Educator," *The Massachusetts Nurse* (July-August 1984), p. 7; *History of the Anne Strong Club for Nurse Instructors of Boston* (1955); unpublished material, M. Adelaide Nutting Historical Nursing Collection, Teachers College, Columbia University; Sylvia Perkins, *A Centennial Review: The Massachusetts General Hospital School of Nursing, 1873-1973* (1975); *Public Health Nurse* (October 1925), pp. 493-494; Alice A. Weston, "Anne Hervey Strong," *Trained Nurse and Hospital Review* (August 1930), pp. 187-189.

JOELLEN WATSON HAWKINS

STRUTHERS, LINA LAVANCHE {ROGERS} (c. 1870, Albion Township, Pell County, Ontario, Canada--June 10, 1946, Toronto, Ontario, Canada). *First school nurse.* Married Dr. William E. Struthers, chief medical inspector of schools, Toronto, July 9, 1913 (died April 20, 1928); no children. EDUCATION: Attended Weston High School, Jarvis Collegiate Institute, Toronto, Ontario, Canada; 1894, graduated from Hospital for Sick Children, Toronto, Ontario, Canada; 1894-1986, post-graduate course, Royal Victoria Hospital, Montreal, Quebec, Canada. CAREER: 1896-?, head nurse and night superintendent, Royal Victoria Hospital, Toronto; 1899, superintendent, Grady Hospital, Atlanta, Georgia; c. 1899-1902, nurse, Henry Street Settlement, New York City; 1902-1908, superintendent of school nurses, New York City; 1908-1910, school nurse, Pueblo, Colorado; 1910-1913, superintendent of school nurses, Toronto, Ontario, Canada.

CONTRIBUTIONS: Lina Rogers was the first school nurse in the United States, having been chosen for this role by Lillian Wald (q.v.) of the Henry Street Settlement. Medical inspection in schools had been instituted in 1897, but it was not until 1902, at an informal meeting of the chairman of the board of education, the health commissioner, and Lillian Wald that the issue of school nurses was discussed. At that time, Wald offered one of her Henry Street nurses, Lina Rogers, who was very concerned about the health of school children and was familiar with children from her work at Henry Street. At the time of her appointment, Rogers was a resident of the Henry Street Settlement House, and she received supplies from the settlement rather than from the city. She did experimental work as a demonstration school nurse beginning on October 1, 1902, and continuing into November. She began with four downtown schools enrolling 10,000 children. As her work load increased, she needed help, and Yssabella Waters (q.v.), another Henry Street nurse, assisted her for some time. Confronted with a number of recurrent problems, Rogers began to prepare courses of treatment for conditions such as dermatological problems. These were submitted to the city's board of health and became part of the school department's regulations. Children who had to be excluded from school were reported to principals and visits made to their homes. One of the problems that quickly arose was that local dispensaries could not cope with the number of children who were found to need medical treatment. The experiment was a huge success, however, and on November 7, 1902, the board of health appointed Rogers as a permanent school nurse.

As a result of the experiment, twelve more nurses were appointed by the board of health on December 1, with Rogers in charge in the newly created office of superintendent of school nurses. Because the city now assumed financial responsibility for the medical inspection of school children, dressings were provided by the board of education rather than by the Henry Street Settlement. Nurses' offices, then called dressing rooms, were established in the various schools, often in the basement, and when the nurse arrived, she would report to the principal and then set up her clinic in the dressing room. Teachers would be informed of the presence of the nurse, and children would be sent for medical inspection and for treatment. Once all children were inspected in one school, the nurse would proceed to the next (most of the nurses were assigned to serve four or five schools) schools. After covering all the schools, the nurse would be ready to make home visits. By March 1903, twenty-five nurses were covering one hundred schools. Later in that year, the work of the school nurses was permanently established with 125 public and four parochial schools served and with 219,239 pupils enrolled and being inspected and treated. Under Rogers' leadership, the program was such a success that the principals reported that conditions in the schools were 100 percent better and that the average daily attendance had increased by 75 percent.

Rogers' pioneer work had an influence on other cities. By 1908, Baltimore, Boston, Grand Rapids, Los Angeles, Philadelphia, and Seattle had nurses engaged in school work, and other cities were experimenting with the idea. In order to share this important work, Rogers reported on it in the *American Journal of Nursing* and at the eleventh annual convention of the Nurses' Associated Alumnae (later the American Nurses' Association) in 1908. In 1917, she published a book, *The School Nurse*, an extensive treatise on the duties and responsibilities of the school nurse. This book detailed the qualifications of such nurses, outlined their duties, and gave details of nursing assessment and interventions for common conditions such as lice and scabies. It also included examples of record-keeping methods, as well as information about home visits and working with parents.

Rogers' reputation spread quickly through the medium of nursing journals and also through conventions of various professional organizations. In 1908, she assumed a similar role in Pueblo, Colorado, and then she returned to Toronto in 1910 to assume a position similar to that she had held in New York, as superintendent of school nurses. School nursing had been instituted by the Toronto Board of Education on April 24, 1910, and Rogers was invited to organize it. On May 6 of that year, she was given two assistant nurses and, in September, two medical inspectors, followed by two more nurses on November 3. This staff then cared for twenty schools enrolling 12,000 children. By 1911, a chief medical inspector, Dr. W. E. Struthers, later to become Rogers' husband, was appointed and thirteen additional nurses hired. This allowed visits by a nurse or medical inspector to each school every day. Some improvements Rogers was responsible for included the use of paper hand towels and obtaining audiometers to test the hearing of the children. By 1912, more nurses and more physicians had been added, so daily service at each school by both a doctor and nurse was possible. Health teaching was an important part of the role of the school nurse and included drills in such hygienic practices as nose blowing and tooth brushing. Rogers emphasized in her book that the major objective in school health was to teach children how to be and stay healthy.

In 1912, she read a paper on school nursing at the International Congress of Nurses (the meeting of the International Council of Nurses) in Cologne, Germany. She was also instrumental in the founding of the first post-graduate course for school nurses, under the supervision of the board of education of Toronto. She was president of the Canadian Public School Nurses' Association for several years, and in 1912 she was treasurer of the Graduate Nurses' Association of Ontario and in 1913 she became a member of its board of directors.

Although no longer actively practicing nursing after her marriage to Dr. Struthers, she continued to write and lecture on the subject of school nurses, in both Canada and the United States, as well as in Europe. She served as president of the editorial board of *Canadian Nurse*. When the National Organization for Public Health Nursing was established in 1913, Rogers was a natural choice to head its committee on school nursing, a position she held until 1916. In addition to her service to national nursing organizations in both Canada and the United States, she was president of the Nurses' Club of Toronto and the Toronto School Nursing Association and was a life member of the United Church Missionary Society. She was instrumental in founding the first open air schools for Toronto children suffering from tuberculosis, at Victoria and then at High Park.

WRITINGS: *The School Nurse* (1917); numerous articles in professional journals.

REFERENCES: *American Journal of Nursing* (March 1903), pp. 448-450 and (September 1908), pp. 966-974; *Canadian Nurse* (August 1910), pp. 333-335, (February 1911), p. 62, (April 1911), p. 164, (May 1911), p. 221, (March 1912), p. 129, (July 1912), pp. 345, 359, and 366-367, (October 1912), pp. 539-544, (August 1913), pp. 539 and 558, (November 1913), p. 733, (March 1914), p. 152, (January 1915), p. 48, (February 1915), p. 104, (January 1918), p. 816, (August 1921), pp. 277-279, and (August 1946), p. 691; M. Louise Fitzpatrick, *The National Organization for Public Health Nursing, 1912-1952* (1975); Minnie Goodnow, *Nursing History* (7th ed., 1943); Lina Rogers, "An Address," *Canadian Nurse* (March 1906), pp. 32-34, "School Nursing in New York City," *American Journal of Nursing* (March 1903), pp. 448-450, "Some Phases of School Nursing," *American Journal of Nursing* (September 1908), pp. 966-974, *The School Nurse* (1917), and form filled out on the occasion of the centennial of the Toronto Academy of Medicine (1934), William Boyd Library of the Academy of Medicine, Toronto; *Toronto Star Weekly* (October 4, 1913); *Toronto Telegram* (June 10, 1946); Lillian D. Wald, *The House on Henry Street* (1915); Thomas Denison Wood, M. Adelaide Nutting, Isabel M.

Stewart, and Mary L. Read, *The Ninth Yearbook of the National Society for the Study of Education, Part II, The Nurse in Education* (1910).

JOELLEN WATSON HAWKINS

SULLIVAN, ELIZABETH ELEANOR (May 17, 1890, Newburyport, Massachusetts--October 17, 1941, West Roxbury, Massachusetts). *Nursing educator; pediatric nurse.* Daughter of Maurice J. Sullivan, hatter, and Ann (Mansfield) Sullivan. Never married. EDUCATION: Attended high school in Newburyport and Haverhill, Massachusetts; 1913, honors graduate of Massachusetts General Hospital Training School for Nurses, Boston; 1919-1920, post-graduate studies at Teachers College, Columbia University, New York City; 1932, B.Ed., 1933, M.Ed., and 1938, Ph.D. in sociology, Boston College, Chestnut Hill, Massachusetts. CAREER: January-June 1913, head nurse of the children's ward, Massachusetts General Hospital; 1914-1915, supervisor (and maybe head nurse), Huntington Hospital, Boston; March-August 1915, instructor and first assistant, Children's Hospital, Boston; September 1915-July 1919, superintendent of nurses, Children's Hospital, Boston; September 1920-1934, nonresident visiting instructor, various nursing schools in greater Boston, principally Faulkner Hospital, Jamaica Plain, and Anna Jacques, Newburyport, as well as teaching sociology at Boston College (part time); 1936-1941, supervisor of schools of nursing, Massachusetts State Board of Registration, Boston.

CONTRIBUTIONS: Elizabeth Sullivan was one of the early members of the nursing profession to hold an earned doctorate. Her dissertation at Boston College focused on the ethical and social implications of modern nursing, based on an ideological approach to the subject. Throughout her career, she was devoted to the improvement of nursing education, first as a superintendent of nurses at Children's Hospital, then as a visiting instructor of science in nursing schools and in the department of sociology at Boston College, and finally as the first supervisor of schools of nursing for the Massachusetts State Board of Registration. She sought to improve the quality of nursing education in both Massachusetts and at the national level through her participation in nursing organizations, notably the National League of Nursing Education and the American Nurses' Association. She also was an active member of the American Sociological Society.

In addition to her contributions to nursing education, Sullivan furthered the development of pediatric nursing. When she graduated with honors from the Massachusetts General Hospital Training School for Nurses, she became head nurse on Ward H, the hospital's children's ward.

She was the recipient of a scholarship from Dr. Fritz Talbot to promote efficiency and interest in pediatric nursing, which enabled her to travel to New York, Philadelphia, and Baltimore to observe nursing in children's hospitals in those cities. Her interest in pediatric nursing led to her appointment to the nursing staff at the Children's Hospital (Boston) and to her assumption of the post of superintendent (1915-1919). She left Children's Hospital to pursue post-graduate training at Teachers College of Columbia University, and that experience apparently led her to recognize the desirability of a bachelor's degree and ultimately a doctorate. To that end, she enrolled at Boston College and taught part time for many years while she studied and earned her bachelor's, master's and doctorate. Stella Goostray (q.v.) was a probationer (beginning nursing student) at Children's Hospital when Sullivan taught the principles and practice of nursing and when she became superintendent. Goostray remembered Elizabeth Sullivan as a marvelous teacher and one who obviously had a major impact on her own future career.

When Sullivan became the first person to hold the position as state supervisor of schools of nursing, she viewed her work as supportive and educational rather than as supervisory or punitive. She can be credited with many of the improvements in training programs of a large number of nursing schools in the state and with assisting schools in meeting modern standards, rather than with forcing them to close. The need for a full-time person to serve as inspector, in the same capacity as that of the New York State inspector, led to a number of years of work on the part of nursing leaders in Massachusetts before the position was established and Sullivan was finally appointed. Her charge was to evaluate schools and help them maintain or surpass the standards set by the board. Her experiences as an administrator and teacher uniquely qualified her to provide the guidance necessary without instilling terror in superintendents and instructors, especially those of hospital programs, many of which did not meet the expectations of modern nursing education.

While engaged in this important work, Sullivan's productive life was cut short by her untimely death from metastatic cancer. She had a lengthy illness, during much of which she continued to work. A memorial mass was held at St. Ignatius Chapel of Boston College, and she was buried in her home town of Newburyport.

WRITINGS: *Problems in Solutions* (1932).

REFERENCES: American Journal of Nursing Collection, Nursing Archives, Mugar Memorial Library, Boston University; *Boston Globe* (October 18, 1941); Stella Goostray, *Fifty Years of the School of Nursing, the Children's Hospital, Boston* (1940), and *Memoirs: Half a Century in Nursing* (1969); Sylvia Perkins, *A Centennial Review: The Massachusetts*

General Hospital School of Nursing, 1873-1973 (1975); *The Pilot* (newspaper of the Boston Archdiocese, October 25, 1941); *The Quarterly Record* (Massachusetts General Hospital, 1941), p. 28.

JOELLEN WATSON HAWKINS

SUTLIFFE, IRENE H. (November 12, 1850, Albany, New York--December 30, 1936, New York City). *Nurse-educator.* Daughter of George Washington Sutliffe and Charlotte (Ramsey) Sutliffe. Never married. EDUCATION: Attended Cathedral School, Albany, New York; 1878-1880, attended New York Hospital School of Nursing, New York City, graduating in 1880. CAREER: 1880-1886, established school of nursing and was superintendent, Hamot Hospital, Erie, Pennsylvania; 1886, developed the Long Island College Hospital School of Nursing, Brooklyn, New York; 1886-1902, director of the New York Hospital School of Nursing; 1898, brief period of service during the Spanish-American War, heading the nursing service at Camp Black, Hempstead, Long Island, New York; 1908, established social services at the Hudson Street Hospital, New York City; 1909, established social services at the New York Hospital; 1916, organized an emergency hospital for the treatment of polio during an epidemic.

CONTRIBUTIONS: The reputation of Irene Sutliffe rests primarily on the years she directed the nursing school at the New York Hospital. She was a beloved early leader of nursing education, much appreciated by her friends and colleagues, as indicated by the extensive obituary in the *American Journal of Nursing* (February 1937). Her younger twin sisters and several of her nieces also became nurses, and her sister Ida succeeded her at the Long Island College Hospital School. Sutliffe's administrative abilities must have been apparent even during her student years; soon after her graduation, she was called upon to establish and administer the Hamot Hospital, and from there she went on establish the school of nursing of the Long Island Hospital, Brooklyn, New York. The esteem with which she was regarded by those at her own training school was evident from the fact that just six years after her own graduation she was appointed to lead the New York Hospital School of Nursing.

Sutliffe was director of that school during the time when nursing education was in its infancy. Curricular offerings were meager, textbooks for nurses nonexistent, and techniques not at all uniformly accepted. Although frail, she managed with but one assistant to run a hospital nursing service as well as a training school. One of her early accomplishments was to establish an affiliation with the Sloane Maternity Hospital, because she understood the importance of such experience for the beginning nurse. In 1890, she created what has been called the first diet kitchen in the country, a fact which demonstrates her understanding of the significance of nutrition in health as well as sickness. An important legacy of her leadership at New York Hospital was the quality of the students who graduated; many became directors of nursing services at large hospitals in the New York metropolitan area, and others became known internationally. Some of these nursing leaders trained under her supervision were Lydia Anderson (q.v.), Mary Beard (q.v.), and Lillian Wald (q.v.). Many of Sutliffe's accomplishments were completed in spite of strong opposition from the medical staff of the hospital, which was more interested in patient care than in educating student nurses.

Sutliffe's vision for nursing was broader than her own sphere of influence at the New York Hospital. In 1890 she attended a meeting in Chicago where she was appointed honorary vice-chairperson of the committee of five of the nursing sub-section of the International Congress of Charities and Correction. In 1893 she attended the World's Fair held in Chicago, and she participated in the meeting which led to the development of what was to become the National League of Nursing Education. At that meeting, she read a paper in which she strongly advised that the profession organize in order to maintain high ideals and standards. Her belief in the value of organization was shown by her support of the founding of the alumnae association of her school, and later by the New York Hospital Nurses' Club.

In 1932 Sutliffe was made a member of the Society of the New York Hospital and given the title of dean emeritus. In new quarters where the hospital moved, by the East River, she was assigned an apartment in the nurses' residence where she spent her last years. She was nursed by two of her graduates during the years just before her death. In 1887 she had adopted a baby girl who had been abandoned in a vacant lot near the hospital. The child died three years later, and it was next to her that Sutliffe was buried.

REFERENCES: M. Adelaide Nutting Collection, Teachers College, Columbia University (microfiche number 0934); *American Journal of Nursing* (February 1937), pp. 215-218 and (April 1937), p. 451; Jane E. Mottus, *New York Nightingales: The Emergence of the Nursing Profession at Bellevue and New York Hospital, 1850-1920* (1981); Meta Rutter Pennock, ed., *Makers of Nursing History* (2d ed., 1940).

LORETTA P. HIGGINS

T

TAYLOR, EUPHEMIA JANE (April 18, 1874, Hamilton, Ontario, Canada--May 20, 1970, Hamilton, Ontario, Canada). *Psychiatric nurse; educator; administrator.* Never married. EDUCATION: Graduated from Hamilton Collegiate Institute, Hamilton, Ontario; attended Wesleyan Ladies College, Hamilton (two years); 1907, received diploma from Johns Hopkins School of Nursing, Baltimore, Maryland; 1908, studied at Teachers College, Columbia University, New York City; c. 1923, continued studying the social and preventive aspects of nursing by attending courses offered through the Department of Public Health, Yale University School of Medicine, New Haven, Connecticut; 1926, B.S., Teachers College, Columbia University. CAREER: 1907-1908, head nurse, private wards, Johns Hopkins Hospital; 1909, junior instructor, Johns Hopkins School of Nursing; 1912-1917, director of nursing services, Henry Phipps Clinic, Johns Hopkins Hospital; 1917-1918, director, Camp Meade (Maryland) unit of the Army School of Nursing; 1919-1922, associate principal of the School of Nursing, Johns Hopkins Hospital; 1922, first executive secretary of the National League of Nursing Education; 1923-1926, superintendent of the Connecticut Training School (which became the Yale School of Nursing); c. 1926-1944, professor of nursing in psychiatry, Yale School of Nursing; 1934-1944, dean of the Yale School of Nursing; 1944, retired.

CONTRIBUTIONS: Euphemia (Effie) Taylor was the second dean of the Yale School of Nursing which was created following the Rockefeller Foundation study, *Nursing and Nursing Education in the United States* (1923). She advanced the concept of the patient-centered methods of nursing care. Dean Annie Goodrich (q.v.) had considered this method of nursing care in her earlier years and was able to develop this at Yale with the cooperation of the faculty, and particularly Taylor. Taylor applied her understanding of patient needs by reorganizing the nursing student assignments at Yale. Students cared for small groups of patients, rather than be assigned to specific tasks or procedures.

As chairperson of the Mental Hygiene Section of the American Nurses' Association, Taylor was instrumental in changing the prevailing viewpoint of nursing to see that good nursing care of the physically ill patient also involved attention to the emotional and intellectual life of the patient. In 1937, she was elected president of the International Council of Nurses (ICN). Her ability to establish natural and friendly relationships with many kinds of people helped her to keep the ICN intact in spite of the economic and political upheavals of World War II. In the early years of the United Nations, she was the official ICN observer to the U.N.

From 1932 to 1936, she served as president of the National League of Nursing Education, and while she was president, the influential *A Curriculum Guide for Schools of Nursing* (1937) was being prepared. She also was the chairperson of the Subcommittee on Administration of Curriculum, one of the committees which determined the content of the 1937 *Guide*. In the early years of her professional career, she was secretary of the Alumnae of Johns Hopkins School of Nursing, and secretary of the Maryland State Nurses' Association. In later years, she was a member of the Nursing Committee on Historical Source Material in Nursing of the Connecticut League for Nursing. She was an early advocate of equality for women, as early as 1929 writing in the *American Journal of Nursing* that "a major problem in considering interprofessional relations between men and women in hospitals is 'responsibility without representation' and 'equal work with unequal pay.'"

In 1926, she received an honorary master of arts degree from Yale University. She received American Red Cross recognition in 1955 for her work during the Connecticut floods of that year, and in 1959 she received the Florence Nightingale Medal from the International Red Cross. The Effie Taylor Memorial Fund was established at the Yale School of Nursing in 1970, used to assist international students enrolled in the nursing program.

WRITINGS: Numerous articles for the *American Journal of Nursing*, including "A Challenge to League Members" (January 1933), p. 47; "Course of Study in Practical Psychopathology" (April 1922); "Conferences with Head Nurses" (June 1922); "The School of Nursing at Yale University" (January 1925); "Some Specialist" (January 1930); "A Mental Hygiene Concept in Nursing" (July 1932); "The Right of the School of Nursing to the Resources of the University" (December 1934); "What the International Council of Nurses Does" (1949); and "The International Council of Nurses" (1950).

REFERENCES: *American Journal of Nursing* (July 1970), p. 1568; Kathleen Buckwalter and Olga Church, "Euphemia Jane Taylor: An Uncommon Psychiatric Nurse," *Perspectives in Psychiatric Care* (1979), pp. 125-131; *The Canadian Nurse* (August 1970), p. 21; Connecticut Nursing Association, *Nursing News* (September 1970); Nursing Archives, Mugar Memorial Library, Boston University; *Nursing Research* (July-August 1970), p. 323; Mary M. Roberts, *American Nursing: History and Interpretation* (1954); Isabel M. Stewart, "Effie Jane Taylor, R.N.," *American Journal of Nursing* (July 1939), pp. 733-737.

ALICE HOWELL FRIEDMAN

THOMPSON, DORA E. (November 20, 1876, Cold Springs, New York--June 23, 1954, San Francisco). *Military nurse.* Never married. EDUCATION: 1897, graduated from New York City Hospital Training School, Blackwell's Island, New York; post-graduate course in operating room nursing. CAREER: 1897-1901, private duty nursing; 1902-1905, member, Army Nurse Corps, serving at Letterman General Hospital, San Francisco; 1905-1911, chief nurse, Letterman General Hospital; 1911-1914, assigned to the Philippines; 1914-1919, superintendent, Army Nurse Corps; 1919, resigned as superintendent, but after an extended leave, was appointed assistant superintendent of the Army Nurse Corps, serving until her retirement on August 31, 1932.

CONTRIBUTIONS: Dora Thompson was the first superintendent of the Army Nurse Corps to move to that rank from a position in the corps, succeeding Isabel McIsaac (q.v.) in that post. Thompson was particularly well suited for her position; she was able to handle many details and was intimately acquainted with army regulations, having served in the Army Nurse Corps for twelve years before being appointed superintendent. She was chief nurse at San Francisco's Letterman General Hospital at the time of the 1906 earthquake which devastated the city, and she worked tirelessly to help the victims of the quake and the fire which followed it. She was commended for her service during the emergency.

Thompson was superintendent of the Army Nurse Corps during World War I, when the Army Nurse Corps grew from fewer than 400 nurses to 21,480 at the end of the war. Thompson established procedures which served to control the process by which Red Cross nurses were assigned to army duty. At that time, the Red Cross nurses were the army reserves, assigned during wartime to fill specific needs. Her responsibilities included assigning nurses to their posts, forming them into hospital units, and allocating them where they were most needed. In addition to taking care of such things as hotel reservations and transportation for army nurses, Thompson had many public relations duties, which were so important in the recruitment of nurses during wartime. To that end, she maintained her visibility, by marching in parades, giving speeches, and so forth.

In order to ensure adequate care of the wounded, she sent nurses to take courses in anesthesiology. She also established the Army School of Nursing, which served to increase the supply of nurses by providing basic training to young women who wanted to serve their country as nurses but who were not registered nurses at the beginning of the war. She insisted that professional dietitians were part of the health care team in military hospitals. Cognizant of the problems in ward administration, Thompson changed regulations to clarify the role of the head nurse, making her fully responsible for the management of the ward and answerable only to the ward surgeon. For her exceptionally meritorious service and untiring devotion to duty during the war, she was awarded the Distinguished Service Medal. At the conclusion of the war, she resigned her position and took an extended leave. Upon her return she was appointed assistant superintendent of the Army Nurse Corps and was sent to the Philippines, as she requested. When army nurses were given relative rank, she became a captain.

WRITINGS: "Nursing as It Relates to the War: The Army," *American Journal of Nursing* (July 1918), pp. 1058-1060.

REFERENCES: *American Journal of Nursing* (February 1920), pp. 421-422; M. Adelaide Nutting Collection, Teachers College, Columbia University (microfiche number AN 0368); information provided by the U.S. Army Center of Military History, Washington, D.C.

LORETTA P. HIGGINS

THOMS, ADAH B. {SAMUELS} (January 12, 1863? Virginia--February 21, 1943, New York City). *Nursing leader; pioneer Black nurse.* Daughter of Harry Samuels and Melvina Samuels. Married a Dr. Thoms, a practicing physician; married Henry Smith, c. 1923; no children. EDUCATION: Elementary and normal schools of Richmond, Virginia; in 1890s, studied elocution at Cooper Union, New York City; 1900, graduate of nursing course given at Woman's Infirmary and School of Therapeutic Massage, New York City; 1903-1905, attended Lincoln Hospital and Home Training School for Nurses, New York City; 1917, took special course in public health nursing given by Henry Street Visiting Nurse Service and also took courses at New York School of Philanthropy (later New York School of Social Work), Hunter College, and New School for Social Research, all in New York City. CAREER: Taught school in

Richmond, Virginia prior to entering nursing; 1900-1903, worked as a nurse in New York City and as head nurse of St. Agnes Hospital, Raleigh, North Carolina; 1905, operating room nurse and supervisor of surgical division, Lincoln Hospital and Home, New York City; 1906-1923, assistant director of nurses, Lincoln Hospital, often serving as the acting director of the training school as well.

CONTRIBUTIONS: Adah Thoms' greatest contribution to nursing was her work to improve and increase opportunities for black nurses. In 1908, under her leadership, the Alumnae Association of Lincoln School for Nurses invited fifty-two nurses to attend a three-day meeting, beginning August 23, at St. Mark's Methodist Church in New York City, a meeting which led to the organization of the National Association of Colored Graduate Nurses (NACGN); on August 25, Thoms was elected treasurer of the organization. From 1916 to 1923, she served as the president of the association. She worked toward an eventual merger with the American Nurses' Association, a goal finally achieved in 1951, after her death.

Throughout her life, Thoms worked for better employment opportunities for black nurses in hospitals and public health agencies, and to raise the admission standards in nursing schools. Largely through her influence, the NACGN associated with the National Urban League and the National Association for the Advancement of Colored People (as early as 1916) in a collaborative effort to improve the status of black Americans. As president of the Alumnae Association of Lincoln Hospital and Home and as a member of the NACGN, Thoms represented her school and association at the International Council of Nurses convention in Cologne, Germany, in 1912, one of only three black delegates. The presence of those early black nursing leaders encouraged the membership of others, from Africa, South America, and the Caribbean.

During World War I, as president of the NACGN, Thoms waged a battle with the American Red Cross and with the Army Nurse Corps for the admission of black nurses. Jane Delano (q.v.) agreed with her, but the surgeon-general refused to authorize the use of black nurses until the war had ended. Finally, in July 1918 the first black nurse was enrolled in the American Red Cross, and in December of that year, the first black nurses were assigned to duty during the influenza epidemic. Eighteen black nurses were appointed to the Army Nurse Corps and were stationed at Camp Grant, Illinois, and Camp Sherman, Ohio, with full pay and rank. Although patients at the hospitals of those military bases were not segregated, the black nurses were assigned to separate quarters. After 1920, Thoms urged black nurses to exercise the right of suffrage and to convince their patients to do so, as part of the movement toward equal opportunity for American women.

After her retirement in 1923, Thoms continued to work with the American Nurses' Association (ANA), the National Organization for Public Health Nursing (NOPHN), and the NACGN, with the eventual goal of the integration of black nurses into the ANA and NOPHN. She was also an active member of the board of the Harlem Branch of the YWCA, the Harlem committee of the New York Tuberculosis and Health Association, and the New York Urban League. She served her community through her work at St. Mark's Methodist Church and the Hope Day Nursery, the latter providing care for children of black working women, the only facility of its kind in New York City at that time. In 1936, she was the first recipient of the Mary Mahoney Medal of the NACGN.

Toward the end of her life, she lost her sight due to diabetes, and in 1943 she died of arteriosclerotic disease at Lincoln Hospital. In 1976, she was elected to the American Nurses' Association Hall of Fame.
WRITINGS: *Pathfinders: A History of the Progress of Colored Graduate Nurses* (1929), the first recorded history of black nurses in America.
REFERENCES: *American Journal of Nursing* (May 1929), p. 560 and (April 1943), p. 419; Mary Elizabeth Carnegie, *Blacks in Nursing, 1854-1984, The Path We Tread* (1986); Jessie L. Marriner, "Public Health Nurses of the Negro Race in Alabama," *Public Health Nurse* (June 1923), pp. 304-307; *Notable American Women*, pp. 455-457; Herbert R. Northrup, "The ANA and the Negro Nurse," *American Journal of Nursing* (April 1950), pp. 207-208; Meta Rutter Pennock, ed., *Makers of Nursing History* (1940); Mabel Keaton Staupers, *No Time for Prejudice* (1961); Adah B. Thoms, *Pathfinders* (1929); *Trained Nurse and Hospital Review* (March 1943), p. 213.

JOELLEN WATSON HAWKINS

THOMSON, ELNORA ELVIRA (November 4, 1878, Illinois--April 24, 1957, San Francisco). *Nurse-educator.* Daughter of John Calvin Thomson and Mary Eliza Thomson. Never married. EDUCATION: 1909, graduated from Presbyterian Hospital School of Nursing, Chicago; for six years studied psychology with tutors; advanced work at the school of civics and philanthropy, University of Chicago. CAREER: c. 1909-1911, chief nurse, Elgin State Hospital, Elgin, Illinois; 1911-1918, director and executive secretary of the Illinois Society for Mental Hygiene; 1918-1919, director of public health nursing, American Red Cross tuberculosis commission to Italy; 1919-1920, director, department of public health nursing, Chicago School of Civics and Philanthropy; 1920-1923 and 1925-1933, professor of applied sociology and director of health and

nursing education, Portland School of Social Work, University of Oregon; 1923-1925, director of the far western office, American Child Health Association, San Francisco; 1933-1944, professor of nursing education and director, department of nursing education, University of Oregon Medical School, Portland, Oregon; 1944, lecturer, public health nursing and history of nursing, University of California, Los Angeles.
CONTRIBUTIONS: Active in professional organizations all of her professional life, Elnora Thomson served as president of the American Nurses' Association from 1930 to 1934. During her term in office, she led the association to consider its responsibility to graduate nurses in the matter of economic security. She supported better distribution of the services of nurses, the professionalization of nurse registries, and protection of the nurse during the Depression, when the Federal Emergency Relief Administration activated a medical care program.

She inaugurated the public health nursing program at the University of Oregon. Later, when there was a reorganization, the department of nursing became an integral part of the University of Oregon School of Medicine. She was the director of this department for thirteen years until her retirement in 1944. She was active in the mental hygiene movement and as a nurse-educator was an early supporter of the inclusion of psychiatric and mental health nursing in the curriculum of the basic nursing education.

Thomson was president of the Illinois State Nurses' Association (1917), president of the Oregon Organization for Public Health Nursing (1923), a member of the board of directors of the National League of Nursing Education and the National Organization for Public Health Nursing, and chapter president of the Oregon branch, American Social Workers' Association. She also was active in Community Chest organizations, the Overseas League, and the Society for Mental Hygiene. In 1941, she served as chairperson of the program committee of the International Council of Nurses (ICN), responsible for planning the 1941 Congress of the ICN which had to be postponed because of World War II.
WRITINGS: Many articles in the *American Journal of Nursing* and the *Annals of the American Academy of Political Science*; her addresses as president of the American Nurses' Association have been published in Lyndia Flanagan, *One Strong Voice: The Story of the American Nurses' Association* (1976).
REFERENCES: *American Journal of Nursing* (May 1957), pp. 718, 782; *American Women, 1935-40* (1940), p. 906; Daisy C. Bridges, *A History of the International Council of Nurses: 1899-1964* (1967), p. 109; Lyndia Flanagan, *One Strong Voice: The Story of the American Nurses' Association* (1976), pp. 87, 297, 450-465.

ALICE HOWELL FRIEDMAN

TITUS, SHIRLEY CAREW (April 1892, Alameda, California--March 21, 1967, San Francisco). *Educator; administrator.* Never married. EDUCATION: Early 1900s, graduated from St. Luke's Hospital School of Nursing, San Francisco; B.S., Columbia University, New York City; M.A., University of Michigan, Ann Arbor; 1938-1939, post-graduate study at the University of Grenoble, France. CAREER: Assistant director, St. Luke's Hospital School of Nursing; 1920-1930, director of the nursing school and nursing services, University of Michigan, Ann Arbor; administrator, Columbia Hospital, Milwaukee, Wisconsin; service with the U.S. Children's Bureau to prevent maternal and infant mortality; 1930-1938, professor and dean, Vanderbilt University School of Nursing, Nashville, Tennessee; 1939-1942, director of nursing, Children's Hospital, San Francisco; 1942-1956, executive director, California Nurses' Association.

CONTRIBUTIONS: Shirley Titus was a nurse whose contributions to the history of the profession were numerous. As executive director of the California Nurses' Association, she led the nurses of her state to higher levels of professionalism. She worked to improve the post war economic conditions of nurses, as well as helping nurses to gain power to define and direct their own practice. Realizing that nurses needed assistance in finding appropriate positions and that employees needed help in locating qualified professionals, she hired a person at the state level to work with the American Nurses' Association professional counselling and placement service. In addition, she was instrumental in obtaining the first collective bargaining contract for nurses, in Oakland, California.

Titus was responsible for establishing the baccalaureate program in nursing at Vanderbilt University. She was appointed professor and dean at Vanderbilt after a decision had been made to reorganize the nursing program into a separate and independent unit, and she successfully implemented that decision and in the process transformed the program into one of the best college-level nursing programs in the country. While she was dean, the school expanded its basic nursing program to include a strong liberal arts component, and it began to offer graduate programs. The new curriculum prepared nurses in the areas of health promotion and disease prevention as well as in the more traditional focus on caring for ill patients.

Through her long career, Titus often espoused ideas which were innovative but which withstood the test of time. She was a champion of the nursing student, warning against exploitation as a source of inexpensive labor. She argued for full-time professional staffs at hospitals, which would eliminate the more traditional dependence upon student nurses to meet staffing needs. She believed that the nursing curriculum should include the liberal arts, and especially the social sciences, as well as a focus on public health nursing. Her ideas were promulgated through articles in a variety of professional journals and through lectures presented at many conferences around the country.

She was active not only in state organizations but also at the national level through the American Nurses' Association, which she served as a member of the board as well as chairperson of various committees. She served as president of the Michigan League of Nursing Education and as a member of the board of directors and vice president of the National League of Nursing Education (NLNE). While serving the NLNE, she prepared the second edition of *A Curriculum for Schools of Nursing*, which had a profound influence on nursing schools around the nation. In 1943, she was elected to the board of directors of the American Journal of Nursing Company. In 1961, the California State Nurses' Association established a scholarship fund in her name. Finally, in 1982, she was elected to the American Nurses' Association Nursing Hall of Fame.

WRITINGS: "An Experiment in Teaching Nutrition to Student Nurses" (with Vivian M. Brown), *American Journal of Nursing* (1923), pp. 754-757; "Meeting the Cost of Nursing Service," *American Journal of Nursing* (March 1927), pp. 165-167; "The Pre-Professional Education of the Nurse," *American Journal of Nursing* (January 1928), pp. 62-66.

REFERENCES: *American Journal of Nursing* (June 1930), pp. 737-739, (March 1934), p. 288, (March 1936), p. 306, (August 1938), pp. 945-946, (November 1938), p. 1269, (February 1942), p. 214, (March 1943), p. 311, (March 1944), p. 306, (August 1961), pp. 87-89, and (May 1967), pp. 1077-1078; Lionne Conta, "Shirley C. Titus, Champion of and for Nurses," *American Journal of Nursing* (June 1930), pp. 737-739; *San Francisco Examiner* (March 22, 1967), p. 59; Shirley Titus Collection, Archives of the California State Nurses' Association, San Francisco.

LORETTA P. HIGGINS

TRACY, SUSAN E. (January 22, 1864, Lynn, Massachusetts--September 12, 1928, Lynn, Massachusetts). *Pioneer in occupational therapy.* Daughter of Cyrus M. Tracy and Caroline M. (Needham) Tracy. Never married. EDUCATION: Graduated from Massachusetts Homeopathic Hospital school of nursing, Boston; post-graduate courses at Teachers College, Columbia University, New York City. CAREER: For seven years, superintendent of the training school at Adams Nervine Asylum, Jamaica Plain, Massachusetts; taught occupational therapy at many institutions, among them Michael Reese and Presbyterian Hospitals, Chicago; Battle Creek Sanitarium, Battle Creek, Michigan, Addison

Gilbert Hospital, Gloucester, Massachusetts, Boston City Hospital, Collis P. Huntington Hospital, Massachusetts General Hospital, and Peter Bent Brigham Hospital, all in Boston, and at Dr. Ordway's sanitarium, Jamaica Plain.

CONTRIBUTIONS: Before the field of occupational therapy existed, Susan Tracy revised previous work in the field, organized it, and was creative in her approach to arts and crafts that benefited the chronically ill. She then taught others about the important benefits of occupational therapy and helped make it an acceptable specialization for nurses and other health-care providers.

Beginning her work in this field about 1906, she first worked with the mentally ill. The first health-care workers who benefited from her knowledge and experience were the nursing students of various New England schools in which she taught. Although patients had previously been put to work making various items, the goal had always been to make products which could be sold, which meant that the patients actually contributed toward the cost of their care and the city or town did not have to appropriate as much to support the public institutions. Tracy changed the focus of patient occupation from the product to the patient. The process of doing became a therapy; the product was not important if the work helped the patient's condition and attitude improved. She assessed each patient's level of ability and tried to plan work to fit the needs and aptitude of the patient.

In addition to teaching her methods, she wrote two textbooks and many articles on the subject of occupational therapy, which became classics in the field and which added to the development of the field by making her ideas readily available world wide.

In 1917, the *Maryland Psychiatric Quarterly* named its January issue the "Susan E. Tracy Number," in her honor. In one of its exhibits, the American Hospital Association provided information about her important work in the field of occupational therapy.

WRITINGS: *Studies in Invalid Occupation: A Manual for Nurses and Attendants* (1910); *Rake Knitting and Its Special Adaptation to Invalid Workers* (1916); many articles in professional journals.

REFERENCES: M. Adelaide Nutting Collection, Teachers College, Columbia University, (microfiche number 2461); Meta Rutter Pennock, ed., *Makers of Nursing History* (1940).

LORETTA P. HIGGINS

TRAVELBEE, JOYCE EVELYN (December 14, 1925--September 2, 1973, Touro Infirmary, New Orleans, Louisiana). *Leader in psychiatric nursing.*

Daughter of Charles R. Travelbee, Sr., and Marie A. (Combel) Travelbee. Never married. EDUCATION: June 1943, graduated from high school; 1943-1946, attended nursing school of Charity Hospital, New Orleans, Louisiana, graduating in 1946; 1949-1956, attended Louisiana State University School of Nursing, graduating with a B.A. in nursing education, 1956; 1957-1959, attended Yale University School of Nursing, New Haven, Connecticut, graduating in 1959 with an M.S. in mental health and psychiatric nursing; 1973, began doctoral program, Heed University, Florida (an unaccredited institution). CAREER: November 1946, staff nurse, DePaul's Sanitarium, New Orleans; November 1946-February 1947, staff nurse, DePaul Hospital, New Orleans; March-October 1947, staff nurse, University Hospital, Minneapolis, Minnesota; February 1948-July 1949, staff nurse, Lakeshore Hospital, New York City; August-December 1949, staff nurse, Willard Parker Hospital, New York City; January 1950-July 1951, staff nurse, U.S. Public Health Service Hospital, New Orleans; August-October 1951, staff nurse, Delgado Hospital, New Orleans; February-June 1952, head nurse, Charity Hospital, New Orleans; November 1952-August 1955, instructor, DePaul Hospital Affiliate School, New Orleans; September 1955-October 1956, instructor, Charity Hospital School of Nursing, New Orleans; October 1956-1965, instructor then assistant professor, Louisiana State University School of Nursing, New Orleans; February-August 1966, instructor, New York University department of nurse education; September 1, 1966-April 30, 1969, associate professor, University of Mississippi School of Nursing; 1969-1971, director of curriculum project, Hotel Dieu School of Nursing, New Orleans; 1971-1973, director of graduate education, Louisiana State University School of Nursing.

CONTRIBUTIONS: Joyce Travelbee's greatest contribution was to the specialty of psychiatric nursing. She was an outstanding educator and a distinguished scholar and theorist. Furthermore, her teaching was based on extensive clinical experience in psychiatric nursing. Beginning her teaching career shortly before graduation from a baccalaureate program, she had a distinguished career as a teacher of psychiatric and mental health nursing at New York University, the University of Mississippi, and Louisiana State University. While at the University of Mississippi, she was chairperson of the curriculum committee and was instrumental in bringing Sister Madeline Clemence there in 1969 for a faculty workshop. Sister Madeline Clemence had in 1962 published an important book on ethics in nursing practice which had a major impact on modern American nursing (*Commitment to Nursing: A Philosophical Investigation*), and since that time she lectured at numerous nursing schools on various aspects of nursing ethics. Travelbee left that position to return to New Orleans where she could be near her mother, who was ill.

Travelbee's books on interpersonal aspects of nursing and interventions in psychiatric nursing represent important contributions to the development of a theory base for nursing practice. She wrote more than a dozen articles focused on behavioral concepts in nursing. Over the course of her career, she presented more than 150 papers on various topics. She conducted workshops on curriculum revision and consulted on integrating mental health concepts into nursing practice. She used theories of interpersonal interaction in the development of her work, and explicitly defined health and illness and the roles and relationship between patient and nurse. Her work was specifically influenced by that of Ida Jean Orlando Pellitier (her instructor at Yale) and Viktor Frankl (the prominent psychiatrist).

Apparently a quiet and private person, Travelbee joined a lay sisterhood, the Third Order of Discalced Carmelites. Her untimely death at the age of forty-seven cut short the contributions of this brilliant scholar.

Over the course of her career, she received several honors, including election as University of Mississippi teacher of the year (1969) and outstanding alumna of Louisiana State University (1970). She was inducted into Kappa Delta Phi and was listed in *Who's Who in American Education--Leaders in American Science* (1968).

WRITINGS: *Interpersonal Aspects of Nursing* (1966, 1971); *Intervention in Psychiatric Nursing: Process in the One-to-One Relationship* (1969); numerous articles in professional journals.

REFERENCES: *American Journal of Nursing* (October 1973); *New Orleans States-Item* (September 1973); *New Orleans Times-Picayune* (September 5, 1973), sect. 1, p. 22; unpublished information provided by Mary Ellen Doona, Boston College, Chestnut Hill, Massachusetts, Jeannette Waits, School of Nursing, University of Mississippi Medical Center, and Theresa Lausinger, director of staff development at St. Elizabeth's Hospital, Danville, Illinois; unpublished biographical sketch (undated), Louisiana State University Medical Center School of Nursing, New Orleans, Louisiana.

JOELLEN WATSON HAWKINS

TRUTH, SOJOURNER (c. 1797, Hurley, Ulster County, New York-November 26, 1883, Battle Creek, Michigan). *Civil War volunteer nurse.* Daughter of James (also known as Bomefree or Baumfree) and Elizabeth (also known as Betsy, Ma-Ma, Mau-Mau, or Betts), slaves of Charles Hardenbergh. She was one of eleven children and was named Isabelle (also called Belle). Married Thomas (slave), about 1816; at least 4 surviving children, three of whom were sold from her before emancipation on July 4, 1827. EDUCATION: Never learned to read or write. CAREER: When her master died, her elderly parents were freed and she was sold, passing from one owner to another until 1810, when she was sold to John J. Dumont; 1810-1827, served the Dumont household in New Paltz, New York. 1827, fled, seeking refuge with Isaac and Maria Van Wagener, who gave her their name and her freedom; 1827-1829, engaged in a successful legal battle to secure the return of her son, Peter, who had been illegally sold; 1829, moved to New York City with her son; 1829-1833, worked as a domestic in New York City; between 1829 and 1831, preached with Elijah and Sarah Pierson and joined their household, spending Sundays at Magdalene Asylum teaching domestic skills to the girls; 1833, joined Robert Matthews (Matthias) in Sing Sing, New York, where they attempted to create the new kingdom of God at Zion Hill (she became involved in a scandal over the death of Elijah Pierson, and was accused of having poisoned him; she won a libel suit related to this charge); 1834-1843, maid, cook, and laundress, New York City; 1843, claimed that mysterious voices had commanded her to take the name Sojourner Truth and to travel east to preach; June 1, 1843, began a preaching career, travelling to Long Island (New York), and to Connecticut, and in the winter of 1843 to the Florence section of Northampton, Massachusetts; 1843-1846, joined the Northampton Association of Education and Industry, a communal farm and silk factory, working as chief laundress; 1846-1850, when the association collapsed, remained in Northampton as servant and guest of abolitionist George W. Benson; between 1846 and 1850, with the help of Olive Gilbert, wrote a narrative of her life, and in 1850 embarked on lecture tours, speaking on the abolition of slavery and raising money for the cause through the sale of her picture and her book; 1850, added women's rights to her concerns when she served as a delegate from Massachusetts to the first national women's rights convention in Worcester; 1851, at a women's rights convention at Akron, Ohio, uttered her famous response, "Aren't I a woman," to arguments by white male preachers that women were inferior; 1859-1864, supported herself through domestic work and continued with her anti-slavery and women's rights work, lecturing through the East and Midwest; November 1863, collected donations for the first Michigan Regiment of Colored Soldiers, and on Thanksgiving Day she brought a carriage full of food to the soldiers at Camp Ward, Detroit; 1864, convinced that she had important work to do, traveled to Washington, D.C., and in October met with President Abraham Lincoln and was approached by Reverend Henry Highland Garnet, who asked her to help raise money for the Colored Soldiers' Aid Society; after visiting the tents and barracks which housed the newly freed slaves (freedmen), began

work at Freedmen's Village, receiving in December 1864 an official commission from the National Freedmen's Relief Association, appointing her as counselor to the freed people at Arlington Heights, Virginia; 1865-1867, served as a volunteer nurse in Freedmen's Hospital, Washington, D.C., and worked for the Freedmen's Relief Society; 1869-1875, campaigned for a Negro state in the West; 1877, travelled through the Midwest and lectured on behalf of a number of causes, including women's rights, temperance, prison reform, and the rights of working men; July 1878, served as a Michigan delegate to the thirtieth anniversary of the First Women's Rights Convention; 1879, spent time in Kansas where she urged blacks to take advantage of the Homestead Law; retired to Battle Creek, Michigan, where she received hundreds of visitors (her funeral was reported to be the largest in the history of that town).
CONTRIBUTIONS: Although she is better known for her work on behalf of the abolition and women's rights movements, Sojourner Truth served as a volunteer Civil War nurse and served the newly freed slaves through her work for the Freedmen's Relief Society. In the fall of 1865, she was invited by the Bureau of Refugees, Freedmen, and Abandoned Lands (Freedmen's Bureau) to help the surgeon in charge of Freedmen's Hospital. She served there until the winter of 1867. In 1986, a commemorative stamp in her honor was issued by the U.S. Postal Service.
WRITINGS: *The Narrative of Sojourner Truth, a Northern Slave Emancipated from Bodily Servitude by the State of New York in 1828. With a Portrait* (1850, reprinted in 1853 with an introduction by Harriet Beecher Stowe; 1875, reprinted by Frances W. Titus, with additions from Sojourner Truth's "Book of Life").
REFERENCES: Jacqueline Bernard, *Journey toward Freedom: The Story of Sojourner Truth* (1967); Mary Elizabeth Carnegie, *Blacks in Nursing, 1854-1984: The Path We Tread* (1986); Arthur H. Fauset, *Sojourner Truth* (1938); *Notable American Women*, pp. 479-481; Hertha Pauli, *Her Name Was Sojourner Truth* (1967); Harriet Beecher Stowe, "Sojourner Truth, the Libyan Sibyl," *Atlantic Monthly* (April 1863), pp. 473-481.

JOELLEN WATSON HAWKINS

TUBMAN, HARRIET (1821, on the Brodas plantation, Dorchester County, Bucktown District, Maryland--March 10, 1913, Auburn, New York). *Civil War volunteer nurse.* Daughter of Benjamin Ross and Harriet (Rit) Greene, slaves; named Araminta and later chose to use her mother's name. Married a free Negro, John Tubman, c. 1844; no children. After her husband's death (1867), married Nelson Davis, Civil War veteran, 1869; no children. EDUCATION: None. CAREER:

Beginning as a young child, served as a maid, field hand, cook, and child's nurse for her master, or was hired out to others, at one time to a weaver; also worked with her father, as a woodcutter; 1847-1849, worked for Anthony Thompson, a Methodist clergyman; upon his death, fled to Philadelphia and worked there in a hotel; 1850-1860, worked on the Underground Railroad, bringing family members and others to freedom in the North; between journeys, worked as a cook in Philadelphia; in the nineteen trips she made to the Eastern Shore of Maryland, she brought out more than eighty slaves (some accounts range as high as 300), including her own siblings and her aging parents, the latter in June of 1857; at one point, there was a $40,000 reward posted for her capture by slave holders in Maryland; during her exploits, became acquainted with Thomas Garrett, a Quaker abolitionist, Frederick Douglass, the leading black abolitionist, and white abolitionists such as Wendell Phillips and John Brown, and began to participate in abolitionist rallies; reported to have assisted John Brown in finding recruits and money for his raid on the federal arsenal at Harper's Ferry, Virginia (Brown was known to refer to her as "General Tubman"); for her work on the Underground Railroad, became known as the Moses of her people; 1858 or 1859, purchased from Senator William H. Seward a small farm in Auburn, New York; 1862-1865, at the urging of Governor John Andrew of Massachusetts, William Lloyd Garrison, Dr. Samuel Gridley Howe, and other leading abolitionists, began to serve the Union army during the Civil War; with an endorsement from Governor Andrew, presented herself to General David Hunter at the headquarters of the Department of the South, Beaufort, South Carolina; as a spy, raider, and scout, led many expeditions behind Confederate lines; receiving no pay and holding no rank, she supported herself by baking pies and gingerbread and making root beer, which were sold for her by an escaped slave who resided in the contraband camp; accompanied many expeditions into the South, for the Negroes would trust her; went with several gunboats up the Combahee River, and rescued nearly 800 slaves who had escaped from plantations and who sought freedom with the Northern army; as a spy, she was fearless, braving territory behind enemy lines and bringing back information about troop positions and movements; spring and summer 1865, worked as a nurse or matron at the Colored Hospital, Fort Monroe, Virginia; 1865-1913, returned to Auburn, New York after the war, caring for her elderly parents and taking in orphans and homeless elderly persons; the Harriet Tubman Home for Indigent Aged Negroes thus came into being, and it continued for a number of years after her death; denied a pension for her war service, for which she began her fight in the late 1860s, she was assisted by the publication of a sketch of her life in 1869, written for her by a friend, Sarah Bradford; 1897, succeeded in securing her pension, when Congress rewarded her with $20 a month, ironically not for her work, but for being a widow of a Union veteran; became a champion for the rights of others who were oppressed, including women; became a leader in the women's suffrage movement, speaking at meetings with Susan B. Anthony and Elizabeth Cady Stanton; worked for the establishment of schools for free blacks in the South and in Auburn, New York.

CONTRIBUTIONS: Although she is better known for her work on the Underground Railroad and for her involvement in the abolition and women's rights movements, Harriet Tubman served as a Civil War nurse at the Colored Hospital, Fort Monroe, Virginia (spring and summer 1865). Her nursing service included bathing the wounded men, caring for their wounds, and through her knowledge of the medicinal qualities of roots, she reportedly cured men of dysentery. In addition, she was reported to have nursed hundreds who suffered from smallpox and malignant fevers. After her return to Auburn, New York, she established what in effect was a nursing home, the Harriet Tubman Home for Aged or Indigent Negroes.

At the end of the 19th century, Queen Victoria sent her a Diamond Jubilee medal, a silk shawl, and an invitation to the British Court. She died of pneumonia in 1913 at her home in Auburn, New York and was buried in the Fort Hill cemetery there, with military honors. In 1914, she was honored in Auburn with a special ceremony during which the mayor, Charles W. Brister, and Dr. Booker T. Washington delivered tributes, and a bronze tablet was dedicated in her memory. On February 1, 1978, a U.S. postage stamp was issued in her honor, commemorating Black History Week, with the original artwork for the stamp presented to Hampton Institute. In that same year, NBC television ran a two-part special on her life, "A Woman Called Moses."

WRITINGS: Book written for her by Sarah H. Bradford, *Scenes in the Life of Harriet Tubman* (1869).

REFERENCES: Bradford, *Scenes in the Life of Harriet Tubman* (1869), and *Harriet Tubman, The Moses of Her People* (2d ed., 1886); Mary Elizabeth Carnegie, *Blacks in Nursing, 1854-1984: The Path We Tread* (1986); Marcy Heidish, *A Woman Called Moses* (1976); Joan Marlow, *The Great Women* (1979); *Notable American Women*, pp. 481-483; *National Cyclopedia of American Biography*, IX :547; Judith Nies, *Seven Women: Portraits from the American Radical Tradition* (1977); Dorothy Sterling, *Freedom Train: The Story of Harriet Tubman* (1954).

JOELLEN WATSON HAWKINS

TUCKER, KATHARINE (c. 1885, probably Newton Lower Falls, Massachusetts--June 6, 1957, Philadelphia). *Public health nurse.* Never married. EDUCATION: Graduated from Newton High School; 1907, A.B., Vassar College, Poughkeepsie, New York; 1910, graduated from Newton Hospital School of Nursing. CAREER: 1911, tuberculosis worker, University of Pennsylvania social service department, Philadelphia; 1912, head worker in the social service department, New York Dispensary; 1913-1916, social service director, committee on mental hygiene, New York State Charities Aid Association; 1916-1929, general director, Visiting Nurse Society, Philadelphia, Pennsylvania; 1929-1935, general director, National Organization for Public Health Nursing; 1935-1949, director, University of Pennsylvania department of nursing education; 1949, retired.

CONTRIBUTIONS: From the earliest days of her career, Katharine Tucker showed an interest in and affinity for public health nursing. Just six years after graduating from nursing school, she became the director of the visiting nurse society of Philadelphia. From there she became the head of the National Organization for Public Health Nursing (NOPHN), and her last position, again a prestigious one, was as director of the department of nursing education at the University of Pennsylvania. Under her leadership at the University of Pennsylvania, an advanced course in maternity nursing was instituted (1942) as either part of the bachelor's degree program or as a special course of study.

In addition to holding positions of high visibility and responsibility, Tucker was active in various nursing organizations. From 1918 to 1919 she was president of the Pennsylvania State Organization for Public Health Nursing. She was first vice-president of the NOPHN from 1916 to 1918 and served as chairperson of the education committee during those same years. From 1919 to 1920 she served as president of the organization. In 1937, she became a member of the board of directors of the National Society for the Prevention of Blindness. In 1942, during World War II, she became chairperson of the committee on supply and distribution, under the auspices of the Nursing Council on National Defense. The mission of the committee was to ensure the distribution of nurses for both the armed forces and the civilian population. She was also a consultant to the subcommittee on nursing of the health and medical committee, office of defense, health, and welfare services, a subcommittee which dealt with the same problem, the distribution of nurses during the time of emergency.

WRITINGS: *Survey of Public Health Nursing, Administration, and Practice* (with Hortense Hilbert, 1934); "Public Health Nursing for the Tuberculosis Patient," *Public Health Nurse* (February 1929), p. 66; editorial, *Public Health Nurse* (April 1929), p. 173; "The Curriculum

Study," *Public Health Nursing* (May 1941), pp. 311-314; "Public Health Nursing in National Defense," *Public Health Nursing* (December 1941), pp. 697-704; "Curriculum Guide Nears Completion," *Public Health Nursing* (February 1942), pp. 89-90.
REFERENCES: *American Journal of Nursing* (September 1935), p. 893, (December 1937), p. 1405, (March 1938), p. 355, (April 1942), pp. 450 and 461, (July 1942), p. 822, and (August 1957), p. 1046; M. Louise Fitzpatrick, *The National Organization for Public Health Nursing, 1912-1952* (1975); Anne L. Hansen, "Katharine Tucker," *Public Health Nurse* (January 1929), pp. 1-2; *National League of Nursing Education Biographical Sketches* (1940); *New York Times* (June 7, 1957), p. 23; *Public Health Nursing* (December 1949), p. 683.

LORETTA P. HIGGINS

TYLER, ADELINE {BLANCHARD} (December 8, 1805, Billerica, Massachusetts--January 9, 1875, Needham, Massachusetts). *Civil War nurse; Episcopal deaconess.* Daughter of Jeremiah Blanchard, farmer, and Mary (Gowen) Blanchard. Married John Tyler, 1826; several stepchildren. EDUCATION: Attended a neighborhood academy, Billerica; 1853-1854, studied nursing at Deaconess Institute, Kaiserwerth, Germany. CAREER: Taught school in Boston; Sunday school teacher, Episcopal Church of the Advent, Boston; volunteer worker for several charitable agencies; c. 1854-1856, apparently worked as a private duty nurse in Boston; 1856-1860, founder and superintendent, St. Andrews Infirmary, Baltimore, Maryland; 1860-1861, taught nursing in her home; 1861-1864, Civil War nurse; 1864-1865, travel in Europe; 1865-1868, may have taught nursing in her home; 1868-1869, nurse with the Midnight Mission, New York City; 1869-1872, superintendent, Children's Hospital, Boston; 1872, retired due to breast cancer.
CONTRIBUTIONS: Adeline Tyler was one of the earliest trained nurses in the United States, a pioneering deaconess nurse, and a hospital superintendent. Trained in Kaiserwerth, Germany, she was invited in 1856 to go to Baltimore to establish an infirmary under the auspices of the Episcopal Diocese. On September 21, 1856, St. Andrew's Infirmary was opened, receiving its first patients. A move to the property of Washington Medical College, Baltimore, on October 7, 1857, enabled the infirmary to expand its services and become part of the Church Home and Infirmary of the City of Baltimore. That institution was officially opened on February 9, 1858, with Tyler in charge of the institution and its staff of deaconesses. When a man was appointed as her superior in

1860, however, she resigned, remaining in Baltimore to instruct candidates for deaconess life in her home.

The outbreak of the Civil War changed the nature of her work. On April 19, 1861, the Sixth Massachusetts Voluntary Infantry was attacked by mobs while passing though Baltimore. She removed the injured soldiers from the police station, where they were being held in protective custody, and treated them at the Church Home and Infirmary. In September, she was appointed superintendent of the Camden Street federal military hospital in Baltimore, a short-lived position for she disagreed with authorities over the distribution of supplies and food; she wanted to serve Confederate as well as Union soldiers. Her military nursing career was not at an end, however. Surgeon-General William A. Hammond in 1862 summoned her to become head nurse of National Hospital, Chester, Pennsylvania. In July 1863, she was at Naval School Hospital (later called U.S. General Hospital, Division No. 1), Annapolis, Maryland. Once again demonstrating her abilities in organizing nursing and improving sanitary conditions, in that position she also undertook the task of providing better and more appropriate food for the wounded through the establishment of a special diet department.

Ill health forced her to resign on May 27, 1864, and she had a respite in Europe with her sister, returning in November 1865. After her return, she spent a brief time working with the Midnight Mission in New York City, a service agency with close Episcopal ties founded in 1868 to serve prostitutes.

She was once again lured into hospital nursing, however, in 1869. This time the call came from a Unitarian institution. At the urging of Dr. Francis H. Brown, founder of the Children's Hospital of Boston, she accepted the position of lady superintendent. Her devotion to the institution was cut short when she resigned in 1872 due to breast cancer. Her Episcopal influence on the religious life of the hospital left its mark; her successor was a member of the Anglican Sisterhood of St. Margaret, East Grinstead, England, and members of the order were affiliated with the hospital and its school of nursing (founded in 1889) for years after her death.

One more trip to England was possible, and then she was forced to retire. As a tribute to her work as an Episcopal deaconess, she was elected an associate of the Sisters of St. Margaret and thereafter known as Sister Adeline Tyler. She received official recognition several times during her life, first when the Massachusetts legislature voted to thank her for the care rendered to the Sixth Massachusetts Volunteer Infantry in 1861. When she retired from the Ladies Aid Society and from the board of managers of the Children's Hospital, she received gifts and honors in recognition of her work on behalf of the hospital.

REFERENCES: L. P. Brockett and Mary C. Vaughan, *Woman's Work in the Civil War: A Record of Heroism, Patriotism and Patience* (1867); unpublished material, Deaconess History Project, Episcopal Women's History Project, New York City; Stella Goostray, *Fifty Years: A History of the School of Nursing, The Children's Hospital Boston* (1940); *Notable American Women*, pp. 491-493.

JOELLEN WATSON HAWKINS

U

URCH, DAISY DEAN (June 9, 1876, Clarkston, Michigan--June 10, 1952, Winona, Minnesota). *Nurse-educator*. Daughter of George Urch and Mary (Morrison) Urch. Never married. EDUCATION: c. 1896, received Michigan teaching certificate following attendance at normal school; 1913, graduated from Illinois Training School for Nurses, Chicago; 1927, B.S. and M.A., Teachers College, Columbia University, New York City. CAREER: c. 1896-1901, taught in a country school near Clarkston, Michigan; 1901-c. 1910, taught at Munising Public Schools, Michigan (serving as principal for seven of those years); 1913-1914, private duty nursing, Chicago; 1914-1917, head nurse, supervisor, assistant superintendent, and instructor, Illinois Training School, Chicago; 1917-1919, chief nurse, Base Hospital Number 12, France; 1919-1921, instructor, City Hospital School of Nursing, New York City; 1921-1922, instructor, Illinois Training School, Chicago; 1923-1925, inspector of schools of nursing, state of California; 1927-1933, director, Highland School of Nursing, Oakland, California; 1934-1936, educational director, Minnesota Board of Examiners of Nurses; 1936, professor of nursing education, College of St. Teresa, Winona, Minnesota; 1937, director of the department of nursing education, College of St. Teresa.

CONTRIBUTIONS: Daisy Urch was recognized as an unusually good executive in her work as a nursing school administrator. She worked hard to combat the exploitation of student nurses and to give them better educational opportunities. She was a versatile and well-educated nurse who willingly and capably filled the roles expected of a member of the nursing faculty of the 1920s and 1930s. Her early experience as a schoolteacher (and principal) undoubtedly played a major role in her training, as she was aware of the methods of education which could be adapted to a nursing school environment. After almost fifteen years of public school teaching, she entered nursing school at the age of thirty-four, following a sister and a friend as students at the Illinois Training School for Nurses, in Chicago. She apparently felt unfulfilled with her life as a schoolteacher, which precipitated her decision to enter nursing school and to change her career. After two years as a private duty nurse in Chicago, she returned to her alma mater as a head nurse and instructor, and soon she became assistant superintendent of the school.

In 1917, with the entrance of the United States into World War I, she became chief nurse for the Northwestern University Base Hospital which served in France. Her unit was one of the six which were sent to Europe shortly after the United States entered the war. At that time, Urch, along with many other nursing leaders, was a member of the American Red Cross, which then constituted the unofficial reserve of the Army Nurse Corps. Her unit, which served in Camier, Argonne, and Dijon, received special mention in the Haig dispatches, the reports prepared by Sir Douglas Haig, the British general. His dispatches covered the most important features on the western front, and served as a report to the British people. Being mentioned in the Haig dispatches was a great honor, much like receiving a medal for extraordinary service.

After the war, she served in important positions in New York City, Chicago, and Oakland, California, and as inspector of schools of nursing for the state of California. From 1934 to 1936, she was educational director for the Minnesota State Board of Examiners of Nurses, and from that position she was recruited to become professor of nursing education and director of the department of nursing of the College of St. Teresa, Winona, Minnesota.

She was active in many nursing organizations, serving in a leadership capacity. She was president of the California State League of Nursing Education, and president and member of the board of directors of the California State Nurses' Association. When she moved to Minnesota, she served as president of the Minnesota League of Nursing Education and as a member of the board of directors of the Minnesota State Organization for Public Health Nursing. On the national scene, she served as a member of the board of directors of the National League of Nursing Education (NLNE), as a member of the NLNE committee on accreditation, and as chairperson and member of the NLNE committee on state board problems (1937).

REFERENCES: *American Journal of Nursing* (1952), p. 478; Sister M. Domitilla, "Daisy Dean Urch," ms. in the American Journal of Nursing Collection, Nursing Archives, Mugar Memorial Library, Boston University; Sir Douglas Haig, "Dispatches," (D544 A2, 43); Philip and Beatrice Kalisch, *The Advance of American Nursing* (1978), p. 299; Grace

Fay Schryver, *A History of the Illinois Training School for Nurses, 1880–1929* (1930).

ALICE HOWELL FRIEDMAN

V

VAIL, STELLA {BOOTHE} (c. 1890, Illinois--c. 1926, Philadelphia). *Public health nurse.* Married. EDUCATION: 1913, graduated from Children's Hospital School of Nursing, Columbus, Ohio. CAREER: 1913-1915, worked with the mentally ill; 1915, social worker at Music School Settlement, New York City; 1916, community health nurse, Cheney Silk Mills; 1918, nurse in charge of pneumonia ward, Camp Lewis, Washington; investigated Seattle canneries, posing as a worker; Red Cross hygiene instructor in Idaho, working with the Nez Perce tribe; created marionette troop to teach health and hygiene to children; lectured to health workers at the University of Michigan and to medical students at New York University.

CONTRIBUTIONS: Stella Boothe Vail used her creative talents to implement a unique method for teaching health promotion and disease prevention. In a short thirteen-year career, her creativity was evident in a variety of positions in which she developed unique methods to advance the public health. She uncovered damaging health practices in industry, made a statistical study of influenza cases at Camp Lewis, and taught health and hygiene to the Indians. Her fame, however, was associated with her use of marionettes, sophisticated graphic design, and clever scenery, as her troop performed at countless fairs, exhibitions, and conventions. In addition to entertaining their audience, the result was to emphasize the importance of hygiene and public health, as well as to describe the work of nurses, especially visiting nurses.

One of the first of her major exhibitions was in Seattle, at a nursing convention in 1922. At that convention, many people learned of her work and as a result she received many assignments and invitations to perform all over the country. She planned and executed the nursing exhibit at the Sesquicentennial Exposition in Philadelphia, and although the results of her work did not lend themselves to being quantified, at the very least she delighted, educated, and informed both the general public as well as members of her own profession.

Earlier in her career, she used her acting ability to get a job, as Susie Brown, a drab, tired worker, and that enabled her to investigate the health practices of the Seattle canning industry. Vail also was an early industrial nurse, working with the community to develop health and recreational programs, including mothers' clubs and clinics for children and pregnant women.

She wrote a number of children's books, many of which taught children about health by imaginative story-telling. While preparing an exhibition for the major nursing organizations, she suffered an attack of appendicitis, underwent emergency surgery, and never regained consciousness, dying three days after the operation.

WRITINGS: "Mary Gay Books": *A Bedtime Adventure*; *Mary Gay's Stories*; *The Morning Circus*; and *Jimmie and the Junior Safety Council.*

REFERENCES: *American Journal of Nursing* (October 1926), p. 789; Elise Van Ness, "Telling the World about Nursing," *American Journal of Nursing* (October 1926), pp. 775-779; Meta Rutter Pennock, *Makers of Nursing History* (1928, 1940).

LORETTA P. HIGGINS

VAN BLARCOM, CAROLYN CONANT (June 12, 1879, Alton, Illinois--March 20, 1960, Arcadia, California). *Maternity nursing leader; midwife.* Daughter of William Dixon Van Blarcom, financier, and Fanny Emelie (Conant) Van Blarcom, linguist and pianist. Never married. EDUCATION: Taught by her mother at home, as she suffered both rheumatic fever and rheumatoid arthritis as a child (her mother died when Carolyn was fourteen years old, and she apparently then lived with her grandfather and other relatives); 1896-1898, chaperone for young students, Hasbrourch Institute, Jersey City, New Jersey, and continued her education there; 1898-1901, attended Johns Hopkins Hospital Training School for Nurses, Baltimore, Maryland, graduating in 1901. CAREER: 1901-1908, supervising nurse, instructor in obstetrical nursing and the care of infants and children, and second assistant superintendent of nurses, Johns Hopkins Hospital Training School; 1908, helped reorganize St. Luke's Hospital Training School, St. Louis, Missouri; (her career was interrupted for 3 years due to ill health); served the nursing and purvey departments, Maryland TB Sanatorium, Sabillisville, Maryland, and the sanatorium at New Bedford, Massachusetts; 1909-1916, secretary of the New York State Committee for the Prevention of Blindness (which

became a national institution); 1916-1917, undertook the same position for the Illinois Society for the Prevention of Blindness; 1917-January 1918, represented the American Red Cross Service in the Atlantic Division; 1920s, health editor of the *Delineator* and wrote and worked on behalf of women and their infants; early 1930s, retired due to ill health.
CONTRIBUTIONS: Although plagued by ill health throughout her life, Carolyn Van Blarcom contributed more to the good health of women and their infants than almost any other nurse of her generation. As secretary of the New York State Committee for the Prevention of Blindness, she undertook a vigorous campaign to end ophthalmia neonatorum, the leading cause of blindness of newborns, caused by intrapartum transfer of the gonorrhea organism from the mother to the infant's eyes. At the time she was practicing, both the cause and prevention were known, but the prevention was not consistently practiced, particularly by midwives, who were in attendance at 50 percent of births. In 1911, she received a grant from the Russell Sage Foundation to conduct a study of midwifery practices in sixteen countries, including England and the United States. She collected information from fourteen countries through the mail and visited England for her investigation of the Midwives' Act, including examination of the laws regarding training, licensure, control, and supervision and the history of midwifery in that country. The report, published in 1913 as *The Midwife in England*, demonstrated that the United States was the only country she surveyed that had no provision for systematic training and licensing of midwives.

Van Blarcom was the first nurse in the United States to be licensed as a midwife, and she is best known as a reformer of midwifery. She was the first person to make a national survey of city and county laws regarding midwifery practice. Following her study, she undertook the cause of the health of mothers and babies through various channels. She wrote extensively, addressing issues concerned with health for the lay public and those concerned with the roles of professionals for medical journals. She was instrumental in the establishment of the Bellevue School of Midwifery in New York City, which provided training between 1911 and 1935 for midwives in an attempt to either make them eligible to practice or to improve their practice and thus improve the health of the women and infants for whom they cared. She served with Lillian Wald (q.v.) and a physician on a subcommittee to establish the course of training for the school. She also served as the chairperson of the midwifery committee of the National Organization for Public Health Nursing. She even arranged for Mary Breckinridge (q.v.) to go to London to be trained as a midwife. Carolyn Van Blarcom was honored for work in midwifery by being named an honorary member of England's Midwives' Institute.

After graduating from the Johns Hopkins Hospital Training School, she demonstrated her remarkable administrative abilities in two posts in tuberculosis sanatoriums. She is credited with turning two dismal and disorganized institutions in well-funded model hospitals. Her reputation as an executive led to her appointment to the New York Committee for the Prevention of Blindness and, after eight years with that organization, to a similar position with the Illinois Society for the Prevention of Blindness.

Feeling the call to serve her country when it entered World War I, Van Blarcom left the Illinois Society to represent the American Red Cross Nursing Service in the Atlantic Division, consisting of New York, New Jersey, and Connecticut. Living in New York, she became a member of the New York chapter of the American Red Cross and director of nursing for the Atlantic Division. She was a chief organizer and participant in the first historic parade of Red Cross Army and Navy nurses down Fifth Avenue, New York City, on October 10, 1917. In that year she also served as an ex-officio member of the Committee on Equipment and undertook a speaking tour of the United States in December 1917 and January 1918 to interest nurses in war service with the Red Cross. Once again ill health forced her resignation, however, on January 15, 1918.

Van Blarcom would not let illness stand in the way of her contributions to the welfare of women and children. Having begun her work as an instructor in obstetrical nursing, she spent one and a half years studying the scope and methods of training in maternity nursing in the United States and Canada in preparation for writing a textbook. First published as *Obstetrical Nursing* in 1922, this book eventually went through six editions, was translated into many languages, and was used in Europe, Australia, and China. The letters, brimming with accolades for the book from physicians, nurses, and laypersons, fill a scrapbook among her personal papers in the Johns Hopkins Archives.

Her writing was hardly confined to texts. During the 1920s, she served as health editor of the *Delineator*, a popular women's magazine, and she wrote *Getting Ready to Be a Mother* (1922), which went through four editions, and *Building the Baby* (1929). On July 3, 1924, she addressed the Third English-Speaking Conference on Infant Welfare in Caxton Hall, London, England, on the subject of maternity care in the United States, one of only four Americans invited to speak at this conference called by order of the king and queen. At the 1925 Congress of the International Council of Nurses in Helsinki, she delivered a paper describing conditions of midwifery in the United States. The role of the nurse in prenatal care was the subject of another paper, delivered in January 1926 at the Third Annual Conference of State Directors in

Charge of the Local Administration of the Maternity and Infancy Act, Washington, D.C.

Her twelve practical pamphlets on pregnancy, delivery, and care of the newborn had perhaps the widest impact of all her work, for they were distributed by the thousands by state and local health departments. She had a remarkable ability to synthesize information from the health care sciences and make it meaningful to women, as those pamphlets so clearly demonstrate.

Besides the work of her pen, her forced retirement in the 1930s was filled with service. She chaired the Literature Group of the American Women's Association and during World War II served briefly in training nurses' aides for the American Red Cross chapter in Pasadena, California. On behalf of Johns Hopkins, she secured a bequest for the E. Bayard Halsted Fund for Medical Research, was an adminstrative assistant in civil defense, chaired the Health and Sanitation Committee of the Women's Civil League, and organized and chaired the Pasadena Committee for Maternal Welfare. She was a member of the Women's Auxiliary and a member of the committee on nurses' scholarships and nursing recruitment for Huntington Hospital. After the war, however, her health continued to deteriorate, and apparently after a great deal of suffering, in 1960 she died in Arcadia, California, of bronchopneumonia.

WRITINGS: *The Midwife in England* (1913); *Obstetrical Nursing* (1922, 5 subsequent editions); *Getting Ready to Be a Mother* (1922); *Building the Baby* (1929); numerous pamphlets and articles in lay and professional journals.

REFERENCES: *American Journal of Nursing* (June 1960), p. 784; Daisy Caroline Bridges, *A History of the International Council of Nurses, 1899-1964, the First 65 Years* (1967); Lavinia L. Dock, Sarah E. Pickett, Clara D. Noyes, Fannie F. Clement, Elizabeth G. Fox, and Anna R. Van Meter, *History of American Red Cross Nursing* (1922); "Honors for Carolyn Van Blarcom" *Johns Hopkins Nurses Alumni Magazine* (May 16, 1901), pp. 79-81; Ethel Johns and Blanche Pfefferkorn, *The Johns Hopkins Hospital School of Nursing* 1889-1949 (1954); *Johns Hopkins Nursing Alumnae Magazine* (May 1916), pp. 79-81; Portia B. Kernodle, *The Red Cross Nurse in Action 1882-1948* (1949); *Notable American Women: The Modern Period*, pp. 703-704; Meta Rutter Pennock, ed., *Makers of Nursing History* (1928), pp. 86-87; Carolyn Conant Van Blarcom, *Obstetrical Nursing* (1922), *Obstetrical Nursing* (2d ed., 1928), and typed addendum for biography for *Biographical Cyclopedia of American Women*, n.d., in Nightingale Room, Welch Library, Johns Hopkins Medical Institutions, Baltimore; Helen Varney, *Nurse-Midwifery* (1980).

JOELLEN WATSON HAWKINS

VREELAND, ELLWYNNE MAE (November 28, 1909, Stockbridge, Massachusetts--December 12, 1971, Riviera Beach, Florida). *Nurse-researcher.* Daughter of William L. Vreeland and Edith M. (Block) Vreeland. Never married. EDUCATION: 1929-1934, attended Massachusetts General Hospital School of Nursing, Boston, graduating April 4, 1934; 1942, B.S. and 1949, M.A., Teachers College, Columbia University, New York City; 1935, 1937, attended University of Vermont; 1938-1939, attended University of Rochester. CAREER: 1934-1935, staff nurse and operating room assistant, Saranac Lake General Hospital, New York; 1935-1936, staff nurse, Stony Wold, Lake Kushaqua, New York; 1936-1939, staff nurse, night charge and emergency division, Strong Memorial Hospital, Rochester, New York; 1940-1942, director of nurses, Schenectady County Tuberculosis Hospital, Schenectady, New York; 1943-1945, assistant director of the nursing division, Albany Hospital, Albany, New York, and Russell Sage College, Troy, New York; 1945-1968, commissioned officer, U.S. Public Health Service; 1945-1948, nursing education consultant, U.S. Public Health Service; 1949-1955, chief nurse, education division of nursing research, U.S. Public Health Service; 1955-1968, chief of research grants division, U.S. Public Health Service.
CONTRIBUTIONS: Ellwynne Vreeland was a strong voice for nursing in the U.S. Public Health Service (USPHS) and in the federal government as a whole. As the first chief of the Research Grant and Fellowship Branch of the Division of Nursing Resources, she developed a program of support for extramural research and for research training in nursing. Through her work, she laid the foundation for federal support for post-graduate education and for nursing research. She convinced various officials in the USPHS of the need for graduate education in nursing and for federal funding for nursing research. She also served on the editorial board of *Nursing Research.*

Entering the USPHS uniformed corps (as well as being an enrolled Red Cross nurse) during World War II, she served as education consultant to the Cadet Nurse Corps. After the war, she was assigned to the Division of Nurse Resources and in 1955 was appointed chief of the Research and Fellowship Branch, Division of Nursing Resources. During this time she was also awarded a Rockefeller Fellowship for graduate study. In 1962, she became chief of the Research and Resources Branch, Division of Nursing and in 1964, nursing research consultant, Intramural Research Branch, Division of Nursing. She retired in 1968.

Over the course of her career, she received numerous awards. As a result of her service during World War II, she received the American Campaign Medal as well as the National Defense Medal. In 1961 she received a medal and citation from the Massachusetts General Hospital. In 1966, she received the U.S. Public Health Service Meritorious Service

Award. In 1970, Teachers College of Columbia University bestowed upon her its Distinguished Achievement Award in Research and Scholarship. In 1984, she was inducted into the American Nurses' Association Hall of Fame.

WRITINGS: Numerous articles in professional journals, including "Fifty Years of Nursing in the Federal Government Nursing Services," *American Journal of Nursing* (October 1950), pp. 626-631; *Cost Analysis for Collegiate Schools of Nursing* (part 1, 1956, part 2, 1957); numerous reports and government publications.

REFERENCES: *American Journal of Nursing* (December 1971); unpublished materials, Nursing Archives, Mugar Memorial Library, Boston University; *Who's Who of American Women* (1st ed., 1959), p. 1317, (3d ed., 1964-1965), p. 1049, and (4th ed., 1966-1967), p. 1192.

JOELLEN WATSON HAWKINS

W

WAECHTER, EUGENIA HELMA (March 29, 1925, Crespo, Argentina--January 12, 1982, Redwood City, California). *Pediatric nurse; nurse-researcher.* Daughter of missionary parents. Never married. EDUCATION: 1942, graduated from Meissner High School, Bunker Hill, Illinois; 1942-1944, attended St. John's College, Winfield, Kansas, receiving A.A., 1944; 1944-1947, attended Lutheran Hospital School of Nursing, St. Louis, Missouri, graduating in August 1947; September 1948, B.S. in biological science and public health nursing, University of Chicago; 1959, M.A. in pediatric nursing, University of Chicago; September 1963-September 1964, studied advanced maternal-child nursing, University of California, San Francisco; September 1964-June 1968, doctoral studies at Stanford University, receiving Ph.D. in child development and education in June 1968. CAREER: November 1948-June 1954, public health nurse, Montgomery County Health Department, Hillsboro, Illinois; June 1954-March 1955, supervising nurse, Montgomery County Health Department; March 1955-June 1958 and September 1959-August 1963, nursing consultant, University of Illinois Division of Services for Crippled Children, Olney, Illinois; September 1964-June 1966 and September 1967-September 1968, lecturer, School of Nursing, University of California, San Francisco; September 1968-July 1973, assistant professor, July 1973-January 1982, associate professor and then acting chairperson and professor, family health nursing, University of California, San Francisco.

CONTRIBUTIONS: Eugenia Waechter was a pioneer in both nursing research and in the area of pediatric nursing. One significant study, "Death Anxiety in Children with Fatal Illness," her initial work, was completed in 1968. It was the first controlled study done directly with children who were terminally ill. Her research program focused on chronic and life-threatening illness in children, the concerns of school-age children with life-threatening conditions, and the concerns of other family members. Numerous investigators replicated her work, contributing to theory building for the profession to which she was so deeply committed. At the time of Waechter's untimely death, she was involved in a federally funded investigation of the responses of children who were found to have cancer. Her work on the care available to children and their families had an enormous impact on the development of a theory base for the profession, and on the work of other researchers.

Waechter's service to the University of California was exemplary. She taught or participated in many courses in maternal child health, child development, family study, and research. She served on numerous dissertation committees and as a faculty member for qualifying examinations of graduate students. Her committee service to the School of Nursing, her department, and the university was immense. Clearly she was well-respected among her peers and colleagues and valued for her leadership. Often she served as coordinator or chairperson of a unit of the school.

Along with teaching, research, service to the university, and writing, she also made significant contributions to the profession. She served as a member of the review panel for *Nursing Research* from 1973 to 1982 and on the editorial board of the *Journal of the Association for Child Care in Hospitals* and on the association's executive board from 1976 to 1978. She was a member of the Society for Research in Child Development, the Foundation for Thanatology and its professional advisory board, the American Nurses' Association (ANA), the American Association for Child Care in Hospitals, the council of nurse-researchers of the ANA, the Cooperative Graduate Education in Nursing Council, the Western Society for Research in Nursing, and the executive board of the San Francisco Faculty Association.

Waechter's presentations, speeches, and papers span the decades from 1965 to 1982. She was known across the United States and around the world, having presented papers and workshops from California to New York and in Canada, Nigeria, Turkey, and Yugoslavia. Widely sought as a consultant, she shared her expertise and experience, particularly with groups whose concern was children and especially children with terminal illnesses. She was a compassionate and scholarly clinician, committed to the children and their families. Indeed, she seemed to have dedicated her research in the hope that her work might help nurses to provide meaningful care to others.

Her publications span decades and represent important contributions to the literature and knowledge about children, their experiences with death, and pediatric nursing. With her colleague

Florence Blake (q.v.), she published two editions of *Nursing Care of Children* (Blake had published seven editions) that were translated into Polish, Portuguese, and Spanish. Subsequent editions include other colleagues as co-authors, and the book has continued after her death to be widely used as a classic in the field. Waechter also contributed to three audiovisual presentations concerned with pediatric nursing, the death of a child, and fear and pain as experienced by children.

At the time of her death due to smoke inhalation from a fire in her home, she was acting chairperson of the department of family health care nursing, University of California, San Francisco, and was completing the tenth edition of *Nursing Care of Children.* Colleagues characterize her as an outstanding scholar and a humanitarian, whose work was on the cutting edge of knowledge in her field. Her work lives on through that of her colleagues and students. She was a leader who will continue to have a profound impact on pediatric nursing practice and on the development and evolution of pediatric nursing.

Over the course of her career, she received numerous awards, beginning with her graduation from St. John's College with highest honors (1944). She received the first honors scholarship awarded by the Lutheran Hospital School of Nursing (1947), and graduated cum laude from the University of Chicago (1959) and Stanford University (1968). She was included in numerous biographical directories, including *Who's Who in Child Development Specialists* (1976), *Personalities of the West and Midwest* (1977 and 1979), *Personalities of America* (1978), *Dictionary of International Biography* (1978), *Notable Americans of 1978-79*, *Community Leaders and Noteworthy Americans* (1979), *International Who's Who in Education* (1979), *International Register of Profiles* (1979), *International Who's Who of Intellectuals* (1979), *The International Who's Who in Community Service* (1979, 1980), *The World Who's Who of Women* (1979), *Men and Women of Distinction* (1979), *Who's Who of American Women* (1981-1982), and the *Directory of Distinguished Americans* (1981). Her textbook received the *American Journal of Nursing* Book of the Year Award in 1976. Her curriculum vitae is included in the Archives of the Missouri Nurses' Association as a nurse who made a significant contribution to the profession. She was the first selected guest lecturer for the Fitzman Chair for Nursing Education, Children's Health Center, Minneapolis, Minnesota (1978). In 1978, she was elected as a fellow of the American Academy of Nursing and selected by the doctoral students of the graduating class of the University of California, San Francisco, for recognition for her work and dedication to the university and to doctoral education. She was elected to the Society for Adolescent Medicine in that year. In 1979, she was invited as a distinguished fellow by the American Platform Association and invited to become a fellow of the International

Biographical Association of Cambridge, England, entitled to use F.I.B.A. (Fellow of the International Biographical Association) after her name. The text, *The Child and Family Facing Life Threatening Illness: A Tribute to Eugenia Waechter*, edited by Tamar Krulik, Bonnie Holaday, and Ida Martinson, was published in 1987 and contains work written by Waechter.
WRITINGS: Numerous articles in professional journals; *Nursing Care of Children*, 1970, 1976, 1985.
REFERENCES: *American Journal of Nursing* (May 1982), p. 862; biographical directories listed above; unpublished materials provided by Bonnie Holaday, School of Nursing, University of California, San Francisco.

JOELLEN WATSON HAWKINS

WALD, LILLIAN D. (March 10, 1867, Cincinnati, Ohio--September 1, 1940, Westport, Connecticut). *Public health nurse; social reformer.* Daughter of Max D. Wald, dealer in optical goods, and Minnie (Schwarz) Wald. Never married. EDUCATION: 1891, diploma, New York Hospital School of Nursing, New York City; 1892, enrolled but did not complete medical studies, Women's Medical College, New York City. CAREER: 1891-1892, nurse, New York Juvenile Asylum, New York City; 1893-1933, nurse and director, Henry Street Settlement, New York City.
CONTRIBUTIONS: Lillian Wald was a leader of the public health nursing movement in the United States. With her classmate, Mary Brewster, she lived and worked as a visiting nurse on the Lower East Side of New York City. Their residence was first known as the "nurses' settlement" and later as the Henry Street Settlement. As a settlement house worker, she helped to improve the daily life of the immigrants who lived on the Lower East Side. She helped them to learn English and to qualify for their citizenship papers. She loved children and provided space for their play and other activities. She sought adequate funding for nursing services from community leaders, including Jacob Schiff, Felix M. Warburg, and Mrs. Solomon Loeb, who became benefactors of the settlement. Wald was instrumental in setting up playgrounds in a city where children had no place to play except in the streets or in crowded tenements. She demonstrated the value of public health nursing in the city schools, by persuading Mayor Seth Low's reform-minded administration to assign a Henry Street nurse to one of the public schools. This nurse, Lina (Rogers) Struthers, (q.v), gave treatments to school children, made visits to their homes, and authorized the return to school of children who had recovered from communicable disease.

Many nursing leaders received training at the Henry Street Settlement House, including Lavinia Dock (q.v.) and Adelaide Nutting (q.v.). Wald was exceptionally tolerant of others, and in August 1908, when the founders of the National Association of Colored Graduate Nurses met in New York City, she and the Henry Street nurses gave them a welcoming luncheon. Wald developed innovative financial arrangements for nursing care, such as reimbursement from the Metropolitan Life Insurance Company for nursing services provided to their industrial policyholders. She encouraged the development of visiting nurse services for rural communities, and urged that public health nursing be included in the training of nurses. She taught courses in public health nursing at Teachers College of Columbia University, and was instrumental in securing funding for that program through the largesse of her friend, Helen Hartley Jenkins. In 1912 she was founder and first president of the National Organization for Public Health Nursing.

Wald was interested in labor conditions, and in 1904 she founded (with Florence Kelley) the National Child Labor Committee. She was a moving force in the passage of the act creating the federal Children's Bureau in 1912. Following the tragic fire at the Triangle shirtwaist factory, in which so many young women from her neighborhood died, she worked to secure inspection of factories and enforcement of municipal regulations for health and safety. Her study of the labor camps for workers building the barge canal and the aqueduct for the New York City water system resulted in the formation of the New York State Bureau of Industries and Immigrations. With her friend Jacob Riis, she fought for reform of the tenement laws, and with others she organized the Joint Board of Sanitary Control to enforce basic sanitary rules on the Lower East Side. She was a pacifist, and in 1914 (with Jane Addams, Florence Kelley, and others) she organized the American Union Against Militarism. Yet, in 1917 when the United States entered World War I, she was a strong contributor to the country's war effort, serving as a member of the Committee on Nursing of the General Medical Board of the Council of National Defense and also was a member of the Committee for the Vassar (nurse) Training Camp, Poughkeepsie, New York. Her interest in international affairs led her to join with Florence Kelley and Jane Addams of the forerunner of the Foreign Policy Association, which through one of its branches became the Civil Liberties Union. She travelled widely, and during an around-the-world tour in 1910, her visit to China and Japan were covered by the *New York Times* in a front-page story.

Wald received numerous awards in recognition of her work on behalf of humanity. In 1912, she received an honorary doctor of laws degree from Mt. Holyoke College, and in 1930 Smith College gave her another honorary doctorate. She received the gold medal of the National Institute of Social Services (sponsored by the Rotary Club). In 1937, she received a distinguished service certificate of the city of New York, and on December 2, 1940, there were memorial tributes from President Franklin D. Roosevelt, two of New York's mayors (Lehman and LaGuardia), former governor Alfred E. Smith, as well as leaders of America's health and social service agencies. In 1971 Wald was elected to the Hall of Fame for Great Americans, at New York University, and in 1976 she was inducted as a charter member of the American Nurses' Association's Hall of Fame.

WRITINGS: *The House on Henry Street* (1915); *Windows on Henry Street* (1934); a number of articles in *Survey*, *American Journal of Nursing*, and *Public Health Nursing*; introduction to *Public Health Nurse in Action* (1941).

REFERENCES: *American Women, 1935-1940* (1940), p. 937; R. L. Duffus, *Lillian Wald, Neighbor and Crusader* (1938); Irving Howe, *World of Our Fathers* (1976); *Notable American Women* (1971), pp. 526-529; Mary M. Roberts, *American Nursing: History and Interpretation* (1955); Helen Huntington Smith, "Rampant But Respectable," in *New Yorker* (December 14, 1929); Adah B. Thoms, *Pathfinders* (1929); Edward Wagenknecht, *Daughter of the Covenant* (1983); Robert Woods and Albert J. Kennedy, *The Handbook of Settlements* (1911) and *The Settlement Horizon* (1922); Edna Yost, *American Women in Nursing* (1947); Lillian Wald's papers and documents from the Henry Street Settlement are at the American Jewish Archives, Cincinnati, Ohio, the manuscript and archive division of the New York Public Library, and the rare book and manuscript division of Columbia University's Butler Library.

ALICE HOWELL FRIEDMAN

WATERS, YSSABELLA GERTRUDE (February 22, 1862, Groton, Massachusetts--August 16, 1938, Groton, Massachusetts). Daughter of Charles H. Waters and Mary (Farnsworth) Waters. *Spanish-American War Nurse; public health nurse.* Married but divorced after her husband left her; the court authorized her to return to her maiden name. EDUCATION: 1895-1897, attended Johns Hopkins Hospital Training School for Nurses, Baltimore, Maryland, graduating in 1897. CAREER: 1897-1898, nurse at Henry Street Settlement, New York City; 1898-1899, nurse during the Spanish-American War; 1899-1912, nurse at Henry Street Settlement, New York City (working with Lillian Wald, {q.v.}); 1912-1922, director of statistical work, National Organization for Public Health Nursing; 1917-1919, Red Cross work; 1919, became chief,

Division of Public Health Nursing, Bureau of Information, American Red Cross.

CONTRIBUTIONS: Yssabella Waters is best known for her statistical work for the National Organization for Public Health Nursing (NOPHN) and for her book *Visiting Nursing in the United States*, a leading source book of its day. This book outlined the history, principles, and organization of visiting nurse and public health nursing services and agencies, as well as being a state-by-state directory. Beginning in 1902, at her own expense, she also accumulated annual statistics on public health nurses that were published and distributed through the NOPHN. Her work encompassed not only the activities of nurses in visiting nurse associations and services, but also Red Cross nurses and public health nurses working for hospitals, counties, and other local governmental bodies, as well as for businesses and schools. In 1905, at the International Conference of Charities and Corrections, she presented a statistical report on the status of organizations and nurses engaged in public health work.

When the NOPHN opened an office in New York City in 1912, Waters was one of the three occupants, making more formal the statistical work she had been carrying on for the past ten years. For the next twelve years, she served as statistician for the new organization. When in 1915 the NOPHN moved to larger quarters, she rented her own office in the suite in order to continue her important volunteer work, and she even contributed toward the salary of an assistant. She was responsible for an annual compilation of public health agencies in the United States. In 1919, she published a description of nursing in industry, the result of her survey of such work, as well as a description of the qualifications and responsibilities of such nurses. Another of her tasks for the organization was correspondence and responses to requests for information about public health nursing. She responded to hundreds of letters requesting information each year, providing statistical information, as well as resources and books about public health nursing. Sincerely interested in educational preparation for public health nursing, she contributed to a scholarship fund to enable a nurse to study in preparation for a role as a public health nurse.

In 1915, she was asked to serve on the Endowment Committee of the Johns Hopkins Nursing School, and she served as the secretary of the committee until 1926. In 1916, she was elected president of the Nurse's Club of the New York City area. She was also a member of the Society of Spanish-American War Nurses, serving as vice-president of that organization. During World War I, she organized the public health nursing division of the placement work for the American Red Cross, deferring her retirement until October 1, 1920. She was chosen in 1917 to serve on the Committee on Home Nursing of the section on welfare,

committee on labor, under the Council of Defense. When she retired, she returned to Groton, Massachusetts, where she kept busy with women's clubs, several small clubs, and five churches, as well as her gardening.
WRITINGS: *Visiting Nursing in the United States* (1909); numerous articles and reports in professional journals. REFERENCES: Alan Mason Chesney Medical Archives, Johns Hopkins Medical Institutions; *American Journal of Nursing* (October 1905), pp. 26-31; Lavinia L. Dock, Sarah E. Pickett, Clara D. Noyes, Fannie F. Clement, Elizabeth G. Fox, and Anna R. Van Meter, *History of American Red Cross Nursing* (1922); M. Louise Fitzpatrick, *The National Organization for Public Health Nursing, 1912-1952* (1975); Mary S. Gardner, *Public Health Nursing* (3d ed., 1936); Ethel Johns and Blanche Pfefferkorn, *The Johns Hopkins Hospital School of Nursing 1889-1949* (1954); Johns Hopkins Nurses' Alumni Association, biographical information; *Public Health Nurse* (1919), pp. 658-659, (1920), pp. 886-887, and (1922), p. 491; Ysabella Waters, "Report of the Statistical Department," *Public Health Nurse* (June 1920), pp. 473-475, "Industrial Nursing," (September 1919), pp. 728-731, and *Visiting Nursing in the United States* (1909); *Woman's Who's Who of America* (1914).

JOELLEN WATSON HAWKINS

WHITMAN, WALT{ER} (May 31, 1819, West Hills, Huntington, Long Island, New York--March 26, 1892, Camden, New Jersey). *Civil War volunteer nurse.* Son of Walter Whitman, farmer and carpenter, and Louisa (Van Velsor) Whitman, homemaker. Never married. EDUCATION: Attended public school in Brooklyn, but his studies ended in his eleventh or thirteenth year. CAREER: c. 1830, office boy for a lawyer and then a doctor; c. 1832, became a printer's devil in the office of the *Long Island Patriot* and the *Long Island Star*; 1833-1836, journeyman compositor in Brooklyn and New York, occasionally writing for newspapers; 1836-1841, taught in seven schools on Long Island and edited the *Long Islander* from 1838-1839; 1838-1840, teacher and typesetter in Jamaica, Long Island; 1841-1848, associated with at least ten newspapers or magazines in New York and Brooklyn, including *Aurora*, *Sun*, *Tattler*, *Brooklyn Eagle*, and *Democratic Review*, the last the best literary journal of its day; January 1846, became editor of the *Brooklyn Eagle*, a democratic newspaper, but lost the job in January 1848 due to his vehemence over the slavery issue; February 1848, wrote for the *New Orleans Crescent*, but after three months left to return to Brooklyn via St. Louis, Chicago, and the Great Lakes; 1848-1849, wrote for *Freeman*; 1850, wrote for the *Daily Advertiser*; 1850-1854, wrote for various papers, and 1851-1854 helped his father build houses in Brooklyn; 1855,

published *Leaves of Grass*, the first edition consisting of twelve poems; in 1856, a second edition was ready with twenty-one new poems, and in 1860 a third edition was published, with more than one hundred new poems; 1857-1859, editor of the *Brooklyn Times*; 1861-1862, published in *The Standard* a series of articles on the history of Brooklyn and four articles on the Broadway Hospital, Brooklyn, New York; December 1862, went to Virginia in search of his brother George, who had been wounded in the Civil War; at that point, he decided that he had to be involved with the war effort, and he moved to Washington, D.C., and devoted himself to caring for soldiers in military hospitals in the city; January 1865, became clerk in the Department of the Interior, but was dismissed on June 30 due to the content of poems in *Leaves of Grass*; subsequently served in the Department of Justice and was on the payroll until June 30, 1874; February 1873, suffered a stroke and retired to his brother George's home in Camden, New Jersey, where he lived and wrote until 1884, when he moved to his own house and continued writing until his death in 1892.
CONTRIBUTIONS: Walt Whitman served as a volunteer nurse in the Civil War. December 21, 1862 he recorded in his journal as the first day that he visited military hospitals of the Army of the Potomac. By his own estimate, he is believed to have tended 80,000 to 100,000 soldiers from both sides in the conflict. He cared for 600 cases in the Battle of Gettysburg. In 1864-1865, he was ill with "hospital malaria," or blood poisoning. He worked on his own; there is no evidence connecting him with any organization devoted to nursing the Civil War wounded. As a volunteer nurse, he talked with the wounded, read to them, wrote letters on their behalf, brought them gifts of food, writing, and reading materials, and on occasion assisted with dressings and operations. He raised money in several cities for a fund to enable him to give small amounts to the soldiers, and to support himself during that time period he wrote for various newspapers, including the *New York Times*. There is conflicting evidence of volunteer work in Broadway Hospital in 1862, although only one of four articles for the *Standard* made any direct reference to going around among the sick soldiers. His Civil War experiences are included in *Specimen Days* (1882), as well as in *Memoranda during the War* (1875) and in his letters to his mother during the war years (published posthumously).
WRITINGS: *Leaves of Grass* (10 editions, 1855-1892); *Passage to India* (1871); *Democratic Vistas* (1871); *Memoranda during the War* (1875); *Specimen Days and Collect* (1882-1883); *Two Rivulets* (1876); *November Boughs* (1888); *Good-Bye My Fancy* (1891); letters to his mother during the war, published in 1902.
REFERENCES: Henry Seidel Canby, *Walt Whitman* (1937); *Dictionary of American Biography*, XX: 143-152; Justin Kaplan, *Walt Whitman* (1980);

Edgar Lee Masters, *Whitman* (1937); *National Cyclopedia of American Biography*, I: 255; Walt Whitman, *Specimen Days* (reprint, 1971).

JOELLEN WATSON HAWKINS

WILLEFORD, MARY B. (February 4, 1900, Flatonia, Texas--December 24, 1941, New York City). *Nurse-midwife.* Never married. EDUCATION: A.B., University of Texas, Austin; graduated from Army School of Nursing, Walter Reed Hospital, Washington, D.C.; 1926, completed midwifery course at York Lying-in Hospital, London, and received certificate, English Central Midwives' Board, London, England; M.A. in public health, Teachers College, Columbia University, New York City; 1929, certificate, teacher of midwifery, London, England; 1932, Ph.D., Columbia University. CAREER: 1926-1930, district nurse-midwife, Frontier Nursing Service, Wendover, Kentucky; 1930-1938, assistant director of the Frontier Nursing Service; 1938-1940, maternal and child health consultant, California State Board of Health; 1940-1941, public health nursing consultant, Children's Bureau (of the U.S. Department of Labor), Washington, D.C.

CONTRIBUTIONS: After completing the midwifery course at the York Lying-in, London, England, February 1926, Mary Willeford joined Mary Breckinridge (q.v.), the founder of the Frontier Nursing Service (FNS). Willeford was one of the first nurses to work as a midwife in the hills of Kentucky. When she began her work there, the group was still officially known as the Kentucky Committee for Mothers and Baby, the name which was adopted at the founding meeting in 1925. In *Wide Neighborhoods*, the story of Breckinridge and the FNS, Willeford is frequently referred to as "Tex." Her exceptional ability to ride horses was an indispensable asset as she travelled through the hills of the Appalachian region to the homes of her patients. Adverse weather conditions, frequent flooding, and the absence of roads were constant challenges that she faced on a regular basis.

In addition to practicing as a midwife, Willeford conducted studies of infant and maternal mortality rates in rural areas of the United States, studies which demonstrated the success of the FNS and the approach that Breckinridge had developed toward providing needed services to the rural community. One study Willeford conducted was of the Ozark region, after receiving a request for such a survey by an interested group in St. Louis, Missouri. In 1935, she made a survey of the health on Indian reservations, again an example of the outreach influence of the FNS as well as her capability as a researcher.

After twelve years with the FNA, she was appointed maternal and child health consultant for the California State Department of Health. Two years later, she became public health nurse-consultant to the Children's Bureau. Her activities with the U.S. Children's Bureau were directed to those states in which midwifery services were prevalent. She assisted with the establishment of a school of midwifery at Tuskegee Institute, in Alabama, the school which was established by Booker T. Washington in the hope of advancing the technical knowledge and competency of southern blacks. Willeford provided consultant service to schools of midwifery which requested appropriations under the nursing education section of the Social Security Act. She also acted as a consultant to those states and counties in which midwives were members of the health department staff, and were practicing midwifery or supervising and guiding the work of untrained midwives. She assisted in special studies, such as the one conducted jointly by the U.S. Children's Bureau under the direction of Dr. Mayhew Derryberry, the public health researcher.

Willeford earned one of the earliest doctorates among American nurses. Her Ph.D. dissertation, "Income and Health in Remote Rural Areas," was based on her personal experience in living and working among the people she studied. In the process, she was able to reveal the poverty of the region and also the impact of poverty on the public health. Her study was done during the Great Depression, when many federal commissions were seeking data and remedies for the deprivation among the people who resided in rural mountain regions. She collected her data in Leslie County, Kentucky, by house-to-house enumeration. She analyzed annual family income and medical expenditures, and she demonstrated the degree of poverty in that isolated region. When she died, one of the signers of the tribute from the Frontier Nursing Service was Justice Louis Brandeis, who had spent his youth in Kentucky and who apparently was well-aware of the good work being done in the Appalachian region by Willeford and the staff of the FNS.

Willeford was a charter member of the Kentucky State Association of Nurse-Midwives, which later became the American Association of Nurse-Midwives. She was one of the sixteen who in 1928 formed the association. She also was a member of the American Nurses' Association and the National Organization for Public Health Nursing.

WRITINGS: Many articles on the Frontier Nursing Service in various magazines, including "Frontier Nursing Service," *Public Health Nursing* (1933), pp. 6-10; "Income and Health in Remote Rural Areas," Ph.D. dissertation, Columbia University, 1932.

REFERENCES: *American Journal of Nursing* (1942), p. 231; ; Mary Breckinridge, *Wide Neighborhoods: A Story of the Frontier Nursing*

Service (1952); Nancy Dammann, *A Social History of the Frontier Nursing Service* (1982); unpublished material, Nursing Archives, Mugar Memorial Library, Boston University; Ernest Poole, *Nurses on Horseback* (1932); *The Quarterly Bulletin* (of the Frontier Nursing Service, Winter 1942), pp. 36-37.

ALICE HOWELL FRIEDMAN

WILLIAMSON, ANNE A. (May 3, 1868, small town in western New York--August 11, 1955, South Pasadena, California). *Leader in army nursing and in hospital and social service administration.* Daughter of Charley Williamson and Martha (O'Rourke) Williamson. Never married. EDUCATION: 1886, graduated from high school; 1886-1888, attended Mt. Holyoke College, South Hadley, Massachusetts; 1889-1890, attended Wilson College, Chambersburg, Pennsylvania, graduating in 1890; 1890-1891, attended business school in New York City; 1894-1896, attended New York Hospital Training School for Nurses, graduating on November 6, 1896. CAREER: 1896-1907, private duty nursing; 1898, nurse in the Spanish-American War; 1907-1908, night superintendent and then assistant superintendent, California Hospital, Los Angeles; 1908-1925, director of nurses, California Hospital; 1925-1955, social service director, California Hospital.

CONTRIBUTIONS: Anne Williamson was one of the pioneers in army nursing and in hospital administration and social service. After graduation from college, she became engaged and was studying to be a stenographer when her fiance died of diphtheria in 1893. It happened that Clara Barton (q.v.) was a friend of her mother, and in her moment of grief, Clara's words about service to humankind came back to her. What better way could she serve, Anne concluded, than to become a nurse, especially since the nurse who had cared for her fiance had made a lasting impression on her. She enrolled as a probationer at the training school of New York Hospital, graduating in 1896.

After graduation, Williamson did private duty nursing until illness forced her to take a rest. It was at the end of her convalescence that war with Spain became imminent. She first wrote to Clara Barton, asking to be allowed to serve with the Red Cross. But Barton urged her to wait until war was declared. Impatiently, Williamson then wrote to Surgeon-General George M. Sternberg, offering her services as a trained nurse. When war was declared on April 25, 1898, Anne was among the first to report to Red Cross Auxiliary Number 3. On July 3, 1898, she was called to serve, being told she must supply her own uniforms and that the Red Cross would provide her travelling expenses and pay her twenty-five dollars a month for her services. She set out for Charleston, South Carolina, on July 27 and from there was sent to Camp Chickamauga in Tennessee, where an epidemic of typhoid fever was raging. Williamson wrote extensively about her military experiences and the suffering that the soldiers endured. After her discharge from the service, Williamson went home and soon returned to private duty nursing. Her cases sometimes took her abroad, so she was able to enjoy life on the Continent with some of America's wealthiest families.

Williamson's next major contribution was as superintendent of the California Hospital. It was her mother's move that prompted her to cross the country in October 1907. Once she had made the decision to remain in California, she began the search for work as a private duty nurse, which she had done for the past eleven years. Unable to find private patients, however, Williamson inquired at California Hospital and was offered the position of night superintendent. She soon became assistant superintendent, and when the superintendent resigned in the spring of 1908, Williamson was asked to take her place. Diminutive in size, she had proved that neither her stature nor her lack of experience in hospital nursing could prevent her from assuming a leadership position. She began to make changes to ensure that the work required of the students did not prove a detriment to their nursing education. She reorganized the classwork and made improvements in the living conditions for nurses. Recognizing the need for nurses to have a knowledge of science, she arranged for students to attend classes in chemistry at Polytechnic High School near the hospital.

Williamson's contributions were not limited to leadership in her institution. Shortly after arriving in California, she applied for membership in the local nurses' organization, which later became District 5 of the California State Nurses' Association. In 1912, she was asked by the board of directors to serve as president. In that same year, she went to Sacramento on behalf of the directors of the hospital, to lobby against the eight-hour bill which would have required a larger nursing staff and which would have reduced the hospital's profits. At Sacramento, she met Anna Jamme (q.v.) who supported the eight-hour bill but who was afraid that it might jeopardize passage of the nurse-registration bill which was then being considered by the legislature. The eight-hour bill passed, and Williamson, secretly relieved, returned home and prepared to institute the change in her hospital.

In 1927, she was approached to run for president of the California State Nurses' Association, and to her surprise she was elected. During her two terms as president, permanent headquarters were established for the association, and Jamme was appointed director. In 1929, Williamson was elected to the board of directors, served for four years, and then took the position of parliamentarian. From 1930 to 1932, she again served as president of District 5.

During World War I, she organized two units for nursing service, Navy Base Number 3 and Army Unit Number 512, struggled to maintain adequate nursing on the civilian front, and helped to sell war bonds, a task that included giving brief speeches at movie theaters. Her service to the Red Cross continued after the war, and in 1925 she served as secretary of the local committee on Red Cross nursing service. For many years, she was also a member of the national relief fund committee of the American Nurses' Association. During World War II, then in her seventies, Williamson continued to serve her country through her hospital work and in preparation for emergency service with other nurses in her community.

On the seventieth anniversary of New York Hospital School of Nursing, Williamson flew to New York for the celebration. On the way, her nursing expertise was once more challenged, when she was asked to assess the condition of an infant being flown east for surgery to repair a congenital heart condition. Acting with the wisdom that had sustained her for fifty years, she recognized that the infant could not possibly survive the cross-country flight, and she ordered the pilot to land at the nearest airport. The result was a stop at Pueblo, Colorado, and the baby was rushed to a hospital in that city.

Williamson never retired from her last position at California Hospital. She served the hospital for forty-eight years from 1907 to 1955, when she died. In her autobiography, published in 1948, she detailed her fifty years in nursing and her dedication to the hospital where she spent so many of those years.

WRITINGS: *50 Years in Starch* (1948); numerous articles in professional journals, including "A Backward Glimpse," *American Journal of Nursing* (October 1950), pp. 637-638.

REFERENCES: *American Journal of Nursing* (July 1927), p. 568, (January 1937), p. 97, (July 1943), p. 688, (October 1955), pp. 1178, 1180; Bertha Sanford Dodge, *The Story of Nursing* (1954); Helene Jamieson Jordan, *Cornell University-New York Hospital School of Nursing 1877-1952* (1952); Anne Williamson, *50 Years in Starch* (1948).

JOELLEN WATSON HAWKINS

WOLF, ANNA DRYDEN (June 25, 1890, Gunter, Madras Presidency, India--July 5, 1985, St. Petersburg, Florida). *Nurse-educator*. Daughter of Luther Benaiah Wolf and Alice (Benner) Wolf, Lutheran missionaries. Never married. EDUCATION: 1906, attended Maryland College,

Lutherville, Maryland; 1911, B.A., Goucher College, Baltimore, Maryland; 1912-1915, attended Johns Hopkins Hospital School of Nursing, Baltimore, Maryland, graduating in 1915; 1916, M.A., Teachers College, Columbia University, New York City; 1926, enrolled in Ph.D. program, Teachers College. CAREER: Summers 1908-1911, playground work in the city of Baltimore; 1916-1919, instructor in nursing arts and assistant superintendent of nurses, Johns Hopkins Hospital School of Nursing; summer 1918, taught practical nursing at Vassar Training Camp, Poughkeepsie, New York; 1919-1925, dean of the school of nursing, Peking Union Medical College Hospital, Peking, China; 1926-1931, associate professor of nursing at the University of Chicago, and director of nursing of the University of Chicago Clinics, Albert Merritt Billings Hospital; 1931-1940, director, New York Hospital School of Nursing and of the nursing service, New York Hospital; 1940-1955, director, Johns Hopkins Hospital School of Nursing and director of the Johns Hopkins Hospital nursing service.

CONTRIBUTIONS: Anna Wolf was a leader in nursing education. Her birth to American missionary parents lent to her life a world perspective and gave her both a tolerance for all people and a commitment to service. In 1919, after having served for three years as assistant superintendent of nurses at the Johns Hopkins Hospital School of Nursing, the Rockefeller Foundation invited her to reorganize the school of nursing at Peking Union Medical College Hospital, Peking, China. From 1919 to 1925 she served as dean of the first school in China which prepared women students to care for male patients.

Her return in 1925 took her first to Teachers College where she spent a year of study in the doctoral program. From New York, she became associate professor of nursing at the University of Chicago Clinics, where she organized the nursing service with a full staff of graduate nurses and helped to equip the new hospital, which was part of the University of Chicago Medical Center. In addition, she developed university courses in teaching and administration in schools of nursing.

Returning to New York in 1931 as director of the New York Hospital School of Nursing and the hospital's nursing service, she was challenged by the opportunity to be part of the reorganization of one of the nation's oldest hospitals, which would be relocated in newly constructed buildings. She was selected for that position because she was considered to be a leader who would not only have the wisdom to preserve the best of the past but also to understand the opportunities offered by the new. While in that position, on April 5, 1939, she was a guest of the Columbia Broadcasting System on a program entitled "So You Want to Be a Registered Professional Nurse." True to her reputation, she gave to the program and to her position all the wisdom, foresight, vision, and concern for the patient as well as for the profession. Those characteristics were demonstrated throughout her career.

On November 1, 1940, she returned to Johns Hopkins to serve as the fifth director of its nursing school and nursing service. Under her leadership, an effort was made to move the school of nursing into a closer relationship with the university. In 1944, the school adopted the baccalaureate degree as a criterion for admission, one that would take time to implement completely. A Special Committee for the Consideration of a University School of Nursing was constituted in 1946, reporting on its work in October 1947. The result was the recommendation that students be awarded the bachelor of science degree in nursing after completion of two years of college work and the thirty-two-month program of the Johns Hopkins Hospital School of Nursing. At the same time, the committee recommended re-establishing the high-school diploma as the minimum requirement for admission and a thirty-six-month program for graduation.

The return of World War II veterans resulted in a marriage boom which in turn reduced the available pool of applicants to nursing school. Faced with declining enrollments in nursing schools, Wolf instituted reforms to attract nurses, including higher salary scales and more fringe benefits, as well as a forty-four-hour week for day nurses and forty hours for evenings and nights. In addition, in order to eliminate some of the more menial responsibilities of nurses, she began the training and employment of large numbers of nurses' aides.

Her energies were devoted to other professional activities as well as to her formal positions. She was president of the Maryland League for Nursing (1953-1954), and served as vice-president, board member, and secretary of the National League of Nursing Education, also serving as first chairperson of the Committee on Accrediting. During and immediately after World War II, she was vice chairperson and member of the National Council for War Services (1942-1946), the National Nursing Council (1946-1948), the U.S. Public Health Service advisory committee on nursing education (1942-1948), and the Nursing Advisory Committee of the American Red Cross (appointed in 1938). She served on the advisory boards for both Cook County Hospital School of Nursing and Johns Hopkins Hospital School of Nursing. During the 1940s, she was a member of the Advisory Committee for guiding programs of the Nurse Training Act of 1943, of the Joint Committee of the Structure of National Nursing Organizations, and of the National Nursing Planning Committee, as well as being advisor to the first federal nurse aid program. She retired on July 1, 1955.

Through her career, she received numerous honors, beginning with trustee scholarships while a student at the Johns Hopkins Hospital

School of Nursing and continuing when she graduated with honors. In 1954, she was honored as an outstanding alumna of Goucher College, and on June 12, 1955, just one month before her retirement, Goucher awarded her an honorary doctor of science degree. On June 19, 1955, she was honored by Johns Hopkins with a citation and an award for distinguished service.
WRITINGS: Numerous articles in professional journals.
REFERENCES: Student and school records of the Johns Hopkins Hospital School of Nursing, Alan Mason Chesney Archives, Johns Hopkins Medical Institutions; Harriet M. Frost, "Anna D. Wolf," in *National League of Nursing Education Biographical Sketches, 1937-1940* (1940); Ethel Johns and Blanche Pfefferkorn, *The Johns Hopkins Hospital School of Nursing, 1889-1949* (1954); *Johns Hopkins Nurses Alumnae Magazine* (April 1955), p. 28; Portia B. Kernodle, *The Red Cross Nurse in Action 1882-1948* (1949); Meta Rutter Pennock, ed., *Makers of Nursing History* (1940), p. 117; Faye Whiteside and Margory Upham Kiefer, "Our Director Retires," *Johns Hopkins Nurses Alumnae Magazine* (July 1955), pp. 69-71.
JOELLEN WATSON HAWKINS

WOOD, HELEN (May 13, 1882, Newton Center, Massachusetts--September 23, 1974, Newton, Massachusetts). *Nurse-educator.* Daughter of William Burke Wood and Amelia Adelaide (Votts) Wood. Never married. EDUCATION: Attended the Newton public schools; 1904, B.A., Mt. Holyoke College, South Hadley, Massachusetts; 1909, graduated from Massachusetts General Hospital School of Nursing, Boston; 1913-1914, graduate studies, Teachers College, Columbia University, New York City; 1924, M.A., Teachers College. CAREER: 1909-1911, graduate nurse and anesthetist, Massachusetts General Hospital; summer 1911, nurse, Grenfell Mission, Labrador; 1911-1913, assistant superintendent of nurses, Faulkner Hospital, Boston; 1913-1914, first assistant, Massachusetts General Hospital School of Nursing; 1914-1915, assistant director of nurses and acting superintendent, Children's Hospital, Boston; 1916-1919, acting superintendent of nurses, Massachusetts General Hospital; 1919-1923, director of the Washington University (St. Louis) School of Nursing, and superintendent of nurses, Barnes Hospital and St. Louis Children's Hospital, St. Louis, Missouri; 1923, director of the summer school for nurses, Stanford University, Stanford, California; 1924-1931, director, University of Rochester School of Nursing, Rochester, New York; 1931-1932, acting superintendent of nurses, Massachusetts General Hospital; 1933-1946, director and professor of nursing, Simmons College School of Nursing, Boston; also served as lecturer on ward administration and teaching for the Brown University extension service, Providence, Rhode Island.

CONTRIBUTIONS: Helen Wood's outstanding contribution was in the field of collegiate nursing education. She reorganized the Simmons College one-year certificate program in public health nursing into a five-year basic baccalaureate nursing education which had a strong liberal arts component. She formed strong affiliations with outstanding local health-care facilities, so students continued to have close contact with patients. The program she designed at Simmons reflected her strong belief that students must have a sound scientific foundation for their nursing subjects. She introduced a course in ward management and ward teaching at Simmons. She advocated the hiring of prepared staff members and avoided the reliance upon student nurses for patient care, the practice of that time in virtually every hospital training school. She believed that high-quality nursing education benefited the entire society, and that hospital trustees should take a more active role in employing graduate nurses to provide patient care rather than saving money by relying upon student nurses. She was convinced that directors of nursing schools should be free to do more educational work rather than be responsible for providing the hospital with nursing service.

In 1924, Wood became the first director of the University of Rochester School of Nursing. Her career at the university was in part a response to the Rockefeller Foundation's study of nursing and nursing education known as the Goldmark Report. She had been a member of the committee which conducted the study (1920-1923). At Rochester, she was the one who worked out the details of the organization and the administration of the Strong Memorial Hospital School of Nursing, which had not yet opened, and she was responsible for overseeing nursing research at the university medical center. In 1970, when she was eighty-eight years old, she received an award as the leader who created the University of Rochester School of Nursing. A residence at the university medical center is named for her.

In addition to her service to the University of Rochester and Simmons College, she served her alma mater, the Massachusetts General Hospital (MGH), on two occasions. The first time was during World War I, when the superintendent went to the front with the MGH Base Hospital Number 6, and Wood served as acting director of nurses at the MGH. Her annual report reflected her thinking about the expansion of nursing education which was later reflected in her future career in collegiate nursing education. She pointed out that nurses were not only being prepared for hospital and community work but also to meet the "cry of the sick and suffering of mankind throughout the world." Her second opportunity to serve as acting superintendent was in 1931, when the superintendent, Sally Johnson, was on a sabbatical leave. In both instances, Wood demonstrated that she was a capable administrator and educator who could be relied upon to fulfill the responsibilities demanded by the position.

Her interest in education was matched by her accomplishments as a scholar. She was a member of Phi Beta Kappa. In 1913, when a student at Columbia, she received the Isabel Hampton Robb (q.v.) scholarship. At the 150th anniversary of the MGH (1961), she was awarded a medal in recognition of her outstanding achievements in nursing.

She was an active member of many nursing organizations, including the National and Massachusetts Leagues of Nursing Education, the Massachusetts Nurses' Association, and the local Red Cross committees in Massachusetts. During both world wars, she was active in recruiting nurses for the military, and during World War I, she was chairperson of the Massachusetts Nurse Recruiting Committee. She was a member of the Committee on Grading of Nursing Schools, a forerunner of the national nurse accreditation movement. She served as a representative of the American Nurses' Association from 1926 to 1934. She was a member of two state boards of nurse examiners, in Massachusetts (1917-1920) and Missouri (1920-1923). In the 1940s, she became a director of the Central Directory for nurses (a branch of the Massachusetts Nurses' Association) and supported the concept of a professional registry to assist the public and the nurse in the area of employment of private duty nurses.

REFERENCES: American Journal of Nursing Collection, Mugar Library, Boston University; *American Women, 1935-1940*, p. 1002; records of the alumnae association, Mt. Holyoke College Archives, South Hadley, Massachusetts; Sylvia Perkins, *A Centennial Review of the Massachusetts General Hospital School of Nursing* (1975); personal papers of Helen Wood, Nursing Archives, Mugar Library, Boston University.

ALICE HOWELL FRIEDMAN

WYCHE, MARY LEWIS (February 26, 1858, near Henderson, Granville County, North Carolina--August 22, 1936, Wychewood, near Henderson, North Carolina). *Nurse-educator; organizer.* Daughter of Benjamin Wyche and Sara (Hunter) Wyche. Never married. EDUCATION: Attended Littleton College (now Henderson College), Littleton, North Carolina; June 1889, graduated from Henderson College; 1894, graduated from Philadelphia General Hospital school of nursing; 1901-1903, post-graduate studies in dietetics and massage, Philadelphia. CAREER: July

1894-1898, superintendent of nurses, Rex Hospital, Raleigh, North Carolina; 1898-1899, private duty nursing, Raleigh; 1899-1901, charge nurse for the infirmary of the State Normal and Industrial College, Greensboro, North Carolina; 1901-1902, private duty nursing, Raleigh; 1903-1913, superintendent, Watts Hospital and Training School, Durham, North Carolina; 1913-1915, worked to establish a home for tubercular nurses; 1915-1917, superintendent, Sarah Elizabeth Hospital and Training School, Henderson, North Carolina; 1917-1925 (when she retired), private duty nursing in Greensboro and Raleigh.

CONTRIBUTIONS: Mary L. Wyche was a leader not only in North Carolina nursing but for the entire country. She was in large part responsible for securing the first law for state registration of nurses, which was enacted on March 3, 1903, in North Carolina. When the North Carolina State Nurses' Association was less than a year old, she became chairperson of its first legislative committee, at a time when the committee drafted the first bill, "An Act to Provide for State Registration for Trained Nurses in North Carolina." The bill was presented to the legislature in early 1903. Under the bill, a board of nurse examiners was created, and Wyche was one of the three nurses on the board, serving as its secretary-treasurer for its first six years (1903-1909).

Like many of her contemporaries, Wyche began her career as a schoolteacher. While a student at Henderson College, she taught in its primary department. After graduating, she moved to Chapel Hill to make a home for her younger brothers who would soon be attending the University of North Carolina. She also kept boarders and taught in order to support the household. When her brothers no longer needed her assistance, she thought about a career for herself, and at that time she turned to nursing.

Wyche organized the first nurse-training school in North Carolina, the training school at Rex Hospital, Raleigh. The school opened in October 1894 with five student nurses, only one year after Wyche had herself graduated from the nursing school at the Philadelphia General Hospital. She also was one of the individuals responsible for the creation of the North Carolina State Nurses' Association. Having attended the meeting of the International Council of Nurses, which was held in Buffalo in 1901, Wyche was filled with enthuasiasm for registration of nurses, which would draw a distinction between the trained and untrained, and for the benefits which could result from the formal organization of the nursing profession. Upon her return to North Carolina, she helped organize the Raleigh Nurses' Association (October 1901), by sending postal cards to the other nurses in the city, inviting them to a meeting of the proposed association. Curious to know about the association, every nurse in town attended the meeting. The group then sent questionnaires to every nurse in the state, asking if they were interested in a state-wide organization. Encouraged by the response, Wyche and her colleagues invited the nurses to meet at the North Carolina State Fair, which was held in Raleigh on October 28 and 29, 1902. On October 28, 1902, she and fourteen other nurses, including Mary Rose Batterham (q.v.), organized the North Carolina State Nurses' Association, which was formally incorporated on December 5 of that year. From 1902 to 1907, Wyche served as its president.

In 1910, the Association of Superintendents of Hospitals and Training Schools was formed with seven members, and Wyche was elected as its first vice-president. This organization was part of the state nurses' association, and it met annually with the association. When the organization convened in Winston-Salem in 1916, the members of this education section determined to become the North Carolina League of Nursing Education. The league became a separate organization in 1918, under the by-laws of the National League of Nursing Education, and Wyche was an active member of the state League.

She devoted much of her energy and leadership skills to the Red Cross Nursing Service, serving on the first Red Cross nursing committee in North Carolina, which was organized in 1910. From May 28, 1912, until 1922, she served on the first local Red Cross nursing committee, which was organized in 1911 for the purpose of enrolling nurses. Two other endeavors occupied Wyche. The first was the movement to establish a pre-nursing course at North Carolina College for Women, Greensboro, which eventually led to the establishment of a nursing school at Duke University, Durham. The second was establishment of a home for tubercular nurses. Birdie Dunn, another North Carolina nurse, suggested the idea to the state nurses' association and along with Wyche undertook to secure funds for such an institution. Both of them contributed a great deal of time to the management of the home during its first year, and as a result it was named Dunnwyche in their honor. Wyche served as president of its board of directors. When the home was sold in 1919 in deference to the war effort, the funds were used to establish a state relief fund for nurses.

After her retirement from active hospital and private duty nursing (1925), Wyche devoted her time to collecting information for a history of nursing in North Carolina, which was published posthumously. She spent her last years in her childhood home, Wychewood, where she died in 1936. On her retirement she was named honorary president of the North Carolina State Nurses' Association. In 1932, four years before her death, she was presented a pin recognizing her contributions to the state nurses' association, at a banquet held in Raleigh.

WRITINGS: *The History of Nursing in North Carolina* (1938).

REFERENCES: *American Journal of Nursing* (April 1924), p. 552, and (October 1936), p. 1064; Victor Robinson, *White Caps* (1946); Mary L. Wyche, *The History of Nursing in North Carolina* (1938); unpublished materials, archives of the North Carolina State Nurses' Association, and American Journal of Nursing Collection, Nursing Archives, Mugar Memorial Library, Boston University.

JOELLEN WATSON HAWKINS

Y

YOUNG, HELEN (November 17, 1874, Chatham, Ontario, Canada--November 23, 1966, New York City). *Leader in nursing administration.* Never married. EDUCATION: Attended public schools in Chatham, Ontario; 1893, graduated from the Collegiate Institute, Chatham; 1893-1895, attended the Toronto School of Pedagogy (normal school), receiving a diploma in 1896; 1909-1912, attended Presbyterian Hospital School of Nursing, New York City, graduating in 1912. CAREER: 1896-1899, substitute teacher, and 1899-1909, teacher, Chatham, Ontario; 1912-1915, head nurse, women's surgical ward and then women's medical service, Presbyterian Hospital, New York City; June-August 1915, served at Mrs. Harry Payne Whitney's hospital, Juilly, France; 1917-1919, acting assistant superintendent, Presbyterian Hospital; 1919-1921, instructor, July 1921-1923, acting director, and 1923-1937, director of nursing service and the school of nursing, Presbyterian Hospital; 1937-1942, director of the nursing service, Columbia-Presbyterian Medical Center; 1942, director of nursing emeritus.

CONTRIBUTIONS: Helen Young served Presbyterian Hospital for thirty years, where she exhibited exceptional leadership qualities in both service to the hospital and to the profession at large. During the summer of 1920, Presbyterian offered a five-week course for graduate nurses preparing to be teachers in schools of nursing and who were registered at Teachers College for the summer session. Young, an instructor in practical nursing for Presbyterian, gave demonstrations in nursing techniques. As assistant to Anna Maxwell (q.v.), director of Presbyterian's nursing service, she had an important role in the development of the administration of the nursing service and in the education of students at Presbyterian Hospital. She was involved in the arrangements with the department of nursing and health at Teachers

College for a five-year course leading to a B.S. degree and also for the plan for graduates of approved women's colleges to enroll in the nursing school at Presbyterian.

On July 1, 1921, Young became acting director of the nursing service at Presbyterian, when Maxwell retired. During her tenure as superintendent, several important changes were made. Separate offices were provided for instructors, a standard rate of five dollars an hour was established for lecturers not on the nursing staff, ward helpers were added, instructors were added for ward teaching, the curriculum was increased in length, weekly clinics were started for students on medical and surgical wards, instruction was reorganized in a block system, and an assistant was hired to be responsible for planning clinical assignments for students over the three-year course. Instructors were encouraged to enroll for graduate study at Teacher's College in order to increase the number who would meet both academic and professional requirements for teaching. In 1924, a campaign was undertaken to build a new residence for nurses.

In 1937, the Presbyterian Hospital School of Nursing became the department of nursing of Columbia University. Young was cited at that time for her foresight in establishing high educational standards and for the nursing program in place at Presbyterian Hospital. Thereafter students were enrolled in the university and taught by faculty under the university's department of nursing. Young then became director of nursing service of the Columbia-Presbyterian Medical Center, a position she held until her retirement in 1942, when she was named director of nursing emeritus.

Young also made significant contributions to the profession in other ways. She was a delegate to the 1917 American Nurses' Association convention in Philadelphia and was present when Jane Delano (q.v.) read a message from Red Cross headquarters concerning impending mobilization of base hospitals for service with the British Expeditionary Force. Young was then serving as Red Cross chairperson of her alumnae association, and so when she returned to Presbyterian Hospital following the meeting, she was able to recruit fifty nurses who sailed in May 1917 to provide nursing care for the Allied forces. She was also a member of the National Red Cross Committee and a leader in the enrollment of young nurses in the Red Cross Nursing Service.

Young was a member of the registry committee headed by Mrs. William Church Osborn and of other committees studying the problems of the private duty nurse. She was president of both the New York City and the New York State Leagues of Nursing Education. She was instrumental in the passing of the New York State nurse practice act of 1938. In 1942, she retired. She remained in New York City, continuing to serve as treasurer of the school of nursing alumnae association for many years. In June 1937, Columbia University presented her with the University Medal for Excellence. In October 1953, she received the twenty-fifth anniversary Distinguished Service Award of the Columbia-Presbyterian Medical Center, the only woman recipient.

WRITINGS: Several books, including *Quick Reference Book for Nurses* (1933), estimated to have been used by 100,000 nurses in English-speaking countries; numerous articles in professional journals.

REFERENCES: *American Journal of Nursing* (January 1967), p. 141; Eleanor Lee, *History of the School of Nursing Presbyterian Hospital, 1892-1942* (1942), and "Helen Young," *National League of Nursing Education Biographical Sketch* (1940); *New York Times* (November 25, 1966), p. 37; *Nursing Outlook* (November 1953), p. 649.

JOELLEN WATSON HAWKINS

Z

ZABRISKIE, LOUISE (1887, Preston City, Connecticut--December 12, 1957, New York City). *Leader in maternity nursing; nurse-author.* Never married. EDUCATION: 1910-1913, attended New York Hospital School of Nursing, New York City, graduating in 1913; post-graduate study at Teachers College, Columbia University, New York City, and New York University, New York City. CAREER: 1913-1916, night supervisor, New York Lying-in Hospital; 1917-1919, public health nurse, Nashville, Tennessee; 1919-1920, staff nurse, 1920-1923, assistant field director, and 1923-1939, field director, Maternity Center Association, New York City; 1939-1957, director, Maternity Consultation Service, New York City; c. 1952, lecturer, New York University School of Education.

CONTRIBUTIONS: Louise Zabriskie devoted her entire career to the improvement of care for mothers and their babies. She was one of the pioneers in advocating the importance of prenatal care. She wrote for both professionals and laypersons. Her *Mother and Baby Care in Pictures* (1935) went through four editions, and she had a regular column in *My Baby* magazine. She was a mentor for students and colleagues, and her advice was sought by physicians, government officials, sales representatives, and parents. She maintained a voluminous correspondence, sharing freely of her wisdom, courage, strength, and unflagging interest in mothers and babies. Those who worked closely with her commented on her ability to synthesize information and ideas and her use of detail in broad critical assessments. Her talks, lectures, and writings reflect the soundness of her ideas and wisdom.

Her last position was as organizer and director of the Maternity Consultation Service, based in New York City, where she was a pioneer example of a nurse as entrepreneur. This service provided classes for parents in a number of settings in New York City. She also continued as a regular lecturer in the school of education at New York University until she reached the mandatory retirement age.

Zabriskie served on the boards of a number of organizations, including the National Council on Family Relations, the National Nursing Council of the Frontier Nursing Service, the executive board of the Yorkville Civic Council, and the nursing committee of Planned Parenthood Federation of America. She was a member of the American Nurses' Association, the National League of Nursing Education, and the National Organization for Public Health Nursing. Few who knew this woman realized that for thirty-five years she labored under a severe handicap, caused by cervical fractures sustained in an automobile accident in 1922.

WRITINGS: *Nurses Handbook of Obstetrics* (1929, and nine subsequent editions; *Mother and Baby Care in Pictures* (1935, and three subsequent editions; countless articles in professional and lay journals, pamphlets on antepartum care.

REFERENCES: Alan Mason Chesney Medical Archives of Johns Hopkins Medical Institutions; *American Journal of Nursing* (October 1935), p. 978, (June 1958), pp. 803-804; Cordelia W. Kelly, *Dimensions of Professional Nursing* (1962); unpublished materials provided by New York University School of Education, Health, Nursing, and Arts Professions.

JOELLEN WATSON HAWKINS

APPENDICES

APPENDIX A

Listing by Place of Birth

ARGENTINA

Waechter, Eugenia Helma

AUSTRALIA

Banfield, Emma Maud

AUSTRIA

Deutsch, Naomi

CANADA

Damer, Annie
Darche, Louise
Davis, Mary E. P.
Gretter, Lystra E.
Harmer, Bertha
Hibbard, M. Eugenie
Hodgins, Agatha Cobourg
Hogan, Aileen I.
Logan, Laura R.
McCrae, Annabella
Macleod, Charlotte
Nutting, M. Adelaide
Pope, Amy Elizabeth
Robb, Isabel Adams (Hampton)
Sirch, Margaret Elliot (Francis)
Stewart, Isabel Maitland
Struthers, Lina Lavanche (Rogers)
Taylor, Euphemia Jane
Young, Helen

DENMARK

Nelson, Sophie C.

ENGLAND

Amy Margaret, Sister
Batterham, Mary Rose
Browne, Helen E.
Carr, Ada M.
Fisher, Alice
Gladwin, Mary Elizabeth
Kimber, Diana Clifford

INDIA

Beeby, Nell V.
Wolf, Anna Dryden

IRELAND

Anthony, Sister

ITALY

Fitzgerald, Alice Louise Florence

LITHUANIA

Goldman, Emma

NORWAY

Fedde, Elizabeth

SCOTLAND

Cumming, Kate

UNITED STATES

California

Cooke, Genevieve
Ellis, Rosemary
Titus, Shirley Carew

Connecticut

Deming, Dorothy
Foley, Edna Lois
Johnson, Sally May
Zabriskie, Louise

Georgia

Collins, Charity E.

Illinois

Geister, Janet M.
Hay, Helen Scott
Thomson, Elnora Elvira
Vail, Stella (Boothe)
Van Blarcom, Carolyn Conant

Indiana

Dreves, Katherine
Lounsbery, Harriet (Camp)
Scott, Alma (Ham)

Iowa

Bowman, Josephine Beatrice
McIsaac, Isabel

Kansas

McCleery, Ada Belle

Maine

Alline, Anna Lowell
Burgess, Elizabeth Chamberlain
Dix, Dorothea Lynde
Parsons, Marion Gemeth
Ropes, Hannah Anderson (Chandler)

Maryland

Clayton, S. Lillian
Frederick, Hester King
Grace, Sister Mary Gonzaga
Hasson, Esther Voorhees
Noyes, Clara Dutton
Pfefferkorn, Blanche
Tubman, Harriet

Massachusetts

Barton, Clarissa Harlowe

Freeman, Ruth Benson
Gardner, Mary Sewall
Goostray, Stella
Hawkinson, Nellie Xenia
Hickey, Mary A.
Hitchcock, Jane Elizabeth
Livermore, Mary (Rice)
Mahoney, Mary Eliza P.
McNaught, Rose
Markolf, Ada Mayo (Stewart)
Palmer, Sophia French
Parsons, Sara E.
Soule, Elizabeth Sterling
Stimson, Julia Catherine
Strong, Anne Hervey
Sullivan, Elizabeth Eleanor
Tracy, Susan E.
Tucker, Katharine
Tyler, Adeline (Blanchard)
Vreeland, Ellwynne Mae
Waters, Yssabella Gertrude
Wood, Helen

Michigan

Domitilla, Sister Mary
Knapp, Bertha L.
Roberts, Mary May
Sly, Sarah
Urch, Daisy Dean

Minnesota

Gowan, Sister Mary Olivia
Haupt, Alma Cecelia
McIver, Pearl
Sargent, Emilie Gleason

Mississippi

Newsom, Ella (King)

Missouri

Beck, Sister M. Berenice
Berthold, Jeanne Saylor
Cushman, Emma D.

New Hampshire

Beard, Mary
Hall, Carrie M.
Maher, Mary Ann
Shaw, Clara (Weeks)
Smith, Martha Ruth

New Jersey

Deane, Elizabeth M.
Goodrich, Annie Warburton
Maass, Clara Louise

New York

Anderson, Lydia Elizabeth
Arnstein, Margaret Gene
Austin, Anne L.
Butler, Ida Fatio
Christy, Teresa Elizabeth
Crandall, Ella Phillips
Dakin, Florence
Delano, Jane Arminda
Dewitt, Katharine
Gage, Nina Diadamia
Goodnow, Minnie

Grant, Amelia Howe
Gray, Carolyn Elizabeth
Hubbard, Ruth Weaver
Jamme, Anna C.
Kinney, Dita (Hopkins)
Maxwell, Anna Caroline
Richards, Linda Ann Judson
Robinson, Alice Merritt
Sanger, Margaret Louise
Schutt, Barbara Gordon
Sutliffe, Irene H.
Thompson, Dora E.
Truth, Sojourner
Whitman, Walter
Williamson, Anne A.

North Carolina

Davis, Frances Reed (Elliott)
Dolan, Margaret (Baggett)
Wyche, Mary Lewis

Ohio

Bickerdyke, Mary Ann (Ball)
Howell, Marion Gertrude
Kemble, Elizabeth L.
Leete, Harriet L.
McClelland, Helen Grace
Sellew, Gladys
Wald, Lillian D.

Pennsylvania

Alcott, Louisa May
Angela, Mother
Brinton, Mary Williams
Dock, Lavinia Lloyd
Francis, Susan C.
Fulmer, Harriet
Heide, Wilma (Scott)
Holman, Lydia
Jones, Elizabeth Rinker (Kratz)
Kennedy, Cecila Rose
Lally, Grace B.
Phillips, Harriet Newton
Reiter, Frances
Riddle, Mary Margaret
Rinehart, Mary Ella (Roberts)

Rhode Island

Drown, Lucy Lincoln
Gabriel, Sister John

South Carolina

Pember, Phoebe Yates

Tennessee

Breckinridge, Mary

Texas

Osborne, Estelle
Willeford, Mary B.

Vermont

Sanborn, Katharine Anne Alexis

Virginia

Cabaniss, Sadie Heath
Minnigerode, Lucy
Minor, Nannie Jacquelin
Northam, Annie Ethel
Powell, Louise Mathilde
Thoms, Adah B. (Samuels)

West Virginia

Blanchfield, Florence Aby

Wisconsin

Blake, Florence Guinness
Bunge, Helen Lathrop
Cannon, Ida Maud
Eldredge, Adda
Flikke, Julia
Fox, Elizabeth Gordon

UNKNOWN

Brown, Amy Frances
Draper, Edith A.
Franklin, Martha M.
Gorman, Alice Amelia
Gregg, Elinor Delight
Muse, Maude Blanche
Simpson, Cora E.
Travelbee, Joyce Evelyn

APPENDIX B

Listing by State Where Prominent

Alabama

Cumming, Kate

Alaska

Deane, Elizabeth M.

Arizona

Sanger, Margaret Louise

California

Berthold, Jeanne Saylor
Bickerdyke, Mary Ann (Ball)
Cooke, Genevieve
Deutsch, Naomi
Ellis, Rosemary
Fox, Elizabeth Gordon
Jamme, Anna C.
Parsons, Marion Gemeth
Pope, Amy Elizabeth
Sirch, Margaret Elliot (Francis)
Thompson, Dora E.
Titus, Shirley Carew
Urch, Daisy Dean
Waechter, Eugenia Helma
Williamson, Anne A.

Colorado

Goodnow, Minnie
Struthers, Lina Lavanche (Rogers)

Connecticut

Arnstein, Margaret Gene
Blanchfield, Florence Aby
Butler, Ida Fatio
Foley, Edna Lois
Franklin, Martha M.
Goodrich, Annie Warburton
Gorman, Alice Amelia
Grant, Amelia Howe
Harmer, Bertha
Parsons, Sara E.
Richards, Linda Ann Judson
Taylor, Euphemia Jane

District of Columbia

Arnstein, Margaret Gene
Beck, Sister M. Berenice
Bowman, Josephine Beatrice
Butler, Ida Fatio
Davis, Mary E. P.
Deutsch, Naomi
Flikke, Julia
Fox, Elizabeth Gordon
Freeman, Ruth Benson
Goodnow, Minnie
Gowan, Sister Mary Olivia
Gregg, Elinor Delight
Hay, Helen Scott

Hickey, Mary A.
Kinney, Dita (Hopkins)
McIver, Pearl
Minnigerode, Lucy
Sellew, Gladys
Stimson, Julia Catherine
Thompson, Dora E.
Vreeland, Ellwynne Mae
Whitman, Walter

Georgia

Collins, Charity E.
Cumming, Kate
Newsom, Ella (King)

Idaho

Vail, Stella (Boothe)

Illinois

Angela, Mother
Beeby, Nell V.
Blake, Florence Guinness
Bowman, Josephine Beatrice
Christy, Teresa Elizabeth
Clayton, S. Lillian
Dock, Lavinia Lloyd
Draper, Edith Augusta
Eldredge, Adda
Ellis, Rosemary
Foley, Edna Lois
Fulmer, Harriet
Hawkinson, Nellie Xenia
Hay, Helen Scott
Knapp, Bertha L.
Livermore, Mary (Rice)
Logan, Laura R.
McCleery, Ada Belle
McIsaac, Isabel
Robb, Isabel Adams (Hampton)
Sellew, Gladys
Thomson, Elnora Elvira
Waechter, Eugenia Helma
Wolf, Anna Dryden

Indiana

Angela, Mother
Scott, Alma Ham

Iowa

Christy, Teresa Elizabeth

Kansas

Bickerdyke, Mary Ann (Ball)

Kentucky

Breckinridge, Mary
Browne, Helen E.
Willeford, Mary B.

Louisiana

Grace, Sister Mary Gonzaga
Travelbee, Joyce

Listing by State Where Prominent

Maryland

Barton, Clarissa Harlowe
Carr, Ada M.
Davis, Frances Reed (Elliott)
Dock, Lavinia Lloyd
Fitzgerald, Alice Louise Florence
Frederick, Hester King
Freeman, Ruth Benson
Northam, Annie Ethel
Nutting, M. Adelaide
Robb, Isabel Adams (Hampton)
Taylor, Euphemia Jane
Tyler, Adeline (Blanchard)
Wolf, Anna Dryden

Massachusetts

Alcott, Louisa May
Amy Margaret, Sister
Barton, Clarissa Harlowe
Beard, Mary
Cannon, Ida Maud
Carr, Ada M.
Davis, Mary E. P.
Dix, Dorothea Lynde
Drown, Lucy Lincoln
Goodnow, Minnie
Goostray, Stella
Gorman, Alice Amelia
Hall, Carrie M.
Hickey, Mary A.
Jamme, Anna C.
Johnson, Sally May
Logan, Laura R.
McCrae, Annabella
Macleod, Charlotte
McNaught, Rose
Maher, Mary Ann
Mahoney, Mary Eliza P.
Maxwell, Anna Caroline
Nelson, Sophie C.
Parsons, Marion Gemeth
Parsons, Sara E.
Richards, Linda Ann Judson
Riddle, Mary Margaret
Robinson, Alice Merritt
Smith, Martha Ruth
Strong, Anne Hervey
Struthers, Lina Lavanche (Rogers)
Sullivan, Elizabeth Eleanor
Tracy, Susan E.
Tyler, Adeline (Blanchard)
Wood, Helen

Michigan

Austin, Anne L.
Blake, Florence Guinness
Davis, Frances Reed (Elliott)
Gretter, Lystra E.
Richards, Linda Ann Judson
Sargent, Emilie Gleason
Sly, Sarah
Truth, Sojourner

Minnesota

Clayton, S. Lillian
Domitilla, Sister Mary
Dreves, Katherine (Densford)
Fedde, Elizabeth
Freeman, Ruth Benson

Gladwin, Mary Elizabeth
Gowan, Sister Mary Olivia
Haupt, Alma Cecelia
Jamme, Anna C.
Powell, Louise Mathilde
Urch, Daisy Dean

Mississippi

Cumming, Kate
Newsom, Ella (King)
Travelbee, Joyce

Missouri

Cushman, Emma D.
Logan, Laura R.
McIver, Pearl
Osborne, Estelle Geneva Massey Riddle
Sellew, Gladys
Stimson, Julia Catherine
Wood, Helen

Montana

Gabriel, Sister John

New Jersey

Dakin, Florence
Dix, Dorothea Lynde
Gorman, Alice Amelia
Maass, Clara Louise
Shaw, Clara (Weeks)

New Mexico

Hogan, Aileen I.

New York

Alline, Anna Lowell
Anderson, Lydia
Arnstein, Margaret Gene
Austin, Anne L.
Bunge, Helen Lathrop
Burgess, Elizabeth Chamberlain
Christy, Teresa Elizabeth
Crandall, Ella Phillips
Damer, Annie
Darche, Louise
Delano, Jane Arminda
Deming, Dorothy
Dewitt, Katharine
Dock, Lavinia Lloyd
Eldredge, Adda
Fedde, Elizabeth
Freeman, Ruth Benson
Geister, Janet M.
Goodrich, Annie Warburton
Grant, Amelia Howe
Gray, Carolyn Elizabeth
Harmer, Bertha
Hitchcock, Jane Elizabeth
Hogan, Aileen I.
Kimber, Diana Clifford
Lally, Grace B.
Leete, Harriet L.
Lounsbery, Harriet (Camp)
McNaught, Rose
Maxwell, Anna Caroline
Muse, Maude Blanche
Noyes, Clara Dutton

Nutting, M. Adelaide
Osborne, Estelle Geneva Massey Riddle
Palmer, Sophia French
Pfefferkorn, Blanche
Pope, Amy Elizabeth
Reiter, Frances
Richards, Linda Ann Judson
Robinson, Alice Merritt
Sanborn, Katharine Anne Alexis
Sanger, Margaret Louise
Sirch, Margaret Elliot (Francis)
Smith, Martha Ruth
Stewart, Isabel Maitland
Sutliffe, Irene H.
Thoms, Adah B. (Samuels)
Tubman, Harriet
Van Blarcom, Carolyn Conant
Vreeland, Ellwynne Mae
Wald, Lillian D.
Whitman, Walter
Wolf, Anna Dryden
Wood, Helen
Young, Helen
Zabriskie, Louise

North Carolina

Batterham, Mary Rose
Dolan, Margaret (Baggett)
Holman, Lydia
Kemble, Elizabeth L.
Nahm, Helen Emilie
Wyche, Mary Lewis

Ohio

Anthony, Sister
Austin, Anne L.
Berthold, Jeanne Saylor
Bunge, Helen Lathrop
Clayton, S. Lillian
Crandall, Ella Phillips
Ellis, Rosemary
Gladwin, Mary Elizabeth
Gray, Carolyn Elizabeth
Hodgins, Agatha Cobourg
Howell, Marion Gertrude
Leete, Harriet L.
Logan, Laura R.
Pfefferkorn, Blanche
Powell, Louise Mathilde
Robb, Isabel Adams (Hampton)
Roberts, Mary May
Sellew, Gladys

Oregon

Gabriel, Sister John
Thomson, Elnora Elvira

Pennsylvania

Aikens, Charlotte
Banfield, Emma Maud
Blanchfield, Florence Aby
Brinton, Mary Williams
Clayton, S. Lillian
Delano, Jane Arminda
Fisher, Alice
Francis, Susan C.
Goodnow, Minnie
Grace, Sister Mary Gonzaga
Gray, Carolyn Elizabeth
Heide, Wilma (Scott)

Hubbard, Ruth Weaver
Jones, Elizabeth Rinker (Kratz)
Kennedy, Cecila Rose
McClelland, Helen Grace
Phillips, Harriet Newton
Schutt, Barbara Gordon
Sutliffe, Irene H.
Tucker, Katharine

Rhode Island

Carr, Ada M.
Gardner, Mary Sewall
Goodnow, Minnie
Parsons, Sara E.

Tennessee

Gorman, Alice Amelia
Newsom, Ella (King)
Titus, Shirley Carew

Vermont

Markolf, Ada Mayo (Stewart)
Robinson, Alice Merritt

Virginia

Cabaniss, Sadie Heath
Minor, Nannie Jacquelin
Pember, Phoebe Yates (Levy)
Powell, Louise Mathilde

Washington

Gabriel, Sister John
Soule, Elizabeth Sterling
Vail, Stella (Boothe)

West Virginia

Lounsbery, Harriet (Camp)

Wisconsin

Beck, Sister M. Berenice
Blake, Florence Guinness
Bunge, Helen Lathrop
Eldredge, Adda

APPENDIX C

Listing by Specialty or Occupation

Anesthesiology

Hodgins, Agatha Cobourg

Education

Alline, Anna Lowell
Amy Margaret, Sister
Anderson, Lydia
Arnstein, Margaret Gene
Banfield, Emma Maud
Beard, Mary
Beck, Sister M. Berenice
Berthold, Jeanne Saylor
Blake, Florence Guinness
Brown, Amy Frances
Bunge, Helen Lathrop
Burgess, Elizabeth Chamberlain
Cabaniss, Sadie Heath
Christy, Teresa Elizabeth
Clayton, S. Lillian
Crandall, Ella Phillips
Cushman, Emma D.
Dakin, Florence
Darche, Louise
Davis, Frances Reed (Elliott)
Davis, Mary E. P.
Delano, Jane Arminda
Dock, Lavinia Lloyd
Dolan, Margaret (Baggett)
Domitilla, Sister Mary
Dreves, Katherine (Densford)
Drown, Lucy Lincoln
Eldredge, Adda
Ellis, Rosemary
Fisher, Alice
Frederick, Hester King
Freeman, Ruth Benson
Gabriel, Sister John
Gage, Nina Diadamia
Gladwin, Mary Elizabeth
Goodnow, Minnie
Goodrich, Annie Warburton
Goostray, Stella
Gorman, Alice Amelia
Gowan, Sister Mary Olivia
Grant, Amelia Howe
Gray, Carolyn Elizabeth
Gretter, Lystra E.
Hall, Carrie M.
Harmer, Bertha
Hawkinson, Nellie Xenia
Hay, Helen Scott
Hibbard, M. Eugenie
Hodgins, Agatha Cobourg
Hogan, Aileen I.
Howell, Marion Gertrude
Jones, Elizabeth Rinker (Kratz)
Kemble, Elizabeth L.
Kimber, Diana Clifford
Knapp, Bertha L.
Logan, Laura R.
McCleery, Ada Belle

McClelland, Helen Grace
McCrae, Annabella
McIsaac, Isabel
Macleod, Charlotte
Maher, Mary Ann
McNaught, Rose
Maxwell, Anna Caroline
Muse, Maude Blanche
Noyes, Clara Dutton
Nutting, M. Adelaide
Osborne, Estelle
Palmer, Sophia French
Parsons, Marion Gemeth
Parsons, Sara E.
Pfefferkorn, Blanche
Pope, Amy Elizabeth
Powell, Louise Mathilde
Reiter, Frances
Richards, Linda Ann Judson
Riddle, Mary Margaret
Robb, Isabel Adams (Hampton)
Robinson, Alice Merritt
Sanborn, Katharine Anne Alexis
Sellew, Gladys
Shaw, Clara (Weeks)
Simpson, Cora E.
Smith, Martha Ruth
Soule, Elizabeth Sterling
Stewart, Isabel Maitland
Strong, Anne Hervey
Sullivan, Elizabeth Eleanor
Sutliffe, Irene H.
Taylor, Euphemia Jane
Thomson, Elnora Elvira
Titus, Shirley Carew
Travelbee, Joyce
Tucker, Katharine
Urch, Daisy Dean
Wolf, Anna Dryden
Wood, Helen
Wyche, Mary Lewis
Young, Helen

History of Nursing

Austin, Anne L.
Christy, Teresa Elizabeth
Goodnow, Minnie
Goostray, Stella
Stewart, Isabel Maitland

Industrial Nursing

Markolf, Ana Mayo (Stewart)
Vail, Stella (Boothe)

International Relief Work

Arnstein, Margaret Gene
Barton, Clarissa Harlowe
Beeby, Nell V.
Brinton, Mary Williams
Butler, Ida Fatio
Cushman, Emma D.
Deane, Elizabeth M.
Fitzgerald, Alice
Gage, Nina Diadamia
Gardner, Mary Sewall
Gregg, Elinor Delight
Hay, Helen Scott
Kennedy, Cecila Rose
Leete, Harriet L.
Minnigerode, Lucy

Nelson, Sophie C.
Noyes, Clara Dutton
Phillips, Harriet Newton
Simpson, Cora E.

Midwifery

Breckinridge, Mary
Browne, Helen E.
Goldman, Emma
Hogan, Aileen I.
Holman, Lydia
McNaught, Rose
Van Blarcom, Carolyn Conant
Willeford, Mary B.

Military Nursing

Alcott, Louisa May
Angela, Mother
Anthony, Sister
Barton, Clarissa Harlowe
Beard, Mary
Bickerdyke, Mary Ann (Ball)
Blanchfield, Florence Aby
Bowman, Josephine Beatrice
Butler, Ida Fatio
Cumming, Kate
Delano, Jane Arminda
Dix, Dorothea Lynde
Flikke, Julia
Gladwin, Mary Elizabeth
Goodnow, Minnie
Grace, Sister Mary Gonzaga
Harmer, Carrie M.
Hasson, Esther Voorhees
Hay, Helen Scott
Hibbard, M. Eugenie
Hickey, Mary A.
Kinney, Dita (Hopkins)
Lally, Grace B.
Livermore, Mary (Rice)
Lounsbery, Harriet (Camp)
Maass, Clara Louise
McClelland, Helen Grace
Maxwell, Anna Caroline
Newsom, Ella (King)
Parsons, Marion Gemeth
Parsons, Sara E.
Pember, Phoebe Yates (Levy)
Phillips, Harriet Newton
Ropes, Hannah (Chandler)
Stimson, Julia Catherine
Thompson, Dora E.
Tubman, Harriet
Tyler, Adeline (Blanchard)
Waters, Yssabella Gertrude
Whitman, Walter
Williamson, Anne A.

Occupational Therapy

Tracy, Susan E.

Pediatric/Maternal Nursing

Blake, Florence Guinness
Francis, Susan C.
Goostray, Stella
Hogan, Aileen I.
Sellew, Gladys
Sullivan, Elizabeth Eleanor
Waechter, Eugenia Helma
Zabriskie, Louise

Professional Service

Aikens, Charlotte A.
Beeby, Nell V.
Cabaniss, Sadie Heath
Carr, Ada M.
Cooke, Genevieve
Damer, Annie
Darche, Louise
Davis, Mary E. P.
Deming, Dorothy
Dewitt, Katharine
Dock, Lavinia Lloyd
Draper, Edith Augusta
Eldredge, Adda
Fisher, Alice
Franklin, Martha M.
Geister, Janet M.
Heide, Wilma (Scott)
Hitchcock, Jane Elizabeth
Jamme, Anna C.
Lounsbery, Harriet (Camp)
McIsaac, Isabel
Mahoney, Mary Eliza P.
Northam, Annie Ethel
Osborne, Estelle
Palmer, Sophia French
Riddle, Mary Margaret
Roberts, Mary May
Robinson, Alice Merritt
Schutt, Barbara Gordon
Scott, Alma Ham
Shaw, Clara (Weeks)
Sly, Sarah
Stewart, Isabel Maitland
Wyche, Mary Lewis

Psychiatric Nursing

Taylor, Euphemia Jane
Travelbee, Joyce Evelyn

Public Health Nursing

Arnstein, Margaret Gene
Batterham, Mary Rose
Beard, Mary
Breckinridge, Mary
Cabaniss, Sadie Heath
Cannon, Ida Maud
Carr, Ada M.
Collins, Charity E.
Crandall, Ella Phillips
Damer, Annie
Davis, Frances Reed (Elliott)
Deming, Dorothy
Deutsch, Naomi
Dolan, Margaret (Baggett)
Fedde, Elizabeth
Foley, Edna Lois
Fox, Elizabeth Gordon
Freeman, Ruth Benson
Fulmer, Harriet
Gardner, Mary Sewall
Geister, Janet M.
Grant, Amelia Howe
Gregg, Elinor Delight
Gretter, Lystra E.
Haupt, Alma Cecelia
Hibbard, M. Eugenie
Hickey, Mary A.
Hitchcock, Jane Elizabeth

Holman, Lydia
Howell, Marion Gertrude
Hubbard, Ruth Weaver
Leete, Harriet L.
Lounsbery, Harriet (Camp)
Maass, Clara Louise
McIver, Pearl
Maher, Mary Ann
Minnigerode, Lucy
Minor, Nannie Jacquelin
Nelson, Sophie C.
Pope, Amy Elizabeth
Sargent, Emilie Gleason
Sirch, Margaret (Francis)
Strong, Anne Hervey
Struthers, Lina (Rogers)
Tucker, Katharine
Vail, Stella (Boothe)
Wald, Lillian D.
Waters, Yssabella Gertrude
Willeford, Mary B.

Research

Arnstein, Margaret Gene
Berthold, Jeanne Saylor
Bunge, Helen Lathrop
Ellis, Rosemary
Northam, Annie Ethel
Pfefferkorn, Blanche
Reiter, Frances
Vreeland, Ellwynne Mae
Waechter, Eugenia Helma

Social Work

Cannon, Ida Maud
Fedde, Elizabeth

Index

Index

Index

Index

About the Editor-in-Chief

MARTIN KAUFMAN received a doctorate from Tulane University in 1969, where he was a Josiah Macy, Jr., Fellow in the History of Medicine. He developed an interest in the history of medicine and public health as a student of John Duffy, at both the University of Pittsburgh and at Tulane University. Kaufman is author of *Homeopathy in America* (1971), *American Medical Education: Formative Years* (1976), *The University of Vermont College of Medicine* (1979), and articles, essays, and reviews in a large number of journals. He was editor-in-chief of the *Dictionary of American Medical Biography* (2 volumes, 1984). In addition to his work on the history of medicine and public health, he is editorial director of the *Historical Journal of Massachusetts*, director of the Institute for Massachusetts Studies, and professor of history and chairperson of the history department at Westfield State College, Massachusetts. He has edited several books related to the history of Massachusetts, and was editor-in-chief of *A Guide to the History of Massachusetts* (1988).

About the Contributing Editors

ALICE HOWELL FRIEDMAN has recently retired as associate professor at the University of Massachusetts School of Nursing. She received her training at the Massachusetts General Hospital School of Nursing and then studied at Columbia University Teachers College, where she received her bachelor of science degree. Her graduate work was completed at Boston University, where she received a master of science degree in 1967. Before joining the faculty at the University of Massachusetts, Professor Friedman taught at the Boston College School of Nursing, and she served as a staff nurse at the Massachusetts General Hospital and St. Luke's Hospital (New York City), and as supervisor of the Visiting Nurse Association of Boston. She also served as executive secretary of the alumnae association of the Massachusetts General Hospital School of Nursing. Professor Friedman has long been active in professional organizations, having served as vice-president of the Massachusetts Nurses' Association, secretary of the Massachusetts Public Health Association, member of the nominating committee of the American Association for the History of Nursing, and member of the nursing archives associates of the Mugar Memorial Library, Boston University. Since November 1985, Professor Friedman has been editor of the *Journal* *of Nursing History*. In addition to her publications on nursing, she contributed an article to *Nursing History: The State of the Art* (1987, edited by Christopher Maggs).

JOELLEN W. HAWKINS is professor of nursing at Boston College, where she is the coordinator of the graduate program in nursing. She studied at Oberlin College, and received her diploma from the Chicago Wesley Memorial Hospital School of Nursing and her bachelor of science in nursing from Northwestern University. Her graduate studies were completed at Boston College, where she received her master's degree in 1969 and her Ph.D. in 1977. Before joining the faculty at Boston College School of Nursing, Hawkins taught at the University of Connecticut School of Nursing, Storrs, Connecticut; at Salve Regina College, Newport, Rhode Island; and at Roger Williams College, Bristol, Rhode Island. Dr. Hawkins has published extensively in her field and is author or co-author of seventeen books, including *Maternity and Gynecological Nursing: Women's Health Care* (1981), *Nursing and the American Health Care Delivery System* (1982), *The Nurse Practitioner: Current Practice Issues* (1983), *Human Sexuality across the Life Span* (1984), *Postpartum Nursing: Health Care of Women* (1985), *An Orientation to Hospitals and Community Agencies* (1986), and *Linking Nursing Education and Practice* (1987). Dr. Hawkins has long been interested in the history of nursing, and she has published articles on aspects of nursing history in various journals, including *Educational Studies*, *Journal of Nursing Education*, *Journal of the Illinois Historical Society*, *Nursing Management*, and the *Journal of Nursing History*. She has received numerous honors, including induction as a fellow of the American Academy of Nursing and receipt of the Massachusetts Nurses' Association distinguished nurse-researcher award.

LORETTA P. HIGGINS is associate professor at the Boston College School of Nursing. She received her training at St. Francis Medical Center, Trenton, New Jersey, and from there went to Boston College, where she received her bachelor's, master's, and doctorate of education. Dr. Higgins is co-author of four books, including *Nursing and the American Health Care Delivery System* (1982) and *Human Sexuality across the Lifespan* (1984). Her recent research has focused upon the contributions of the nursing sisterhoods during the American Civil War, and she presented a paper on that topic before the third annual conference on nursing history, sponsored by the American Association for the History of Nursing.